Common Dilemmas in Family Medicine

EDITED BY

John Fry
General Practitioner
Beckenham, Kent
England

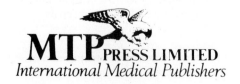

MTP PRESS LIMITED
International Medical Publishers

Published by
MTP Press Limited
Falcon House
Lancaster, England

British Library Cataloguing in Publication Data

Common dilemmas in family medicine.
1. Family medicine
I. Fry, John
362.1'72   R729.5.G4
ISBN 0-85200-470-2

Printed and bound in Great Britain by
Butler & Tanner Ltd, Frome and London

610/FRY

Tralee General Hospital Library

ACC. No._____ Class __610 FRY__

This book must be returned not later than the last date
stamped below.
FINES WILL BE RIGOROUSLY IMPOSED

Contents

List of Contributors

Dr N.N. ANDERSEN
Turpinsvej 2
DK 2610 Rødovre, Denmark

Dr D.M. BARR
Department of Family Medicine
Illinois Masonic Medical Center
836 Wellington Avenue
Chicago, IL 60657, USA

Dr A.T.M. BARTELDS
Nederlands Huisartsen Institut
Postbus 2570
3500 GN Utrecht, The Netherlands

Professor A.O. BERG
School of Medicine
Department of Family Medicine, RF–30
University of Washigton
Seattle, WA 98195, USA

Lt Col T. BOUCHIER HAYES
Senior Medical Officer RMAS & Staff
    College
Camberley, Surrey, UK

Dr D. BROOKS
The Ridings
124 Manchester Road
Hopwood, Heywood OL10 2NN, UK

Dr D.A. COFFMAN
9 Wrottesley Road
Willesden, London NW10 5UY, UK

Dr D. CRADDOCK
5 Warham Road
South Croydon, Surrey CR2 6LE, UK

Dr A.G.O. CROWTHER
32 Kingfield Road
Sheffield S11 9AS, UK

Dr G. DAVIE
PO Box 27399
Sunnyside
Pretoria 0132, South Africa

Dr M.D. D'SOUZA
The Canbury Medical Centre
1 Elm Road
Kingston-upon-Thames
Surrey KT2 6HR, UK

Dr W.E. FABB
12 Westminster Avenue
Bulleen
Victoria 3105, Australia

Dr A. FRASER
149 Upper Heidelberg Road
Ivanhoe
Victoria 3079, Australia

Dr P. FREELING
St George's Hospital Medical School
Cranmer Terrace
London SW7 0RE, UK

Professor J. FROOM
Department of Family Medicine
Health Sciences Center
State University of New York at Stony
Brook
Long Island, NY 11794, USA

Dr J. FRY
133 Croydon Road
Beckenham
Kent BR3 4DG, UK

Dr E. GAMBRILL
Leacroft, Ifield Road
Crawley
Sussex RH11 5BS, UK

Dr D.G. GARVIE
The Surgery
Palmerston Street
Wolstanton
Newcastle, Staffs, UK

Dr E.C. GAWTHORN
11 Lucifer Street
North Balwyn
Victoria 3104, Australia

Professor J.P. GEYMAN
Department of Family Medicine RF–30
University of Washington
Seattle, WA 98195, USA

Dr K. GILL
Huisarts
Zwammerdam, The Netherlands

Dr J. GRABINAR
31 Coniston Road
Bromley
Kent BR1 4JG, UK

Dr P. KERRIGAN
9 The Hoe
Billericay
Essex CM12 9XB, UK

Dr J. LEVENSTEIN
South African Acadamy of Family
    Practice/Primary Care
24/25 Medical House
Central Square
Pinelands 7430, South Africa

Dr S. LEVENSTEIN
163 Koeberg Road
Brooklyn
Cape Town 7405, South Africa

Dr P. B. MARTIN
Westley Hall, Homestead Drive
Basildon, Essex, UK

Dr B. MATTHEWS
9 Royal Crescent
Bath BA1 2LR, UK

Dr B.R. McAVOY
The Medical Centre
Byfield
Daventry
Northamptonshire, UK

Dr A. MOULDS
The Health Centre
Laindon
Basildon
Essex SS15 5TR, UK

Dr N. NØRRELUND
Arhusvej 190
DK 8570 Trustrup, Denmark

Dr A.E. PALLESEN
Skovbuen 59
DK 2610 Rødovre, Denmark

Professor G.J. PISTORIUS
Department of Family Medicine
OFS University
PO Box 339
Bloemfontein 9300, South Africa

Dr B. POLLAK
Beech Cottage, Gibson's Hill
London SW16 3EX, UK

Dr M.E. PRESTON-WHYTE
Uppingham Road Health Centre
131 Uppingham Road
Leicester LE5 4BP, UK

Dr P.M.M. PRITCHARD
Monks' Corner, 31 Martin's Lane
Dorchester on Thames
Oxfordshire OX9 8JF, UK

Professor R.A. ROSENBLATT
School of Medicine
Department of Family Medicine RF–30
University of Washington
Seattle, WA 98195, USA

Dr S. ROTTENBERG
14 Norfolk Place
London W2 1QJ, UK

Dr R.G. RUSSELL
Skinners Cottage
Drayton
Belbroughton, Worcs, UK

Professor S. SCHUMAN
Department of Medicine
Section of Preventive Medicine
Medical University of South Carolina
171 Ashley Avenue
Charlestown, SC 29403, USA

Dr J.A. SMITH
2 Paterson Street
Newlands
Cape Town 7700, South Africa

Dr K.W. SEHNERT
4210 Fremont Avenue South
Minneapolis, MN 55409, USA

Dr R. STEEL
St John's House
28 Bromyard Road
Worcester WR2 5BU, UK

Professor W.L. STEWART
Box J-222, MSB
J Hillis Miller Health Center
Gainesville, FL 32610, USA

Dr A.G. STRUBE
33 Goffs Park Road
Southgate
Crawley, Sussex, UK

Dr G.STRUBE
33 Goffs Park Road
Southgate
Crawley, Sussex, UK

Dr R.B. TAYLOR
Wake Forest University
Bowman Gray School of Medicine
300 South Hawthorne Road
Winston-Salem, NC 27103, USA

Dr M.K. THOMPSON
24 Fryston Avenue
Shirley
Croydon, Surrey, UK

Dr R. WEST
Division of Primary Health Care
Department of Community Health
School of Medicine
The University of Auckland
Auckland, New Zealand

Dr M.J. WHITFIELD
24 Hanbury Road
Clifton, Bristol BS8 2EP, UK

Dr O.W. WILLIAMS
Health Centre
Caebricks Road
Cwmbwrla, Swansea SA5 8NS, UK

DR J.D. WILLIAMSON
91 Dodworth Road
Barnsley
South Yorkshire S70 6HB, UK

Dr K.M.H. YOUNG
Shell UK Ltd
Shell-Mex House
Strand, London WC2R 0DX, UK

Preface

One of the exciting challenges of medicine has been the reaching of decisions based on less than complete evidence.

As undergraduates in teaching hospitals future physicians are taught to think in clear and absolute black and white terms. Diagnoses in teaching hospitals all are based on supportive positive findings of investigations. Treatment follows logically on precise diagnosis. When patients die the causes of death are confirmed at autopsy.

How very different is real life in clinical practice, and particularly in family medicine. By the very nature of the common conditions that present diagnoses tend to be imprecise and based on clinical assessment and interpretation. Much of the management and treatment of patients is based on opinions of individual physicians based on their personal experiences.

Because of the relative professional isolation of family physicians within their own practices, not unexpectedly divergent views and opinions are formed. There is nothing wrong in such divergencies because there are no clear absolute black and white decisions. General family practice functions in grey areas of medicine where it is possible and quite correct to hold polarized distinct opinions. The essence of good care must be eternal flexibility and readiness to change long-held cherished opinions.

To demonstrate that with many issues in family medicine it is possible to have more than one view I selected 10 clinical and 11 non-clinical topics and invited colleagues and fellow-practitioners to enter into a debate-in-print.

Each topic has been selected because each is of some practical importance to family practitioners. Each chapter begins with a brief statement of the issues relating to the topic, there follow 'pro' and 'con' arguments and finally a short commentary attempts to strike a judicial balance.

The prime aim of this rather unusual exercise has been to show that there can be more than one view on the common issues of family medicine and that due attention should be given to the differing opinions.

The target readership audience is all who work in, and those who are interested in, family medicine and its intricacies and dilemmas. In particular this book seeks to stimulate teachers and learners of family medicine. It seeks to encourage them to consider and discuss the varying points of view in their teaching and learning of this growing important and essential field of health care. It is an inevitable level of care in all national health systems and there is much more to be discovered within it.

Therefore, this book is dedicated to the present and future generations of family physicians who faced with dilemmas will endeavour to resolve them for what is best for their patients.

I wish to thank all my co-contributors. They responded most willingly to my rather unusual invitation to engage in this debate-in-print – often arguing a case contrary to their own fondly held beliefs. Not only did they respond but most of them delivered well on time.

My fellow commentators Wes Fabb of Melbourne, Australia, and John P. Geyman of Seattle, USA, shared with me the difficult tasks of judge and jury in presenting the balanced commentaries and critiques.

We all of us debators, commentators and editor hope that our own enjoyable efforts will encourage our readers to pause, ponder, and participate in a continuing debate on these topics.

John Fry
Beckenham, 1982

1 Mild-to-moderate hypertension – to treat or not to treat?

The issues

Hypertension is a sphygmomanometric diagnosis of uncertain causes and nature. Within the spectrum of hypertension there are likely to be different at-risk groups with differing prognoses and differing requirements for treatments. In asking who should be treated, how, where and why, three questions can be asked: Should the elderly, the middle-aged and the young be treated in the same ways? What are the most effective regimes of treatment? What are the objectives of treatment?

Other questions to be posed are: What resources of manpower and money would be required for comprehensive care of all hypertensives? Who treats hypertensives best – family physicians, specialists, or nurses? What is the value of screening? (see also Chapter 17). Are the benefits of long-term care of mild–moderate hypertensives really beneficial?

The case for treatment (1)
Daniel M. Barr

In the 17 years since I started medical school, I have observed the management of hypertension move from therapeutic nihilism to diagnostic nihilism. I expect the current therapeutic shotgun to become more focused as the result of studies currently underway in the United States, United Kingdom and elsewhere (Page, 1979; Relman, 1980). This new

1

rifle approach will be targeted at least to age and sex subgroups of the hypertensive population as well as prevention of specific outcomes in these subgroups (that is, death, myocardial infarction, stroke, renal disease, etc.). It is possible that a more useful clinical rule-of-thumb for selection of patients for work-up of secondary hypertension will emerge from these epidemiological efforts and controlled clinical trials.

A provocative paper by Fry (1974) suggested that observed deaths were not significantly increased over expected death rates in untreated hypertensive patients over age 60 in his practice population. That paper apparently contributed to the debate over treatment of older hypertensives in England, but it has not been prominently recognized by US medical editors and commentators (Page, 1979; Relman, 1980). It also generated considerable controversy for Fry among his general practice colleagues in academia. There is considerable opinion supporting further testing of Fry's conclusions. He may be right!

However, at this time, US practice standards have been strongly influenced by less selective and inconclusive studies undertaken at great expense and by the enthusiastic advocacy of these studies as strong preliminary evidence by at least one prominent medical journal editor (Relman, 1980).

My approach to treating older (over 60) hypertensives can be summarized as follows:

(1) Treat all mild (90–105 mmHg diastolic) hypertensives equally initially if there is no potentially troublesome co-morbidity (in other words, weakness which might be confused by potassium level uncertainty, etc.).

(2) If the diastolic blood pressure does not decrease to 90 mmHg or below in 2–8 weeks, individualize:

(a) if less than 100 mmHg, try increased dosage and/or additional agents without using the more potent drugs with more frequent, severe adverse effects; or

(b) if 100–105 mmHg, be more aggressive and, if necessary, use more potent agents.

The message in these words is that my level of concern about treating down to 90 mmHg or below in patients 60 and over is less than in younger age-groups.

If co-morbidity exists, sometimes I prefer to resolve those problems, if possible, prior to aggressive antihypertensive therapy. I also prefer to avoid those diuretics with clinically apparent greater tendencies to contribute to potassium loss, as I have had a rash of hospitalizations related to catastrophic or disturbing complications of hypokalaemia in apparently well-monitored patients.

I expect to change this approach to treatment in the next 5 years based on studies now under way. In interpreting those studies I will distinguish between *efficacy* (defined in the American way, 'Does it work under ideal circumstances?') and *effectiveness* ('Does it work under the realities of clinical practice?'). Practice of effectiveness studies will continue to be helpful in raising questions in this area, but efficacy studies or controlled clinical trials produce the most unambiguous results to guide practitioners. In the meantime, I will individualize what I do in relation to the biological and psychosocial needs of the patient. In addition, I will be influenced by my practice situation and my own professional and personal characteristics as reflected in part in this commentary.

References

Fry, J. (1974). Natural history of hypertension: a case of selective non-treatment. *Lancet*, **2**, 431–433

Page, I. H. (1979). Two cheers for hypertension. *J. Am. Med. Assoc.*, **242**, 2559–2561

Relman, A. S. (1980). Mild hypertension: no more benign neglect. *N. Engl. J. Med.*, **302**, 293–294

The case for treatment (2)
Eric Gambrill

In this section we are facing what is probably the single most important dilemma in the practice of family medicine which is likely to confront us during the remainder of this century. On the one hand, we have the daunting task of detecting, investigating, treating and following up almost 20 per cent of the population between 40 and 70 years of age; and, on the other, we have the prospect of thousands of people maimed, handicapped and killed by an eminently treatable condition because we, as professionals, have failed to come to terms with the changing patterns of illness and mobilize our resources accordingly. The dilemma is compounded by the fact that we do not have, at this time, unequivocal evidence which ideally would be available in order to prove conclusively that reducing the blood pressure of mild to moderately hypertensive patients will achieve the desired effect. Nevertheless, I hope to demonstrate that on philosophical, humanitarian and economic grounds we should be preparing ourselves to meet this challenge rather than burying our heads in the sand and hoping that it will go away.

THE EPIDEMIOLOGICAL EVIDENCE

It has been well known for over 20 years that even mildly elevated levels of blood pressure are associated with considerable extra risks of early mortality. Figures produced by American insurance societies and published in 1959 (Society of Actuaries, 1959) showed conclusively that male mortality ratios increase with each step upwards in both systolic and diastolic pressure. Indeed, as Table 1.1 illustrates, a man aged 40–69

Table 1.1 Mortality according to variations in initial blood pressure *Build and Blood Pressure Study* **(Society of Actuaries, 1959). Standard and substandard issues combined. Mortality ratios**

(a) Men aged 15–39 at issue

Systolic BP mmHg	Diastolic BP mmHg				
	80	85	90	95	100
120	95	105	115	—	—
132	105	125	150	190	—
142	130	155	185	225	275
152	160	185	225	275	325

(b) Men aged 40–69 at issue

Systolic BP mmHg	Diastolic BP mmHg				
	80	85	90	95	100
120	80	95	110	130	—
132	105	115	130	150	175
142	130	145	165	190	215
152	160	180	200	225	250
162	195	215	235	260	300

Note For all practical purposes, the population represented by insurance company data was an untreated one. This is because people with a pressure over 160/100 were excluded from life insurance altogether and probably no one with pressures below that level would have been given effective treatment over the years to which the figures relate.

years with an initial pressure of 160/100, hardly a dramatically hypertensive figure, was four times more likely to die during the period of the study than another man in the same age-group with an initial pressure of 120/80. Even more sobering are the figures produced by the Metropolitan Life Insurance Company (1961) which showed that both men (and to a lesser extent) women suffered a very significant decrease in their expectation of life even if their initial blood pressure reading was only mildly raised (Figure 1.1). Thus a man aged 35 years with an initial blood pressure of 150/100 could be expected to die $16\frac{1}{2}$ years earlier than a man of equivalent age with an initial blood pressure of 120/80 or less.

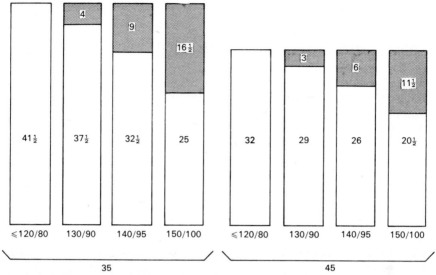

Figure 1.1 Expectation of life associated with various initial blood pressure levels.

While it is true that within these groups individuals with added risk factors such as smoking, obesity, diabetes, family history of cardiovascular disease and belonging to a negroid race fared proportionately worse, whereas other individuals without such risk factors fared proportionately better, nevertheless the contribution of mild hypertension to morbidity and mortality is of major significance.

If the effect of hypertension was merely to cause sudden death in people of retirement age and beyond after a healthy and productive life, then perhaps it might be argued that this is a 'consummation devoutly to be wished', but of course it is not so. Hypertension takes its toll of highly productive people, especially men, in middle-age, with families to support and a vital economic role in society. It does not necessarily kill outright but often causes paralysis and incontinence following a stroke; cardiac failure and angina, with or without a preceding myocardial infarction; and, of course, progressive renal failure and potential blindness in those with more severe degrees of hypertension. It is also possible that a considerable proportion of our increasing population of demented elderly people could have been saved from this fate by better control of their elevated blood pressure at a younger age.

AVAILABLE TREATMENT

All the evidence offered so far relates to untreated hypertension in the community. The reason for this is quite simple – 20 years ago there was no acceptable treatment for mild to moderate hypertension, since the drugs which were available and effective in the immediately life-threatening situation of malignant hypertension had severe and frequent side-effects which made them totally unsuitable for the treatment of asymptomatic mild to moderate hypertension on a long-term basis. The subsequent development of safer and better tolerated drugs during the 1950s and 1960s, culminating in the introduction of thiazide diuretics and later the beta-blockers, has now made prophylactic drug treatment a feasible proposition, and research into the effectiveness of low-salt diets, exercise regimes, biofeedback and meditation has opened up the possibility of alternatives to the pharmacological approach.

Thiazide diuretics are the cheapest and safest hypotensive agents, although they are not without some side-effects and are relatively contraindicated in patients with diabetes, gout and hypokalaemia. Beta-blockers are more expensive and contraindicated in asthma, some types of heart block and uncontrolled cardiac failure or diabetes. Nevertheless, there is some evidence that the beta-blockers may have a cardioprotective effect and therefore reduce the risks of myocardial infarction in hypertensive patients, a beneficial effect of treatment which had not previously been demonstrated.

While it is important for the doctor to be aware of potential side-effects of the drugs, not least because an asymptomatic patient is much more likely to default from long-term treatment if he or she feels unwell while taking the tablets, nevertheless many of the reported side-effects are vague and non-specific. Table 1.2 shows the symptoms reported by a group of elderly patients on treatment for hypertension compared with a control group of hypertensives not on treatment. It is noteworthy that there is little, if any, difference in reported symptoms between the two groups.

Table 1.2 Symptoms in a group of elderly patients on treatment for hypertension compared with a matched group of hypertensives not on treatment

		Treatment group n=99	Control group n=119
1	Headaches	15 (15%)	24 (20%)
2	Tiredness	57 (57%)	61 (51%)
3	Breathlessness	50 (50%)	43 (36%)
4	Light-headedness	28 (28%)	28 (24%)
5	Depression	12 (12%)	22 (18%)
6	Indigestion	26 (26%)	33 (28%)
7	Health worries	26 (26%)	34 (29%)
8	General wellbeing	27 (27%)	24 (20%)

VALUE OF TREATMENT

There is at present a major Medical Research Council clinical trial under way in the United Kingdom, in which general practitioners are vital participants, which is designed to investigate the benefits of treatment at levels of blood pressure between 90 and 109 diastolic; 18 000 patients are included in the study which is, however, not due to report until 1985. In the meantime, we have some evidence from important studies in the United States and Australia which strongly suggest that treatment is worthwhile, at least for certain groups of people with blood pressure measurements within this range.

In the American study, the Hypertension Detection and Follow-up Program, one group of hypertensive patients received very carefully controlled therapy, intensive education, financial assistance and systematic follow-up while the other group were referred to their own physician in the usual way. The group receiving special care showed a steady decrease in cumulative mortality (5.9 per 100) over 5 years compared to the control group (7.4 per 100). Control of blood pressure was consistently better in the special-care group. However, deaths from diabetes and malignancy were also less frequent in this group, perhaps demonstrating an unexpected bonus from the higher level of care provided. Detailed analysis suggests that men over 50 years of age and black women benefited particularly in the special-care group (Hypertension Detection and Follow-up Program Cooperation Group, 1979).

The Australian trial, mounted by the National Heart Foundation of Australia, studied 3427 men and women aged 30–69 years with diastolic phase V pressures of 95–110 mmHg and was stopped in March 1979 because of a significant reduction in mortality in the actively treated group, mainly due to a marked reduction in the incidence of strokes in men with initial readings of 100 mmHg or above (diastolic phase V). The evidence was less clear-cut for younger men and women (Reader, 1980). Thus it would appear that evidence is gradually accumulating that the systematic effective management of hypertension has a great potential for reducing mortality in the large numbers of people with high blood pressure including those with 'mild hypertension'.

I would suggest that people under the age of 69 with sustained levels of diastolic blood pressure above 100 mmHg (diastolic phase V) should be offered treatment. This might involve up to 10 per cent of the adult population. Below this figure, down to 90 mmHg, some doctors would treat and some would merely observe, but it would seem prudent to take other risk factors into account in this group and also not to ignore systolic hypertension since this is also highly predictive of cardiovascular disease in patients below the age of 65. Above the age of 70 years present evidence does not justify routine treatment for patients with no evidence of target organ damage (Figure 1.2).

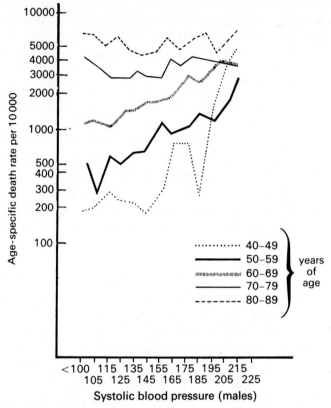

Figure 1.2   Age specific death rates per 10 000 against blood pressure in males

PLAN OF ACTION

How is it possible to contemplate such a policy in view of the limited resources of general practice? Do we have the time? Could it possibly be cost-effective?

The planning and execution of such a programme would require a transformation of traditional general practice from a demand-oriented disease service to a need-oriented health promotion service. It would involve changes in attitudes and work patterns by the doctors and expectations and involvement in their own health care by the patients. In the course of such a transformation many aspects of positive health would be involved beyond the management of hypertension in the community, which may pay increasing dividends in the long term.

It would be necessary to devise screening or case-finding techniques which could detect patients at risk and to develop protocols of minimum essential history, examination and investigations for each case. It would demand efficient record-systems for the monitoring of treatment and the long-term follow-up of patients and it would require effective use to be made of the skills of the practice administrative staff and nurses, since much of the routine work could be devolved by the doctors, leaving them free to concentrate on the difficult problems and to direct the whole system, taking note of advances in therapy and new epidemiological evidence as it becomes available. Pioneers such as John Coope and Julian Tudor-Hart (see Coope, 1980; and Tudor-Hart, 1982) have already shown the way to British general practitioners.

Calculations by George Teeling-Smith (1980) of the Office of Health Economics have demonstrated that treating male patients only over the age of 50 years with diastolic blood pressures consistently over 95 mmHg would possibly avoid up to 12 000 deaths in the United Kingdom by the time the definitive results of the Medical Research Council trial are published in 1985. He estimates that, taking into account the costs of therapy and medical time, the cost of each life saved would be in the order of £6700. However, he further estimates that there would be a 'pay-off' of perhaps £40 000 to the economy for that investment. Although such calculations are dependent on many unquantifiable assumptions they do demonstrate that it is possible to argue an economic case for spending the apparently formidable extra cost of between £80 and £100 million to the National Health Service on such a project over the next 5 years.

References

Coope, J. (1982). Article in *Tutorials in Postgraduate Medicine – General Practice*. E. Gambrill, (ed.). (London: Heinemann)

Hypertension Detection and Follow-Up Program Cooperation Group (1979). Five year findings of the HDFUP. *J. Am. Med. Assoc*, **242**, 23, 2562

Metropolitan Life Insurance Company (1961). *Blood Pressure: Insurance Experience and its Implications*. (New York: Metropolitan Life)

Reader, R. (Chairman) Management Committee (1980). The Australian therapeutic trial in mild hypertension. *Lancet*, **1**, 1261

Royal College of General Practitioners (1980). *Hypertension in Primary Care, Occasional paper No. 12*. (London: Royal College of General Practitioners)

Society of Actuaries (1959). *Build and Blood Pressure Study, Volume 1*. (Chicago, Ill.: Society of Actuaries)

Teeling-Smith, G. (1980). *Office of Health Economics Briefing, No. 12*, London, November

Tudor-Hart, J. (1980). *Hypertension*. (London: Churchill Livingstone)

The case against treatment
John Fry

THE DILEMMA

The dilemma put quite simply is whether 20 per cent of the adult population should be under continuing treatment for raised blood pressure? Should each family physician take on intensive screening of his population as a continuing basis to discover and manage the 200 or so mild to moderate hypertensives in his practice of 2000–2500 persons. This may mean a possible workload of up to 20 extra consultations each week.

Is it all worth while? For whose good are we to undertake this huge commitment? For our patients' better health and longevity? For our own self-satisfaction or increased income? For the public welfare?

I shall demonstrate that there are too many uncertainties over our lack of understanding of the nature and course of high blood pressure to accept positive directness to treat all mild to moderate hypertensives.

THE PRESENT STATE

The dilemma has been created by the advent of the new powerful antihypertensive drugs and diuretics, which are effective in reducing blood pressure without too many unpleasant side-effects.

Before the new antihypertensive therapies there was a selective approach to the clinical problem and only those in need of treatment were treated. Now anyone with a blood pressure over 140/90 is a candidate for lifelong drug-taking.

The pressures for treating all hypertensives have come mainly from epidemiologists, the drug companies, specialists and a few family physicians. They have based their case on population surveys and analyses of public health data. The results from clinical trials of treating mild to moderate hypertensives have been equivocal as to the benefits.

It is not right that family physicians who work with individual patients in relatively small practice populations should accept without question the views of such specialists.

It is not right that we should accept the case as 'all or nothing'. It does not follow that all mild to moderate hypertensives should receive lifelong drugs. Within the mass there are some high-risk groups and some low-risk groups – the former probably need therapy, the latter probably do not.

It is right that family physicians should consider individuals individually and use their *art* based on their own experience and that of fellow family physicians, as well as the *science* provided by mass statistical-survey specialists.

It is my intention to offer courage and support to fellow practitioners in their efforts to treat individual hypertensives individually and to show that there is a case for active non-treatment of mild to moderate hypertensives.

WHAT IS MILD TO MODERATE HYPERTENSION?

It must be accepted that we do not understand the true nature of hypertension. It is a diagnosis of mensuration. Because we have sphygmomanometers and because they record 'blood pressure' we are able to record individual levels. From population surveys it has been decreed that 'high blood pressure' is anything above 140/90 or 160/100 – there is no general agreement over when 'normal' blood pressure becomes 'high'.

Only in a minute (less than 5 per cent) proportion of high blood pressure is a definitive cause ever found; 95 per cent of high blood pressure is 'essential' or of unknown cause.

A SINGLE DISEASE?

In view of our lack of knowledge of the natural causes, course and outcome of high blood pressure it is quite wrong to view it as a single specific disease and make postulates from such a stance.

Eventually when we know much more about hypertension, if we ever shall, it may be possible to pick out subgroups with particular risks and patterns. At present we have to go on what is known and what is not known. Therefore, it is not right for family physicians to accept without question reports and statements from specialists on their experience of hypertension.

The spectrum of hypertension (Figure 1.3) illustrates that only a small proportion of cases is likely to be seen and managed by specialists; the greatest numbers will be managed by family physicians and internists (in the United States). However, it is likely that another equally large proportion – one-half of all hypertensives in the community – are undiagnosed.

The types of cases seen by hypertension specialists and family

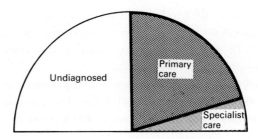

Figure 1.3 The spectrum of hypertension

physicians are very different, mild and moderate being managed by the latter and severe grades being managed by the specialists.

AT-RISK PROFILES

Because of our elementary understanding it is useful to look more broadly and create at-risk profiles for persons with high blood pressure to help in deciding on priorities for long-term care.

The following must be taken into account as *risk factors*:

  (1) cigarette smoking;
  (2) family history of heart disease or strokes;
  (3) age at diagnosis – the prognosis is worse in younger persons;
  (4) sex – the outlook is worse in males;
  (5) race – the prognosis tends to be worse in blacks than whites;
  (6) weight – this is paradoxical as fat ladies tend to have better prognosis than thin ladies, but weight reduction lowers raised blood pressures;
  (7) exercise – regular energetic exercise probably lessens the chances of developing associated ischaemic heart disease;
  (8) diabetes – makes prognosis worse;
  (9) cholesterol/triglycerides – raised levels are poor risk factors;
(10) salt – reducing high salt intake lowers blood pressure levels.

EXPERIENCE IN A FAMILY PRACTICE

There is need for a positive family practice view to be given without any sense of defensive professional inferiority.

For over 30 years I have kept a register of all persons in my practice with high blood pressure levels of more than 140/90 for those under 50 years of age and more than 160/100 in those over 50. During the 30-year period I have records of 1200 hypertensives. All have been followed up with clinical records. Until the early 1970s antihypertensive drugs were not used, therefore this represented *a picture of natural history of high blood pressure in my practice*. The findings that follow are those from the pre-1970 period on some 1000 hypertensives. This has been a continuing survey of clinical observation without the statistical niceties of the Framingham study (United States).

INCIDENCE

During the 30 years the incidence of high blood pressure has totalled 17 per cent in adults over 40. High blood pressure increases with age (Figure 1.4) and almost one-half of all hypertensives are aged 60 or more when first diagnosed – this is an important fact as the prognosis is much better in those over 60.

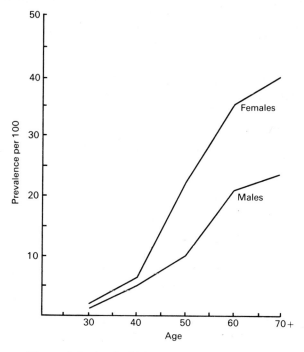

Figure 1.4   Age incidence in high blood pressure

Levels of blood pressure

At diagnosis the levels of diastolic blood pressure (DBP) were as follows:

$$\left.\begin{array}{l}\text{90–99 mm – 23 per cent}\\\text{100–109 mm – 28 per cent}\end{array}\right\}\textit{mild}$$

110–119 mm – 35 per cent   *moderate*

120 mm and over – 14 per cent   *severe*

Changes in blood pressure

It must not be assumed that blood pressure will rise with time in all persons.

In my untreated group over 15 years:

diastolic blood pressure *decreased* spontaneously   in 30 per cent

diastolic blood pressure remained *unchanged*   in 20 per cent

diastolic blood pressure *increased*   in 50 per cent

Note therefore that in almost one in three there is a chance that the diastolic blood pressure will fall spontaneously.

Mortality risks

Standardized mortality rates (SMRs) for untreated hypertensives (pre-1970) in my practice showed an extra risk of 2.5 times greater than expected but the risks were very different at various ages of first diagnosis (Figure 1.5).

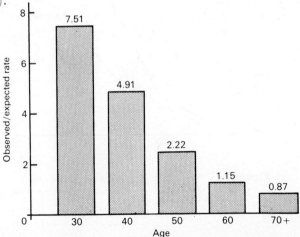

Figure 1.5   Hypertensives – SMRs at ages 30–70+ (from Fry, 1975)

Figure 1.5 shows that standard mortality rates decrease with age and after 60 are not more than expected. Note that one-half of all hypertensives are over 60 when first diagnosed and therefore one must question whether they should all be treated intensively to reduce their diastolic blood pressure.

Strokes and ischaemic heart disease

Similar patterns occur with the incidence of strokes and ischaemic heart disease (IHD) in hypertensives (Figures 1.6 and 1.7 – see p. 16).

There are definite increased risks at all ages for hypertensives to develop strokes but the risks are three times greater in under-60s (Figure 1.6). For ischaemic heart disease the extra risks in hypertensives are twice that expected in the 40–49 age group but no more than expected in those over 50.

Low-risk hypertensives

It is customary to relate prognosis to the levels of diastolic blood pressure, and in my experience this is generally so, but within my series of hypertensives there were 87 who were followed up for 15–25 years with diastolic blood pressures of more than 120 mm. At follow-up 78 per cent were still alive and 58 per cent had no complications of any sort. This group was notable in that females outnumbered males by 2.5:1 and that many of the women were obese.

There is within the spectrum of hypertension, therefore, a 'safe group' that can apparently come to terms with their raised high blood pressure. This group has to be acknowledged and recognized (Fry, 1975).

Treatment – compliance and control

Hypertension is not easy to control in spite of available strong antihypertensive drugs.

In a survey of 100 hypertensives diagnosed and treated with drugs in my practice from 1970–74 until 1981 I found that I was able to control only 50 per cent to a level of diastolic blood pressure below 100 mm, and 25 per cent were still above 110 mm – this in spite of referring the recalcitrant ones to hypertension specialists who were also unable to reduce their blood pressures (Fry, 1981).

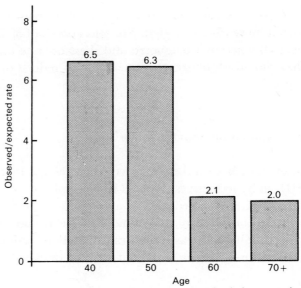

Figure 1.6   Observed/expected ratios of incidence of strokes in hypertension (Fry, 1975)

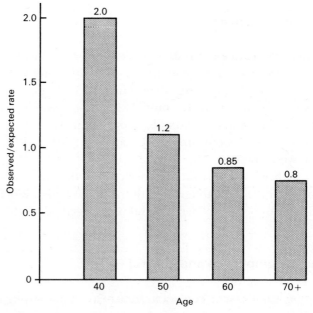

Figure 1.7   Observed/expected ratios of incidence of ischaemic heart disease in hypertension (Fry, 1975)

Less than satisfactory control does not mean that the family physician is inadequate or incompetent or that the patient is wilfully non-compliant.

A rule of halves also has been enunciated by others (Bannan, Beevers and Jackson, 1981), who state that of all hypertensives

(1) one-half are still *undiagnosed*;
(2) one-half of those diagnosed are *not being treated*;
(3) one-half of those being treated are *poorly controlled*;
(4) thus only one-eighth of all hypertensives are *well controlled* (Figure 1.8).

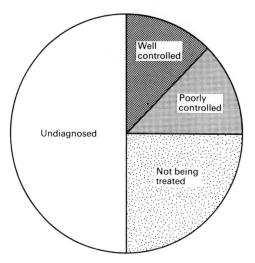

Figure 1.8 Hypertension – rule of halves

THE CASE AGAINST TREATING MILD TO MODERATE HYPERTENSION

My case then rests largely on my own experience in my own family practice over 30 years. It is based also on a cussed reluctance in non-acceptance of the pressures being placed on family physicians by specialists to accept their edicts and directives.

To summarize:

(1) High blood pressure still is full of uncertainties and unknowns.
(2) High blood pressure is present in one in five adults, and treating them all would be a weighty task.
(3) Within the spectrum of high blood pressure there are high-risk and low-risk groups that need to be defined.
(4) It is the low-risk group that make up more than one-half of all hypertensives who do *not* need therapy.

Finally, a compromise is necessary.

(1) All adults should have a blood pressure check at least once every 5 years.

(2) Clear clinical records should be kept including a register of all hypertensives.

(3) Individual care should be organized on assessment of risk factors.

References

Bannan, L. T., Beevers, D. G. and Jackson, S. H. D. (1981). Detecting hypertensive patients. *Br. Med. J.*, **1,** 1211

Fry, J. (1979). *Common Diseases.* 2nd edn. (Lancaster: MTP Press)

Fry, J. (1974). Natural history of hypertension, a case for selective non-treatment. *Lancet*, **2,** 431

Fry, J. (1975). Long surviving hypertension – a 15 year follow up. *J. R. Coll. Gen. Practit.*, **25,** 481

Fry, J. (1981). Self-check: high blood pressure. *Update*, **22,** 1681.

Treatment of mild to moderate hypertension: a critique

John P. Geyman

The preceding three papers have effectively outlined the therapeutic dilemma facing any physician attempting to establish specific indications for the use of antihypertensive drugs for mild to moderate hypertension both in individual patients and for a practice as a whole. These papers reflect a wide spectrum of opinion among family physicians concerning the use of these drugs. Barr represents a relatively aggresive approach to the problem (now largely mainstream opinion in the United States) which favours the use of antihypertensive drugs for all patients less than 60 years of age with mild hypertension (diastolic blood pressure 90–105 mmHg). Gambrill takes a middle course to treatment, and drawing from major studies in several countries, subscribes to the use of antihypertensive drugs for all patients less than 69 years of age with a diastolic blood pressure over 100 mmHg, reserving drug treatment for those patients with a diastolic blood pressure of 90–100 mmHg with risk factors and for those over 70 years of age with evidence of target organ damage. Fry takes a comparatively nihilistic approach to treatment based almost entirely on the experience of 1200 patients with hypertension in his own practice over 30 years, recommending withholding the use of antihypertensive drugs for at least a half of all patients with hypertension. He bases this recommendation on his observation that the mortality rate for his untreated hypertensive patients over 60 years of age was not greater than their expected mortality rate, and that almost one-third of his untreated hypertensive patients were found during follow-up to have spontaneous reduction of their diastolic blood pressure.

Further comment is in order with respect to presently available studies on this subject. The recently completed large-scale study in the United States, the Hypertension Detection and Follow-up Program (HDFP), was designed to compare outcomes of care (that is, 5-year mortality) given in special centres (Stepped Care Group) with care given in community hospitals, clinics, and physicians' offices (Referred Care Group). This study involved more than 10 000 patients, and it was found that the 5-year mortality was 20 per cent lower for the Stepped Care Group with entry diastolic blood pressure 90–104 mmHg compared to the corresponding Referred Care Group (Hypertension Detection and Follow-up Program Cooperative Group, 1979). This study is now being used widely to support the aggressive use of antihypertensive drugs for all patients with mild hypertension (diastolic blood pressure 90 mmHg). Aagaard (1981) points out important methodological reasons which he feels invalidate such a conclusion, including the lack of a double-blind, placebo-control design, and particularly the excellent support system and overall medical care afforded the Stepped Care Group. He thereby supports the view that drug treatment *per se* is generally not effective in reducing morbidity and mortality in patients with mild hypertension, which was the conclusion of the Veterans Administration (VA) Cooperative Study Group on Antihypertensive Agents (1980) and the US Public Health Service (PHS) Cooperative Study (1977), two other large-scale, *placebo-controlled* studies.

In a further analysis of other studies, Kaplan (1981) supports Aagaard's concerns and extends them to the recently completed national blood pressure treatment trials in Australia (The Management Committee, 1980) and Norway (Helgeland, 1980), both *placebo-controlled* studies. He points out that neither study demonstrated benefit of drug therapy for patients with diastolic blood pressure below 100 mmHg, and recommends the following middle course of treatment based on a critical review of available studies:

(1) Use of antihypertensive drugs for patients with diastolic blood pressure above 110 mmHg, or above 100 mmHg with accompanying target organ damage or other cardiovascular risks.

(2) Close follow-up for months without drug therapy for patients with diastolic blood pressure below 110 mmHg without obvious cardiovascular disease or other risk factors.

(3) Continued follow-up at least every 6 months if the diastolic blood pressure remains below 100 mmHg, reserving use of drug therapy for those with persistent diastolic blood pressure above 100 mmHg.

These recommendations seem sound, particularly in view of well-documented observations that repeated measurements of blood pressure frequently show spontaneous reductions, that attention to risk factors (for example, weight control, smoking cessation, exercise programmes) often leads to reduction of blood pressure, and that sodium restriction without drug therapy frequently lowers diastolic blood pressure in patients with mild elevations of blood pressure. Restriction of antihypertensive drugs to these indications would avoid 'over treatment' of perhaps 20 million people in the United States (almost 10% of the population) with diastolic blood pressure in the 90–100 mmHg range (Kaplan, 1981).

Indications for drug therapy and treatment goals do vary with age, especially in patients over 65 years of age. In a recent paper on hypertension in the elderly, O'Malley and O'Brien (1980) present what is probably 'mainstream' opinion on the use of drug therapy in this age group, recommending such treatment for patients with diastolic blood pressure above 110 mmHg, or 100–110 mmHg with complications or systolic values over 180 mmHg. On the other end of the age spectrum, efforts must also be directed to diagnosis, follow-up, and appropriate management of young people with possible hypertension. Based on his long-term studies in his family practice in Georgia, Hames (1974) has found, for example, that the prevalence rate for blood pressure over 140/90 in individuals in the 15–29 age group in one rural county was 34.9% for black males, 31.6% for black females, 19% for white males, and 12.7% for white females.

An active register of all hypertension patients is clearly needed in any family practice. More and better research is needed in family practice settings on this and other common problems. This research requires epidemiological and statistical rigour which is increasingly possible in collaborative research projects involving medical school departments of family practice and practising family physicians. At the same time, however, critical analysis of large-scale clinical studies in non-family settings can also help to establish treatment guidelines for the family physician. With regard to the treatment of hypertension, the family physician clearly has a health promotion role including periodic follow-up, detection and treatment of risk factors, attention to psychosocial problems, and the rational use of antihypertensive drugs for patients with persistent diastolic blood pressure above 100 mmHg.

References

Aagaard G.N. (1981). Hypertension Detection and Follow-up Program: An alternative interpretation. *Am. Heart J.*, **102,** 300

Hames, O.G. (1974). Natural history of essential hypertension in Evans County, Georgia. *Postgrad. Med.*, **56** (6), 119

Helgeland, A. (1980). Treatment of mild hypertension: a five-year controlled drug trial: the Oslo Study. *Am. J. Med.*, **69,** 725

Hypertension Detection and Follow-up Program Cooperative Group (1979). Five-year findings of the Hypertension Detection and Follow-up Program: Reduction in mortality of persons with high blood pressure, including mild hypertension. *J. Am. Med. Assoc.*, **242 (23),** 2562

Kaplan, N.M. (1981). Whom to treat: the dilemma of mild hypertension. *Am. Heart J.*, **101,** 867

The Management Committee. (1980). The Australian therapeutic trial in mild hypertension. *Lancet.* **1,** 1261

O'Malley, K., O'Brien, E. (1980). Management of hypertension in the elderly. *N. Engl. J. Med.*, **302 (25),** 1397

US Public Health Service Hospitals Cooperative Study Group. (1977). Treatment of mild hypertension. Results of a ten-year intervention trial. *Circ. Res.*, **40** (Suppl I), 98

Veterans Administration Cooperative Study Group on Antihypertensive Agents. (1980). Effects of treatment on morbidity in hypertension. II: Results in patients with diastolic blood pressure averaging 90 through 114 mmHg. *J. Am. Med. Assoc.*, **213,** 1143

Commentary

What to do with the mild to moderate ageing hypertensive probably is 'the single most important dilemma in primary care (family medicine) which is likely to confront us for the rest of this century'. The debate rages and is unresolved. However, it is generally agreed that younger hypertensives (under 50 years) *should* be treated. Risks of raised blood pressure vary inversely with age. It is uncertain whether elderly mild to moderate hypertensives (over 60 years) derive any demonstrable benefits from years of antihypertensive therapy. What to do with 50–60-year-old hypertensives is also unclear.

It has to be accepted at present that we do not know the causation of essential hypertension and that use of antihypertensive drugs is empirical. The chief benefit of effective control of hypertension is reduction of mortality from strokes. It is uncertain whether deaths from heart disease are reduced. Until the situation becomes clearer with results of extensive trials it is wise to keep an open mind.

Whatever the final outcome of the debate each family practitioner must consider his or her role in the care of hypertensive patients. How should hypertensives be diagnosed – the most economical way is to record every adult's blood pressure at least once every 5 years. What is the best management of hypertensives? A programme of continuing care and assessment should be evolved, even if drugs are not prescribed.

Each hypertensive should be cared for individually and periodic critical review of effectiveness of therapy should be carried out.

Therapies may require changes – either more drugs or even withdrawal
of drugs – and the blood pressure of some hypertensives may become
normotensive in time.

2 Psychotropic pills or psychotherapy?

The issues

'Psychiatric problems' in family practice are largely 'symptom diagnoses' with descriptive features and few positive signs. Many factors enter into possible causes and management – patient, family and environment; the physician; the disorder; and possible therapies. There are many uncertainties on the natural histories of the varied syndromes.

In asking what treatment for what and with what results, three questions can be posed: Who should treat the patient – the family physician, but when should the patient be referred to a psychiatrist? What are the criteria for selecting pills (and which ones) or psychotherapy? What are the results of the various treatments and how do they compare?

The case for pills
Paul Freeling

Anything to do with psychoemotional problems seems all too often to be considered 'only a matter of opinion'. Judgements as to whether or not the management of a person with psychoemotional problems is appropriate seem to vary with the occupation and training of the professional involved (Smith, 1981). It has been demonstrated that people in England and Wales vary in their opinion as to the nature of problems which it is appropriate to take to a family doctor, and that the variance is related to how well they believe they know their own general practitioner (Cartwright and Anderson, 1981). In the same study a decrease, between 1964 and 1977, was shown in the numbers of both doctors and their patients believing a general practitioner 'was a suitable person to talk to about problems such as children getting into trouble, or difficulties between husband and wife'. The proportion who would turn to their own family doctor had not changed over time and there was no evidence of a change in consulting rates in the 2 weeks preceding the interviews on which Cartwright and Anderson base their report. Nevertheless, 92 per cent of the general practitioners in the 1977 sample thought there was 'a growing tendency for people to seek help for problems in their family lives'. This might be related to the increase, between 1964 and 1977, in the proportion of patients who thought they would consult their own general practitioner about 'a constant feeling of depression for 3 weeks'.

One suspects that the differences in perceptions between doctors and their patients reported by Cartwright and Anderson reflect differences in labelling by the two groups. They may be related to the limited diagnostic vocabulary (Hodgkin, 1979) of primary care physicians and the lack of an accepted taxonomy for patient behaviour representing an integration of clinical medicine and behavioural science (McWhinney, 1972). They may be related also to the factors which have led to eloquent pleas for the adoption by doctors of a biopsychosocial model which would account for 'the reality of diabetes and schizophrenia on human experiences as well as disease abstractions' (Engel, 1977); and what seems certain is that people with psychoemotional problems vary in the ways in which they present themselves to doctors. Some will present with physical symptoms, some will present with other symptoms related to mood and some will present the problems, interpersonal or intrapersonal, by which they see themselves beset. These different presentations may reflect cultural differences as to what is or is not acceptable to present to a doctor; they may represent what the patient thinks has been learnt, from previous encounters, of a particular doctor's preferences between different types of presentation, or they may represent true variation in the psychological susceptibility of individual patients to the psychosocial transitions (Parkes, 1971) that all of us experience. Certainly it has been demonstrated (Brown and Harris, 1978) that previous life experiences and present social factors have a significant predictive value, for example, for the likelihood of women in one part of London developing a depressive illness.

PERCEPTIONS AND DIAGNOSES

The family doctor then may be faced in different consultations by similar complaints representing problems of differing types and severity, or by different complaints representing problems which are similar in type and severity. It is the doctor's responsibility to elicit and elucidate these problems. In some cases at least a descriptive diagnosis must precede the decision as to methods of management. Some of the patients who present a psychosocial problem, or from whom one can be elicited, will be suffering from a complex of symptoms which together form a syndrome representing a defined psychiatric illness amenable to the treatments available to doctors by prescription, practice or by referral.

There is huge variation in the frequency with which family doctors make these defined diagnoses, but apparently considerably less variation in the frequency with which these conditions exist in the patients consulting. At least one study (Zintl-Wiegand and Cooper, 1979) has led to the conclusion that 'differences in rates of psychiatric illness reported by general practitioners are due more to the differing perceptions and diagnostic habits of the practitioners themselves than to real differences in frequency among patients'. The variations between general practitioners in the frequency with which they make psychiatric diagnoses has been studied by others. Marks, Goldberg, and Hillier (1979) have delineated two contributing factors: first a bias towards making psychiatric diagnoses at all, and second the accuracy of those diagnoses when made. Each factor varies considerably. It would seem that doctors in training can have their bias altered and their accuracy increased by being trained in appropriate methods of interviewing (Goldberg *et al.* 1980), but that the least accurate doctors seemed blocked in their learning if they did know what to do for patients in whom they made accurate diagnoses.

CHOICES

A dilemma is 'an argument forcing (an) opponent to choose one of two alternatives unfavourable to him: (a) position that leaves only a choice between equally unwelcome possibilities' (Sykes, 1976). There is no true dilemma facing a general practitioner who elicits a psychoemotional problem from a patient because more than two alternatives face the doctor and, with reasonably accurate diagnosis, the choices do not offer equally unwelcome possibilities. There is a whole spectrum of choices as to management, varying from liquidation of the problem as a problem (the patient recognizes that what he thought was, in fact is not) through elimination of a behavioural pattern or its underlying cause, to adjustment of the patient's environment or state to meet the needs imposed by an otherwise unalterable situation (Dudley, 1970).

There is no need for the selection of one kind of therapy to result in the exclusion of all others. The choices available to the general practitioner in the management of emotional disorder associated with psychosocial problems stem from the general practitioner's correctly holistic view of medicine in which 'the individual is conceived of as a complex dynamic system in an unstable state of equilibrium, acting and reacting to changes within the environment and to changes within the system ... [so that] when we speak of psychological processes and physiological processes, we are speaking of different ways of approaching a phenomenon. The phenomenon is not so divided' (World Health Organization, 1964).

The holistic viewpoint requires not only a consideration of a wide range of problems and selections from a wide range of solutions or therapies, it also requires that the effect of a selected therapy on all parts of the complex dynamic system be considered both before selection and after application. Above all the holistic approach leads us to considering the use of differing therapies simultaneously, as for instance in one recent study (Blackburn *et al.*, 1981) showing that treatment of depression in both hospital and general practice was most effective when it combined cognitive therapy with pharmacotherapy. It is interesting that this finding was not affected by the presence of endogenous factors. The complexity which this approach introduces into doctors' decision-making may have led to creation of a dilemma where none should exist.

What the apparent dilemma directs us towards is the matter of accurate diagnosis of the mood and psychological wellbeing of the patient as a basis for treatment decisions. This point would not need to be made if we were considering the use of pharmacotherapy for pulmonary tuberculosis, since in pulmonary tuberculosis one cause, the infecting organism, is clearly available to be removed, and we have medications of proven effectiveness for doing this. The management of psychoemotional problems in general practice requires a knowledge of the efficacy of the medications available and of their wider effects.

DIAGNOSING PSYCHOEMOTIONAL STATES

It seems sensible to focus, for the purposes of this relatively short essay, on doctors' decisions concerning the presence or absence of marked affective disorder. Where a patient manifests schizophrenia or mania the doctor will have little difficulty in deciding upon diagnosis or upon management. Severe depression (sometimes called psychotic depression) will not usually pose problems as to diagnosis although it may pose problems as to management.

The purposes of a doctor are directed towards helping 'each person in his care to attain optimum development as a whole person' (Royal

College of General Practitioners, 1972). Methods of doing this include helping patients to avoid developing maladaptive responses and to eliminate such responses if they have been developed already. The symptoms related to psychoemotional problems may form complexes which can be categorized as either 'anxiety' or 'depression'. The two complexes may overlap so that some authorities avoid the use of these terms in general practice (Shepherd et al., 1966) and some general practitioners use the term 'mixed anxiety and depression' (Watson and Barber, 1980).

Anxiety can be viewed as a form of arousal which is sometimes helpful to a patient as a drive leading to decision-making and consequent change, while depression can be viewed as a protective response which is unpleasant to experience and which prevents decision-making or change. If such a view is taken then the use of drugs for the treatment of anxiety requires very careful consideration since it may be either adaptive or maladaptive; the use of antidepressants, on the other hand, would require only careful diagnosis and careful monitoring since depression will only be adaptive when a situation is truly hopeless or insufferably sad. In all other situations treatment with antidepressants will probably facilitate an adaptive response helping the depressed person to change his or her view of himself as a 'loser' (Beck et al., 1979) and benefit from a constructive approach to any problems which exist. It will always be difficult to assess the efficacy of drug treatment in the treatment of psychoemotional problems because of the degree to which spontaneous resolution, non-specific factors such as changes in precipitating events, the placebo effect of medication, and support from the social environment or contact with a helping professional, may account for outcome in the treatment of either anxiety or depression (Paykel, 1979).

Nevertheless it seems that where depression is concerned symptom pattern and life stress are only weakly related (Paykel, 1974). The notion that depression associated with identifiable problems does not warrant treatment may be positively dangerous. The terms endogenous and exogenous are certainly less helpful than terms relating to symptom patterns in deciding upon the efficacy of interventions, and most predictor studies have focused on them. For this purpose psychotic depression shows a symptom-pattern including delusions, psychomotor disturbance, absence of mood reactivity, presence of diurnal variation (worse in the morning), early wakening together with absence of obvious stress in a good and stable premorbid personality (Klerman, 1971). Neurotic depressives tend, in this classification, to show milder illness with anxiety, reactivity, evening worsening, initial insomnia, concomitant stress and a vulnerable or neurotic premorbid personality.

GRADING

While each individual has his or her own idiosyncratic focus amongst his symptoms, depressive symptoms form an orderly progression mainly related to severity (Lader, 1981), and it is to severity that decision about treatment must be related. Some general practitioners may find it helpful to adopt, formally or informally, a scale designed for use in epidemiological studies (Raskin, Reatig and McKeon, 1970) which permits the severity of depression to be rated on a 5-point scale from 'very severe' (4) to 'not at all' (0), for three composite items. The first item, 'verbal report' covers: 'says he/she feels unhappy; talk of feelings of worthlessness, helpless or hopeless; complains of loss of interest; may wish he/she were dead; reports crying spells'. The second item 'behaviour', covers 'looks sad; cries easily; speaks in a sad voice; appears slowed down; lacking in energy'. The third item, 'secondary symptoms of depression' covers: 'insomnia; gastrointestinal complaints; dry mouth; recent suicide attempt; lack of appetite; difficulty in concentrating or remembering'. A score of seven or more on this scale would normally imply a depressive experience severe enough to be treated. Its main value, however, would be as a checklist to make sure all diagnostic information has been consciously considered.

WHOM? WHERE? WHAT?

The choices of treatment result from three questions: By whom? Where? With what? 'By whom' lies between specialist doctors, other specialist helpers, and general or family practitioners. 'Where' lies between ambulatory and working in the community, ambulatory and not working in the community, attending a special day centre, or in hospital wards of various types. 'With what' lies, for depression, between electroconvulsive therapy, monoamine oxidase inhibitors, tricyclic and newer antidepressants, social interventions and psychotherapeutic support.

The evidence that psychotic depressives respond better than neurotic ones to electroconvulsive therapy seems most clear cut. Published studies of electroconvulsive therapy nearly all involve inpatients, and on these patients six out of nine comparative studies showed electroconvulsive therapy better overall than tricyclic antidepressants, two found equal effects and one found the drug faster but not otherwise better. Few family doctors would feel competent to prescribe electroconvulsive therapy, but it seems clear that it is sometimes advisable for those depressed patients whom even the more competent would need to refer because of the severity of their illness and, in particular, the failure of other attempts at management.

The moderate and milder depressive experiences will usually respond to tricyclic antidepressants, and the decision whether to use these in association with personal and social support will usually rest upon consideration of duration and persistence of symptoms as well as upon their severity.

DRUGS AND DOSAGE

Once the decision has been taken to give a tricyclic or newer antidepressant drug there can be no excuse for not giving an adequate dosage, and there is much to be said for the doctor restricting himself to drugs with which he is familiar. I personally restrict myself to imipramine 75–150 mg daily, with trimipramine 50–150 mg as an alternative where sleeplessness is a major symptom. I am attempting to become familiar with the newer antidepressants but have yet to be convinced that their claimed advantages outweigh my lack of familiarity with them. It should hardly be necessary to state that all patients prescribed antidepressants must be warned of likely side-effects and also of the temporal delay in response; this is particularly true of the monoamine oxidase inhibitors (MAOI) which most family doctors avoid, as I do, leaving their use to specialists in whose hands they can occasionally be very helpful.

Anxiolytics

Where anxiety is concerned the matter of pills against psychotherapy is of a different order, especially if included under psychotherapy are various kinds of behaviour therapy which are usually too time-consuming for personal use by the family doctor. That there are drugs which are more effective than placebo in relieving the symptoms of anxiety seems widely accepted. The benzodiazepines, in particular, are described as clinically effective, free of serious side-effects and carrying a low potential for suicide (Petursson and Lader, 1981). The use of these drugs is widespread; they constitute a significant proportion of the total prescriptions written by general practitioners in the United Kingdom and some of their trade-names seem to have become part of the public domain. More recently concern has been expressed about the value of their long-term use and it is now suggested that it be avoided (Committee on the Review of Medicines, 1980). It seems that for patients who have been on normal dosage of a benzodiazepine for a year or more, withdrawal of the drug produces effects some of which are similar to the symptoms for which the drugs were originally prescribed. These symptoms tend to disappear within 2–4 weeks after withdrawal of the drugs.

It would seem, therefore, that no doctor should prescribe a benzodiazepine drug for a patient without careful thought and certainly not without careful monitoring. Further, no family doctor should prescribe a benzodiazepine until a careful assessment of the source of anxiety experienced by the patient has been identified, or at least until the situation in which it is experienced has been delineated.

Where anxiety is clearly associated with particular situations, approaches based upon behaviour therapy may be of value. Where anxiety is associated with approach/avoidance conflict, with the patient's need to make choices between decisions each involving outcomes good in some aspects and bad in others, then reduction of anxiety by drugs may be particularly disadvantageous and a counselling approach be more appropriate. When, however, a patient is crippled by paralysing fear, when the symptoms of anxiety are so severe that the patient cannot make even a first approach to a situation or to a decision, then it may be justified to use benzodiazepines to enable the patient to take those first steps. When the doctor does this the patient should be informed of the doctor's purpose and intention and a verbal 'contract' drawn up. I have found that this use of a verbal contract has enabled me to help patients who suffered from quite severe phobias without having to refer them to behaviour therapy.

SUMMARY

The use of drugs in psychosocial problems is not only permissible, but in some cases essential. In general, they are more useful to patients suffering from depression than those experiencing anxiety. In particular, no drug should be given except on the basis of accurate diagnosis nor without due consideration of its wider effects on a patient's life and circumstances. In no case can drug treatment alone excuse a family doctor from the responsibility of caring about, as well as for, his patient and in no case should drugs be used without continuous monitoring for their side-effects and outcomes.

References

Beck, A. T., Rush, A. J., Shaw, B. F. and Emery, G. (1979). *Cognitive Therapy of Depression*. (New York: Guilford Press)

Blackburn, I. M., Bishop, S., Glenn, A. I. M., Whalley, L. J. and Christie, J. E. (1981). The efficacy of cognitive therapy in depression. *Br. J. Psychiar.*, **139**, 181

Brown, G.W. and Harris, T. (1978). *Social Origins of Depression: a Study of Psychiatric Disorders in Women*. (London: Tavistock Publications)

Cartwright, A. and Anderson, R. (1981). *General Practice Revisited*. pp. 51–3. (London: Tavistock Publications)

Committee on the Review of Medicines (1980). Systematic review of the benzo-diazepines. *Br. Med. J.*, **280**, 910–12

Dudley, H. A. F. (1970). The clinical task. *Lancet*, **2**, 1352–54

Engel, G. L. (1977). The need for a new medical model. A challenge to bio-medicine. *Science*, **196**, 4286, 129–136

Goldberg, D. P., Steele, J. J., Smith, C. and Spivey, L. (1980). Training family doctors to recognise psychiatric illness with increased accuracy. *Lancet*, **2**, 521–523

Hodgkin, K. (1979). Diagnostic vocabulary for primary care. *J. Family Pract.* **8**, 1, 129–144

Klerman, G. L. (1971). Clinical research in depression. *Arch. Gen. Psychiatr.*, **24**, 305

Lader, M. H. (1981). *Focus on Depression*. (Middlesex: Bencard)

McWhinney, I. R. (1972). Beyond diagnosis. *N. Engl. J. Med.*, **287**, 8, 384–387

Marks, J., Goldberg, D. P. and Hillier, V. F. (1979). Determinants of the ability of general practitioners to detect psychiatric illness. *Psychol. Med.*, **9**, 337–53

Parkes, C. M. (1971). Psychosocial transitions: a field for study. *Soc. Sci. Med.*, **5**, 101–115

Paykel, E. S. (1974). Recent life events and clinical depression. In Gunderson, E. K. and Rake, R. H. (eds.) *Life Stress and Illness*. pp. 134–63. (Springfield: C. C. Thomas)

Paykel, E. S. (1979). Predictors of treatment response. In Paykel, E. S. and Coppen, A. (eds.) *Psycho-pharmacology of Affective Disorders*. pp. 193–220. (Oxford: Oxford University Press)

Petursson H. and Lader, M. H. (1981). Withdrawal from long-term benzodi-azepine treatment. *Br. Med. J.*, **283**, 643–645

Raskin, A., Reatig, N. and McKeon, J. (1970). Differential response to chlor-promazine, imipramine and placebo. *Arch. Gen. Psychiatr.*, **23**, 164–173

Royal College of General Practitioners (1972). *The Future General Practitioner – Learning and Teaching*. (London: British Medical Journal)

Shepherd, M., Cooper, B., Brown, A. C. and Kalton, G. W. (1966). *Psychiatric Illness in General Practice*. (London: Oxford University Press)

Smith, R. (1981). Psychological problems in general practice. Oxford conference on a 'grey area'. *Br. Med. J.*, **283**, 832–833

Sykes, J. B. (ed.) (1976). *The Concise Oxford Dictionary of Current English*. (Oxford: Oxford University Press)

Watson, J. M. and Barber, J. H. (1980). Depressive illness in general practice. *Health Bull.*, **39/2**, 112–115

World Health Organization (1964). *Psychosomatic Disorders, World Health Organization Technical Reports Series, No. 275*. (Geneva: World Health Organization)

Zintl-Wiegand, A. and Cooper, B. (1979). Psychiatric morbidity and needs for care in general practice. In Hafner, H. (ed.) *Estimating Needs for Mental Health Care*. pp. 69–79. (New York: Springer-Verlag)

The case for psychotherapy
Stanley Levenstein

The most significant finding to emerge from the study of psychotherapy in recent years is that it is the *relationship* (Truax and Carkhuff, 1975; Rogers, 1974) between therapist and patient which is the most important determinant of the outcome of therapy, irrespective of the theoretical orientation or method of the therapist. While I am not suggesting that a wholesale transplantation of the process of psychotherapy on to general practice would be feasible or even desirable, I think it would be foolish to ignore the implications of this finding for the management of our patients with emotional problems.

DOCTOR–PATIENT RELATIONSHIPS

The research data on the importance of the therapist–patient relationship indicated that *empathic understanding* (the ability to think *with*, rather than for or about the patient), *unconditional positive regard* (a deep and genuine caring for the patient as a person) and *genuineness* (as opposed to a façade of interest) were the most important variables affecting the outcome of therapy. When one thinks about it, it is not really surprising, for these are the very ingredients which are missing from the relationships of most patients with emotional problems. Indeed Sullivan's (1953) definition of psychiatry as 'the operational statement of interpersonal relations' implies that most psychiatric problems can be traced back to past and/or current difficulties in interpersonal relationships.

UNHELPFUL CLASSIFICATIONS

It is with these difficulties in interpersonal relationship that our patients present to us daily, be it with overt depressive symptoms, psychosomatic complaints or whatever. An important point arises here, namely that traditional psychiatric classification gives little assistance in helping us to understand what it is that is *really* troubling a patient. For example 'depression' merely describes *symptoms* and not causes, and it is as inappropriate a basis for treatment as is 'dyspnoea' of unestablished causation. This could explain the limited usefulness of antidepressant or anxiolytic drugs – they are designed to treat symptoms and not causes. So far no-one has invented an 'antitrust-problem' drug or an 'antiauthority-figure-problem' or an 'antiproblem with closeness and intimacy', or an 'anti-need-to-be-in-power, and-control of others' drug, etc. These are some of the areas of relationship difficulties which cause personal unhappiness. No 'happiness drug' has yet been invented to counter them.

IDEAL SITUATIONS

The general practitioner is ideally placed to observe the difficulties which patients have in their relationships, as sooner or later they will emerge in their relationship with *him*. For example, a patient with a problem in relating to authority figures may behave excessively obsequiously towards his general practitioner for some time and then launch a most aggressive attack on him for an apparently trivial reason. A patient with a problem in dependency needs may present by trying to assert his independence from the doctor by consulting as seldom as possible, asking for prescriptions to be left with the receptionist, and by poor compliance with doctor's treatment regimes, even at the risk of serious decline in his health.

BALINT GROUPS

It is these kinds of doctor–patient interactions that have been the object of study of Balint groups (Balint, 1971; Balint and Norell, 1973; Levenstein, 1978) since 1950. It was in these seminars composed of general practitioners under the leadership of a psychodynamically orientated therapist that the importance of trying to 'tune in' and listen to what our patients are really trying to say to us first came really to be appreciated. The patient makes certain 'offers' such as headaches, abdominal pain, coping with a restless baby, etc. By developing the necessary sensitivity the general practitioner can come to understand the hidden message behind the offer and therefore respond in an appropriate way. By 'appropriate' I mean in a way that is meaningful to the patient and not just to the doctor, as in the case with giving advice, reassurance, prescribing psychotropic drugs, etc. These latter actions may well have meaning for the general practitioner and may well serve to reduce *his* anxiety, but they are unlikely to help the patient whose problems are in his own world of relationships and not the general practitioner's.

A NON-PILL SOLUTION

What can the general practitioner do for his patient with emotional problems apart from prescribing pills? In accordance with what has been said so far, this question may best be answered by saying that he can offer him a worthwhile *relationship*, one which unlike his other significant relationships, is not characterized by rejection, a need to control and dominate him, lack of understanding of his feelings, etc. Such a relationship is not developed overnight, but this is where the ongoing relationship over time that characterizes general practice has special importance. It may take a long time and a great deal of patience and sensitivity on the part of the general practitioner to establish a trusting relationship with a mistrustful patient. However, once it has been established the patient has achieved something really valuable and certainly more substantial than the temporary relief gained by swallowing some pills, the prescribing of which may well have given him the idea that the doctor regards him as 'ill' or 'neurotic' – a disease instead of a person.

CASE HISTORIES

I would like to illustrate the above points by quoting three examples from my own practice.

MR S. A middle-aged man had presented on a few occasions with depressive symptoms. He was married with three children and worked as an estimator for the municipality. He described himself as a 'compulsive worker'. Antidepressant medication had had only a temporary and limited beneficial effect. He then started developing various psychosomatic symptoms, culminating in attacks of breathlessness and tightness around the chest. On one of these occasions he was taken from work to hospital where extensive investigations failed to reveal any cardiac or other organic pathology. At this stage he at last accepted the psychogenicity of his symptoms.

On coming to see me after discharge from the hospital the patient told me that he had been brought up in an orphanage after the death of his mother when he was 8 years old. He admitted never being able to get close to anybody including his wife and children. He also recognized for the first time that his compulsive working was a defence against confronting his own sense of loneliness and isolation. He said he often wanted to talk to people, but was afraid they would let him down. I replied 'like your parents did?' He said that he now felt free to come and talk to me whenever he felt the need, which he has done at approximately monthly to 2-monthly intervals since. He has had no further psychosomatic 'attacks' nor has he presented with depressive symptoms again. I think he can be regarded as representative of a kind of comparative trial of the effects of psychotropic drugs and 'relationship therapy' having received both forms of treatment.

MISS L. This 18-year-old woman presented with symptoms of 'acute anxiety' – trembling, sweating, hyperventilation, etc. At first she said she did not know what could be causing her symptoms, then, when it became clear that I was really interested, she said she was having a lot of conflict as to whether or not to go on to the pill. She was very attracted to her boyfriend with whom she had been going out for some time, but she feared that he might drop her once he had 'got what he wanted'. She was also in conflict about moral misgivings based on her upbringing on the one hand, and what she felt was her right to lead her own life on the other. Discussion helped her to clarify her main areas of conflict and also to approach her boyfriend openly about the difficulties in their relationship, including the implications of sexual contact for her. She has had no further 'anxiety attacks' or symptoms in spite of (because of?) not having taken any tranquillisers.

MRS V. This married woman of 24 presented with 'postpartum depression' 2 months after the birth of her first baby, requesting medicine to make the baby sleep. She herself was sleeping badly and had been taking antidepressant tablets at night which she had 'borrowed from a friend' for the past 3 weeks to no avail. She was very tearful and said that she was a 'hopeless mother'. Brief discussion revealed that she had been an eldest child herself and that her own mother had lacked confidence in dealing with her. She appeared noticeably more relaxed when it became clear to her that feelings of lack of self-confidence, and also angry and hostile feelings towards the baby, did not meet with my disapproval or rejection. She was encouraged to visit on a *p.r.n.* basis, and her husband was seen in an attempt to involve him in a supportive way as well as to give him a chance to express his feelings about the situation. The woman's depression had improved markedly when I saw her again 10 days later (she had stopped taking the antidepressant pills in the meanwhile), and the baby had begun to sleep better without any medication. This improvement has been maintained in the 4 or 5 months since then.

IMPLICATIONS OF THE CASE HISTORIES

None of the above cases can be described as psychotherapy *per se*, and all the consultations concerning them took place during routine consulting hours ($\pm$ 15 minutes per consultation), but I think it is reasonable to claim that all the patients mentioned benefited from a *psychotherapeutic relationship* with their general practitioner in which they were helped to understand and manage their emotional problems more effectively. Since time is often raised as an excuse for giving pills instead of general practitioner time, it may be mentioned that the same amount of time or more may have been used (a great deal less productively) if these patients had simply been issued with prescriptions, and then returned repeatedly with some symptom or other because their *real* needs were not being met.

I do not wish to imply that there is *no* place for psychotropic drugs in general practice. In the more severely disturbed patients and those who are more defensive or 'closed', psychotropic drugs will have a relatively more important role to play, but pills should always be an *adjunct to* and never a *substitute for* a caring, accepting, relationship. When given as *part* of the treatment, pills can sometimes serve as 'a little bit of the doctor in a bottle' and as such may have a beneficial effect. However, the effects of a psychotherapeutic relationship are more lasting than the 'placebo' effects of pills, because the former makes contact with the real person behind the symptoms while the latter only act on a surface level, with the result that sooner or later the untouched underlying problems will surface again. While patients who have been treated with a psychotherapeutic approach may also manifest with problems again, they will be in a position to 'build on' their relationship with their general practitioner to make more meaningful progress with their difficulties.

Let us remember that *all* people have a need to be understood, accepted, and cared for, and that it is thus not only the better educated, more verbal, and more intelligent among the population who can derive benefit from 'general practitioner psychotherapy'.

Opponents of the psychotherapeutic approach may point out that it cannot solve the patient's problems. In so doing they miss the point, for the purpose of a psychotherapeutic approach is *not* to solve the patients' problems but to help *them* to understand their problems more clearly in order to be in a better position to try to resolve or at least accept their own difficulties. The obsession with 'curing' the patient's psychological (and other) ills seems to be a hangover from the medical school training and the premium it places on dramatic results of treatment, causing especially those in the surgical specialties to be highly revered role-models. This must have provided at least some of the motivation for looking for 'quick cures' such as pills for all sorts of other problems as well. The result has been the mushrooming of pharmaceutical industries all over the world with psychotropics providing a substantial proportion of their income and thus causing ever-increasing pressure on doctors to prescribe them.

Perhaps it would be best to conclude this chapter by putting it into its societal context and pointing out that we are living in an age where technology, for all its undoubted advantages, has had an appallingly dehumanizing effect on people's lives. Medicine has not been spared from this, and it was partly as a reaction to being treated as organ-systems or biochemical processes rather than as human beings that the public clamour for more personalized, primary medical care gained momentum in the postwar era.

A psychotherapeutic approach to our patients is not intended as a cure-all for their problems. However, it is a helping hand from another human being, which is especially important nowadays when people are increasingly being regarded as numbers to be fed into and pushed out of a computer to determine their maximal profitability to the huge technological-economic machine of our times.

References

Balint, M. (1971). *The Doctor, His Patient and the Illness.* 2nd edn. (Surrey: Pitman Paperbacks)

Balint, E. and Norell, J. S. (eds.) (1973). *Six Minutes for the Patient: Interactions in General Practice Consultation.* (London: Tavistock Publications)

Levenstein, S. (1978). A report of three years' experience of a Balint group in Cape Town, South Africa. *S. Afr. Med. J.*, **54,** 121

Rogers, C. (1974). *On Becoming a Person – A Therapist's View of Psychotherapy.* (London: Constable)

Sullivan, H. S. (1953). *The Interpersonal Theory of Psychiatry.* (New York: W. W. Norton)

Truax, C. B. and Carkhuff, R. R. (1975). *Toward Effective Counseling and Psychotherapy.* (Chicago: Aldine)

Commentary

The breadth of psychosocial–emotional disorders is huge yet intensely personal. Both contributors point out the difficulties of applying medically approved labels to the problems that individual patients present and for which they seek help.

Whatever therapy is eventually selected and applied a holistic approach is essential. Much more emphasis has to be given to 'care' rather than attempts to 'cure'. Improvement and recovery depend very much on the patient working out his/her own solutions with considerable help and support from a personal physician who may prescribe psychotropic pills plus psychotherapy. Individual physicians develop their own philosophies towards these common problems. Such philosophies must include some interpretation of what they can see as the nature of the conditions and some skills and expertise, based on experience, of care. It matters little whether there is a greater emphasis towards psychotherapy or towards a more ready use of psychotropic drugs. The essence must be that the patient is helped towards recovery.

Good practice and care of patients demand that there can never be exclusive use of either pills or psychotherapy. The physician should be able to use one or other or both depending on the patient's needs. Absence of much reliable data and knowledge of the natural history and outcome of these common conditions, and of the results of treatments with pills or psychotherapy or both, makes it difficult to decide on values and makes the needs for more research apparent and urgent.

3 Alcoholism – disease or self-inflicted vice?

The issues

Alcoholism comprises a huge and largely hidden collection of medical and social problems. The causal factor is clear and evident, but the effects depend very much on individual, family and community features. Consumption of alcohol is almost a universal social custom – fewer than 20 per cent of adults are strict teetotallers – and its problems and control involve politicians, teachers, lawyers, police, social workers, industrialists as well as physicians. Who should take actions?

Decisions on whether alcoholism should be viewed as a disease or as a self-inflicted vice, aided by social habits and expectations, will influence public policies and actions depending very much on what the public want their elected representatives to do. The medical profession's views on whether alcoholism can be considered as a disease *per se*, or as a bad personal habit akin to smoking that can be changed only through health education, will influence attitudes to treatment and care.

The case for alcoholism as a non-disease (1)
John Fry

In western societies such as the United States or United Kingdom two-thirds of adults regularly consume alcohol and 10 per cent of these have 'drinking problems' or suffer effects of alcoholism. This means that a family physician caring for 2500 persons might expect 75–100 adults with

39

drinking problems. In fact this is a tip-of-the-iceberg phenomenon and only very few of these heavy drinkers surface, mainly because of serious medical or social complications or because they, or more often members of their families, seek treatment.

How can we really accept that 10 million Americans, 2.5 million Britons and 0.5 million Australians with drinking problems are suffering from a disease brought about by their own self-chosen habits. If alcoholism is a disease then so is cigarette-smoking, overeating or drug-taking.

Certainly the effects of excessive consumption of alcohol, tobacco, food and drugs create social and medical problems that have to be managed, but the labelling of these personal habits as 'diseases' creates difficulties and confusion.

ALCOHOLISM AS A DISEASE – DIFFICULTIES CREATED

Suppose we accept alcoholism as a disease, what are the consequences?

(1) Alcoholics must not be *blamed or punished* for what they have done to themselves by drinking too much for too long.
(2) Alcoholics must be allowed to take on the '*sick role*' and all the privileges that such a role entitles the sick person to assume and accept.
(3) Alcoholics must be accepted as '*patients*' by physicians.
(4) Alcoholics must be provided with *therapy* to treat them.
(5) Alcoholics must have *more services and facilities* for early detection, treatment and after-care.
(6) Alcoholics must have *more units, physicians and nurses, counselling services and resources* provided for them.
(7) Alcoholics must be accepted as *being somewhat different from their fellows* as the reason for succumbing to excessive alcohol consumption for too long. Their metabolism, psychology and genetics may be different from the norm.

Unfortunately there is no evidence that alcoholics *are* any different from their fellows in metabolism, psychology or genetics. There is no good evidence for treating alcoholics as patients with more resources, physicians, units or therapies. There have been no good clinical trials to demonstrate the benefits of active professional intervention.

Accepting alcoholism as a disease puts the responsibilities for success on the medical profession. We are expected to develop better treatments and to produce miraculous results. Alcoholics do not appear to be given many responsibilities for their own self-help.

PRESENT STATE

Alcohol is a drug that, like tobacco, has achieved social respectability. It is, nevertheless, a drug of dependence and its ill-effects are directly related to how much has been consumed for how long.

Consumption of alcohol has been going up in all western countries. In the United Kingdom it increased by more than 50 per cent between 1959 and 1974, and probably much more since 1974.

What have been the real effects of this huge increase in alcohol consumption?

(1) Admissions for alcoholism went up 6-fold in Scotland from 1956–76.
(2) Cirrhosis mortality has been increasing everywhere and especially in France and Italy.
(3) Convictions for drunkenness have increased.
(4) Road traffic accidents associated with alcohol are increasing.
(5) Industrial absenteeism and accidents related to alcohol are increasing.
(6) Marital break-ups from effects of alcohol have increased.
(7) Crime and violence are increasing everywhere and some is blamed on alcohol.
(8) Suicide and parasuicide, too, are often related to alcoholism.

Accepting all these facts we have also to accept that the results of medical treatment are less than good and any improvements that do occur are not necessarily the results of the treatment.

WHAT ARE THE IMPLICATIONS?

Alcoholism has become a bigger problem, not because it has become a more difficult disease but because more and more persons are drinking more and more alcohol for more and more time.

The best hope for the future must be with mass community action rather than by considering alcoholism as a disease requiring treatment of individuals.

The problems that have to be faced squarely by politicians rather than physicians are to make consumption of alcohol much more difficult. In Britain the relative price of alcohol is much lower than it was 20 years ago. Taxation of alcohol has lagged well behind inflation. More people are able to afford to consume more alcohol and this has encouraged more alcoholism. We need mass political and economic action to make alcohol harder to consume in such large quantities. However, governments seek votes and electoral popularity and are reluctant to impose such health measures, as they would lose popularity with the consuming public and reap the whirlwind of the huge alcohol industry lobby.

So we have a modern dilemma – how and what public health measures should be taken to control and prevent the effects of self-inflicted vices such as excessive smoking and alcohol consumption, without interfering with personal freedom?

Treating alcoholism as a disease is merely tinkering with the end-results of self-inflicted acts; it will have little effect on the prevention of an increasing modern epidemic.

The case for alcoholism as a non-disease (2)
Benno Pollak

The major advantage of labelling alcoholism as a disease is purely a social one. It legitimizes social support for the rehabilitation of alcoholics instead of punishing and stigmatizing them. By offering medical help it raises the chronic alcoholic's and his family's expectations of possible treatment and cure, and if it should fail it is no longer the patient's fault. Treatment may be harmful where the alcoholic refuses to accept any responsibility for his alcohol abuse and the harm it may bring him and his family.

Although the majority of the medical profession and society still accept the view that alcoholism must be some physical or mental disease, it has never been defined with any precision. Nowhere is there any reliable evidence that it has any pathological entity.

Pharmacologically, alcohol acts as a drug capable of inducing an unlimited variety of acute and chronic reactions, physically and mentally. Longstanding alcohol abuse becomes responsible for widely different disease processes, but only in some cases and not in others. We do not know why alcohol selects its own target organs in this arbitrary way. Similar drinking histories may lead to cirrhosis in some, pancreatitis, peripheral neuritis, cardiomyopathies or brain damage in others. However, in general, cirrhosis is more common in chronic than sporadic drinkers and women are at a greater risk than men.

Claims have been made that alcoholism is more likely to be a mental disorder than a physical one. However, it could not be shown that alcoholics have a personality and mental make-up which is different from the rest of the population. Alcoholics suffer from many psychiatric symptoms such as anxiety depression, paranoia, sleep disturbances, memory defects and intellectual deterioration, etc., but they are mainly *effects* and not *causes* of drinking and disappear with abstinence and alcohol control.

The most influential contribution for a disease concept of alcoholism came from Jellinek (1960), generally regarded as the first important scientist of alcoholism. He saw alcoholism as a disease characterized by a physical and psychological dependence on alcohol generating an overpowering compulsion to drink combined with a total lack of control over it. It has been suggested that abnormal neurophysiological and biochemical reactions were underlying this compulsion to drink; the hallmarks of this 'disease' were its withdrawal symptoms such as 'the shakes', sweats, sleep disturbances, amnesia, feelings of acute anxiety and others. It was the severity of them which kept the chronic alcoholic chained to the bottle whenever he tried to escape from the compulsion. Once this condition had reached an advanced stage, it became chronic and irreversible, and lifelong abstinence its only treatment. This disease concept of alcoholism has been challenged over the last 10–15 years.

Studying the drinking patterns of 'chronic alcoholics' has revealed that a considerable proportion of them change their drinking habits for months or years and resume social, controlled drinking or total abstinence without any treatment. An alcoholic may, for instance, drink heavily in a social group where this is the norm and much less in a new milieu. Some chronic alcoholics experience only mild dependence on alcohol.

I can substantiate these findings from my own observations. Having recorded the drinking habits of some 100 problem drinkers in my practice in 1972, I have met the same patients years later noting that a majority had changed their alcohol intake to more normal and socially acceptable norms. A change of job, marriage, family life, or moving home seem to have played a relevant part in it.

Abnormal drinking is more likely a behaviour disorder than a mysterious disease. No case can be made out for genetic, constitutional, metabolic and other physical and psychological factors which distinguish alcoholics from the general population in any essential ways.

How much a person drinks depends on his early home environment, his subsequent social life and the general socioeconomic and cultural fabric of the society in which he lives. It had been shown that alcoholism grows in proportion to national per capita consumption, the level of which depends on the price and availability of alcohol, and national attitudes to drinking.

In conclusion, the medical profession has been left in a state of confusion about the nature of alcoholism. By restricting its views on the chronic, heavily damaged, dependent alcoholic, the profession has failed to recognize the much larger group of problem drinkers – considered to be 1–2 million in the United Kingdom – who would be much more amenable to be influenced by their doctor's advice. Alcohol abuse should be seen as a social behavioural disorder with medical complications rather than a medical disorder with social complications.

The misuse of alcohol – whatever the reason for it – is no more a disease than the misuse of any other social habit.

Reference

Jellinek, E.M. (1960). *The Disease Concept of Alcoholism.* (New Haven: College and University Press)

The case for alcoholism as a disease
Ken Young

'An endemic disorder of frightening magnitude' reported the Royal College of Psychiatrists in 1979 and then went on to define alcoholism as 'a primary, chronic progressive and sometimes fatal disease, baffling in its complexity. Symptoms can be physical and/or mental. As it advances, alcoholism may be further complicated by a diminishing – or loss – of moral and spiritual values.'

EXTENT AND EFFECTS

The first statement is arresting and should disabuse all those who read it of the thought that the situation is not as bad as the Royal College states, or that it does not change much with the passage of time – the poor may always be with us, but we can assert without any doubt whatsoever that the alcoholic is most certainly with us, and increasingly so in all societies, whether advanced or not, posing no less a problem for a capitalist government as it does for a communist one!

The untold misery it causes cannot be measured; the escalating cost cannot be guessed at; and even more disturbing is the suspicion that the judgement and balance of persons in positions of power and influence may be dangerously impaired before any restraint can be applied.

There is no doubt that the degree of intellectual damage caused by alcohol may be very great before it is recognized, and when this is aggravated by physical malfunction we can readily appreciate the cost to industry, government and, say, the armed forces, from the shopfloor to the boardroom, from the corporal to the colonel.

FALSE DILEMMA

Dilemma, or rather dilemmas, there certainly are, but I do not believe that we should allow an academic argument about the disease theory of alcoholism to prevent or even delay our taking the preventive, ameliorative measures we know are of positive value if only on purely pragmatic grounds.

FAILURES OF ATTEMPTS TO MINIMIZE SALES OF ALCOHOL

Total prohibition has been clearly demonstrated as being at best futile and at worst even increasing the prevalence of alcoholism. Granting licences to purchase alcohol to certified alcoholics, as in India, or making the whole business a furtive and shameful transaction, as in Canada, has done little if anything to reduce its abuse, so although we know that making it expensive does reduce to a small degree the total amount purchased, methods which totally deprive the whole community of alcohol, or which cause humiliation to the individual purchaser will not succeed, and may even exacerbate the problem by increasing social tensions generally.

UNCERTAINTIES

Most communities must continue to live with alcohol while seeking always to mitigate or greatly reduce its harmful effects, and to do this effectively we must know why alcohol is taken in excess; why a given individual cannot abstain; why another becomes more tolerant of alcohol, and so on. These people must be identified *and* as early as possible, and this is a vital point. Anyone can recognize a drunkard, but even a very skilled medical observer will often fail to identify a person with an early alcohol problem. Indeed it has been claimed that only a 'cured' alcoholic can recognize a fellow 'undried' sufferer!

OBJECTIVES

Therefore we must seek to find ways and means of encouraging the incipient alcoholic to seek help on his own initiative and in the certain knowledge that there will be no sanction or criticism as a result, and further that he can expect complete confidentiality if that is his wish – certainly of no less degree than would be his right for *any* disease he might wish to have investigated and treated.

If however, the view still held by so many that failure to control alcohol intake is a sign of moral weakness or lack of willpower, then all attempts to curb, much less to understand, this 'endemic disorder of frightening magnitude' must end in abysmal failure.

It clearly follows that the condition we call alcoholism must be made as respectable and as acceptable to the individual and the society in which he lives as, for example, tuberculosis, cancer and diabetes. After all it was not so long ago that families concealed, out of shame, close relatives suffering from tuberculosis or mental defect, and although the former is now very respectable, the latter has not yet fully reached that laudable state!

MAKING ALCOHOLISM RESPECTABLE

How else, therefore, can we make alcoholism respectable other than by classifying it as a disease? This is not a new idea, for the disease concept was first written about by two famous physicians of the eighteenth and nineteenth centuries – Dr Benjamin Rush, an American, and Dr Thomas Trotter, an Englishman. They wrote about 'inebriety as an illness' and this later resulted in a slogan adopted by many of the Hospitals for Inebriates (in the United States) which declared that 'Intemperance is a Disease'. Sadly, or indeed ironically, these hospitals, movements and enlightened individuals never made much impression on the populace because the incomparably, more powerful temperance movement, then prevalent in the United States, rejected absolutely the idea that alcoholism was a disease, because acceptance of that concept would have been totally at variance with the very basis of the belief that moral weakness was the sole cause of the condition, and for which the cure or correction could only come from the exercise of willpower mediated, of course, by appropriate prayer and the good works of the temperance society involved.

Regrettably too, there was more than a whiff of suspicion that the reclaiming of lost souls, alcoholics in this case, took on a competitive flavour – the game, as might be expected, inexorably going to the more vociferous and well-funded societies. But further discussion on this subject, however interesting, would be controversial and profitless in that it would thereby deflect us from further pursuing the hypothesis that alcoholism is a disease. Indeed, debate about causation and treatment continues to bedevil the care of the alcoholic, so much so that it obscures the dominating influence of government revenue departments and the mighty lobby of brewers and distillers on the question of the control of alcohol purchase and intake.

CONSIDERING ALCOHOLISM AS A DISEASE

Alcohol undoubtedly *causes* many diseases both lethal and crippling in physical and psychological terms, but we are concerned here to examine the causes of the disease that gives rise to alcohol addiction in men, or inability to abstain or even control drinking no matter what the cost to self, work and family.

Alcoholism has too many definitions, whereas disease has none, and this 'multiplicity of hypotheses' has confused the public. And further, the disease concept of alcoholism may be lost in due course by its very vagueness. Therefore it is believed by many workers in the field that the multiplicity of the hypotheses clearly suggests that there is not just one alcoholism, but a whole variety.

The American Medical Association accepted the disease concept of alcoholism in 1956, and although unable to explain the nature of the condition, this fact does not mean that it is not an illness; there are after all many diseases whose nature was unknown for many years, cancer itself being a prime example. Indeed, even now we only know as much about alcoholism as we do about cancer, and that is a great deal less than we know about pneumonia, for instance.

Jellinek, in his book *The Disease Concept of Alcoholism*, contends that, 'Alcoholism is a genus not a species', and he uses a botanical comparison to clarify his thesis, citing the hibiscus flower, of which there are over 200 species, with a genus which comprises herbs, shrubs and trees; so, just as a botanist may ask, 'to which hibiscus are you referring?' we should be able to ask, 'to what sort of alcoholism are you referring?'

Thus we come to the heart of the matter; for it is not enough to list symptoms or signs, or postulate reasons for the alcoholism of an individual; these are too vague, too much in the eye of the beholders and therefore unsatisfactory generally as a basis for matching the appropriate treatment and management to the 'species' of alcoholism involved.

We said at the beginning of this paper that alcoholism was 'a primary, chronic progressive and sometimes fatal disease' but it is no less important to recognize that the disease may not cause any damage to the individual, or society, or both. (Dr Jellinek has termed as alcoholism, 'any use of alcoholic beverages that causes any damage to the individual or society or both'.) It is important to concede, as it were, that alcohol is as basic a substance in our society as bread, and could in truth be seen as no less a necessity than that staple of our civilization. Such a concession would, by acknowledging the undoubted virtues of alcohol, its widespread favour, and beneficent influence on some 80 per cent of the total population, defuse resistance to those seeking to control the abuse of it.

TYPES OF ALCOHOLISM

How then shall we classify these species of alcoholism? Fortunately there are not the hundreds of different species as in the hibiscus family, but some quite clearly definable patterns are recognized and have been classified simply by using the Greek alphabet.

Alpha alcoholism

This is a wholly psychological dependence upon the effect of alcohol to relieve pain of the body or mind, but it does not lead to loss of control or inability to abstain, nor does it unduly impair personal relationships, or appear to progress to any serious degree. The need for alcohol in these circumstances implies an innate illness and the 'undisciplined' use of alcohol may be seen as a symptom of the pathological condition which it relieves. This alpha type has been called 'problem drinking'.

Beta alcoholism

This type of alcoholism may lead to such complications as cirrhosis or polyneuropathy, but strangely enough may occur without either physical or psychological dependence upon alcohol. The drinking is usually heavy, related to social custom, and frequently associated with poor nutritional habits. Withdrawal symptoms are exceedingly rare.

Gamma alcoholism

This is a species of alcoholism where there is an increased tissue tolerance with changes in cell metabolism, and physical dependence with withdrawal symptoms and loss of control. This gamma species predominates in Anglo-Saxon countries and is the only species recognized by Alcoholics Anonymous. It also gives rise to the most severe and serious kinds of alcohol injury. The physical dependence results in craving, and the subsequent loss of control damages personal relationships no less than health, finances and social standing.

Delta alcoholism

This type is very similar to gamma, except that there is a total inability to abstain, rather than a loss of control, and thus withdrawal symptoms arise after only 1 or 2 days of abstinence.

Epsilon alcoholism

This is recognized by many when called dipsomania (Europe), or periodic alcoholism (United States). Little is known about this type of heavy drinking, and diagnosis is extremely difficult because of its episodic nature and relatively easy concealment.

The five groups mentioned cover the vast majority of those suffering from alcoholism, and were described in some detail to make the point that there were recognizably different syndromes of the disease of alcoholism, thus allowing doctors: to diagnose the disease in patients, to offer treatment, and to offer a prognosis at least as optimistic as that pertaining to many cancers. If, however, the disease concept is totally rejected, then the doctor has no part to play, resulting in my view in the epidemic of alcoholism increasing quite inexorably because the majority of sufferers will go undetected, a state of affairs which is to be especially deplored in the case of the young, and therefore more easily rehabilitated patient. There is good reason too for alcoholism to be called the *disease of denial*. It is denied by the patient himself, by his closest family members, his colleagues at work, and even by his own doctor. And it will continue to be denied so long as the sufferer fears that he will be seen as a degenerate drunkard, a weakwilled sinner, or one to be punished rather than helped, for it must be borne in mind that a great many people still have as their image of an alcoholic, the homeless, unrepentant, and unredeemable meths-drinking tramp.

If we add to this huge group of those who deny or genuinely do not believe that they have a problem, the unknown but significant number of those suffering from such diseases as schizophrenia and depression who alleviate their misery with alcohol, and the proven statistic that the risk of suicide in the alcoholic is substantially increased, then truly we have an incontestable case for adopting the disease concept of alcoholism.

By all means continue research into the causes and effects of alcoholism but keep in mind the immeasurable misery and cost of alcoholism to the individual and the community with each day that passes. Treated as a disease, alcoholism would be as respectable and acceptable as cancer, and its victims no less deserving of sympathy and active support in the moral, social, medical and financial sense.

Maybe one day in the distant future some bright researcher will clearly adduce proof that alcoholism is *not* a disease, and thereby bring great joy to many working in remote laboratories insulated from the distractions generated by humanity in the mass, and a few faces may be redder. But what of the countless thousands of sufferers from the disease whose anguish and pain, multiplied by that of their loved ones, has been ameliorated, or even cured by the pragmatist who preferred to treat alcoholism as a disease, rather than by casting stones at the 'sinner'.

Alcoholism – disease or self-inflicted vice: a critique

W.E. Fabb

It seems we have a semantic problem. In the foregoing contributions on the subject of alcoholism, the debate largely revolves around whether or not it is a disease. For, so the argument goes, if it is a disease a patient can adopt the sick role with all its privileges and expect care, not punishment. A further implication of calling alcoholism a disease is that the alcoholic would decline to accept any responsibility for his condition and would be disinclined to accept a role in its remediation.

But does the word 'disease' really carry these implications? We all know patients do accept responsibility for their condition and the need to cooperate in its management, especially if doctors have the inclination and skill to assist them towards such acceptance. Often it is the doctor who creates dependency, not the patient.

So does it really matter whether or not it is a disease? What seems to matter is the extent to which the patient, his or her family and associates, and the doctor and his associates can work together towards the recognition of the condition and its appropriate management. If the labelling (or otherwise) of alcoholism as a disease gets in the way of this process, let us do away with this counterproductive debate.

Whatever it is, alcoholism causes widespread misery. It afflicts directly at least one in ten of the population of developed countries and indirectly possibly two or three times that number, for the alcoholic's behaviour affects his or her family, associates and sometimes 'innocent bystanders' who become the victims of drunk driving. The effects on the individual and his or her family are physical, psychological, social and economic. The effects on the nation are social and economic and amount to billions of dollars in lost productiviy, ill-health and social disruption. In the face of all this, to argue about whether alcoholism is a disease or not seems pointless.

A rational approach to acoholism includes a description of the condition in as many dimensions as possible – biochemical, physical, psychological and social (Dr Young's approach is a beginning), an appraisal of the genetic and environmental determinants of the condition, a detailed account of the many ways in which the condition can be prevented, detected in its early stages and effectively managed at each stage, and a description of how the community's resources can be mobilized to assist the individual and his family. In particular, the way in which the individual, his or her family and associates can contribute in management needs to be spelt out; the results of such cooperative endeavour are well known to all workers in the field.

However, what seems of overriding importance is the attitude of those involved in the detection and management of this distressing condition. Care and concern are essential attitudes, perseverance and a positive approach are necessary, and the capacity to start again in the face of failure is a required characteristic in any health worker who hopes to be successful in this field. What is not helpful is a punitive 'It's your own fault' approach. *That* will not help anyone, not even the doctor.

Commentary

One reason for the 'alcoholism' dilemma is the confusion as to what it is. Within its spectrum there are excessive drinkers, problem drinkers, social drinkers and alpha to epsilon alcoholics – each of them with their own significant problems.

The majority who consume alcohol are social drinkers for whom this is an enjoyable pastime. However, it causes serious ill-effects for those individuals in whom it acts as a drug of addiction or habituation.

The dilemmas facing the family practitioner are that having discovered that his patient is suffering from, or likely to suffer from, the ill-effects of alcohol how far should he or she go in interfering in the personal social habits of the individual, and what actions (if any) should be taken if the individual refuses to accept the practitioner's advice?

A related dilemma is the extent of responsibilities: for the individual, for the family, for the family practitioner and the medical profession, and, finally, for society. There are no easy universally acceptable answers, but the individual, family, professional and social reactions depend on these answers.

The family practitioner must be prepared to help his or her patients with alcoholism. The condition must be made respectable and considered as a 'disease', albeit resulting from a self-inflicted act, as in smoking. However, whatever management the practitioner employs, the results of his or anyone else's care of alcoholics are usually frustratingly poor.

References

FARE. Federation of Acoholic Rehabilitation Establishments

Gitlow, S.E. (1979). The disease of alcoholism. *Cancer Res.* **39,** 2836–2839

Grant, M. and Gwinner, P. (1979). *Alcoholism in Perspective*. (London: Croom Helm)

Jellinek, E.M. (1960). *The Disease Concept of Alcoholism*. (Newhaven: College and University Press)

Madden, J.S. (1979). *A Guide to Alcohol and Drug Dependence*. (Bristol: John Wright and Sons)

Trotter, T. (1804). *Medical, Philosophical and Chemical Thoughts on Drunkenness, and Its Effects on the Human Body*. London

Ward, D.A. (1980). *Alcoholism: Introduction to Theory and Treatment*. (Dubuque, IA: Kendall-Hunt)

Wildman, R.C. (1980). Alcoholism: a disease? an illness? or a sickness? *Nurs. Forum*, **19,** 199–206

4 Acute myocardial infarction – home or hospital care?

The issues

The majority of deaths in developed countries are from heart diseases, and acute myocardial infarction is now the largest component of these.

With a potentially fatal disorder is there any case for home care, or should all persons with acute myocardial infarction be managed in hospital coronary care units? Just as obstetric delivery in the home is safe in retrospect, so the home care of acute myocardial infarctions can be safe only in retrospect. But are there any groups with definitely defined low risks that can be managed at home – if so, by whom and how?

Is hospital care in a busy general ward any better than home care – should all acute myocardial infarctions be treated under full intensive coronary care unit conditions? Finally, what of the various stages of care – can a satisfactory compromise between hospital and home care be achieved?

The case for home care
Brian R. McAvoy

Acute myocardial infarction is still the commonest cause of death in men and women in the western world. In 1979 in England and Wales it accounted for nearly 108000 deaths (Office of Population, Censuses and Surveys, 1979).

A British general practitioner with an average list size of 2500 patients will see nine cases of acute myocardial infarction in a year (Royal College of General Practitioners, Office of Population, Censuses and Surveys, and Department of Health and Social Services, 1974). With careful selection, the majority of these patients can be cared for at home.

The arguments for *home care* can be considered under the following headings:

(1) Medical
    (a) Good prognosis
    (b) Avoidance of transportation risks
    (c) Continuity of care
    (d) Improved rehabilitation and compliance
(2) Social/psychological
    (a) Comfort and familiarity of home
    (b) Reduced stress for spouse
(3) Other
    (a) Cost-effectiveness
    (b) Enhanced job satisfaction for both general practitioner and nurses.

Before developing these arguments it is important to establish that I am not advocating home care for *all* patients with heart attacks. Hospital coronary care units have an important but limited place in the management of acute myocardial infarction patients, providing a higher chance of successful resuscitation than in a general ward (Hill, Holdstock and Hampton, 1977).

Admission to a coronary care unit is indicated for patients in the following categories:

(1) poor social circumstances, such as living alone, or in hostel accommodation;
(2) presence of serious complications – peripheral circulatory failure with hypotension, acute left ventricular failure, arrhythmias;
(3) when the infarct occurs in the street or at the patient's place of work;
(4) when there is pressure from the patient or relatives for admission, for example, a young male patient.

With such selection the specialized services of a coronary care unit can be used to full advantage for those most likely to benefit by them. However, many general practitioners in the United Kingdom keep a significant proportion of their myocardial infarction patients at home. McCormick and Fry (1972) showed that less than one-third of new patients who suffer a myocardial infarction are admitted to hospital. Let us look more closely at the reason for this.

MEDICAL

Good prognosis

Up to 63 per cent of deaths from acute myocardial infarction occur within the first hour (Adgey, 1977). Ventricular fibrillation is present in about 14 per cent of cases within the first 2 hours (Adgey, Allen and Geddes, 1971) and is the mechanism of death in over 90 per cent of those who die suddenly (Adgey, 1977). It is in the relatively small group of patients who have sought help within 1 hour or so of the onset of symptoms that mobile coronary care may have a part to play. Community mortality may have been reduced in some North American cities by the introduction of mobile coronary care (Crampton *et al.*, 1975; Sherman, 1979), but similar studies have not been carried out in the United Kingdom. However, in only 25–40 per cent of cases will the general practitioner be called within the first hour (Mather *et al.*, 1971; McKenzie *et al.*, 1971; Smyllie, Taylor and Cunningham-Green, 1972). The Teesside coronary survey (Colling *et al.*, 1976) revealed a median time for patients coming under care at home or in hospital of about 3 hours, the largest component of this delay being the time between onset of symptoms and calling for medical help. Other studies of admissions to hospitals have shown median delay times ranging from 3 hours 30 minutes to 8 hours 16 minutes (Cochrane, Ghosh and Evans, 1976; Gilchrist, 1971; Hackett and Cassem, 1969; McNeilly and Pemberton, 1968; Moss and Goldstein, 1970; Shaw, Groden and Hastings, 1971; Walsh *et al.*, 1972).

When a patient collapses or has very severe pain or breathlessness, or if the attack occurs in the street or place of work, an ambulance is often summoned via a 999* call, bypassing the general practitioner. This is appropriate and facilitates rapid admission of many of those patients previously identified as requiring treatment in a coronary care unit.

Thus we have a situation whereby most of the patients about whom a general practitioner has to make the decision, home or hospital care, will have had their symptoms for a period of time which takes them beyond the most dangerous stage of their illness, when coronary care facilities would have been most beneficial. Admittedly this is a selected group but as the *Lancet* (1979) stated 'the decision on whether the patient should remain at home or be transferred to hospital should be based mainly on the time after onset of symptoms when the patient calls for aid'.

Three major United Kingdom studies have now shown that home care

* The emergency call number in the United Kingdom.

several hours after a myocardial infarction has no higher mortality than hospital care.

Mather *et al.* (1976) in the Bristol study compared home and hospital treatment in men aged under 70 years who had suffered acute myocardial infarction within the previous 48 hours. Some 455 patients were randomly allocated to receive care either at home or in hospital, initially in a coronary care unit. The mortality rate at 28 days was 12 per cent for the random home group and 14 per cent for the random hospital group; the corresponding figures at 330 days were 20 per cent and 27 per cent. The authors concluded that 'home care is a proper form of treatment for many patients in acute myocardial infarction, particularly those over 60 years and those with an uncomplicated attack seen by general practitioners'.

In the Teesside coronary survey (Colling *et al.*, 1976) nearly 2000 definite or probable cases of myocardial infarction were identified. Of the survivors, approximately one-third were treated at home, one-third were admitted to a coronary care unit, and one-third to a general medical ward. The mortality rates at 28 days were 8.8 per cent for the home group, 12.9 per cent for the coronary care group and 18.7 per cent for the ward group. The authors emphasized that one-third of the patients were treated at home, and these patients had a lower mortality rate than those in hospital, a difference that could not be attributed to age, sex or severity of attack. As the median time for patients coming under care was about 3 hours they maintained that as used at present, coronary care units are unlikely to improve mortality rates.

The third randomized trial was conducted in Nottingham by Hill, Hampton and Mitchell (1978), using a hospital-based team to respond to calls from general practitioners; 349 patients were suspected of having myocardial infarction. The team (comprising a senior house officer and coronary care unit nurse) drove to the patient's home, made its own assessment, excluded some patients on predetermined medical and social grounds and remained with the others for 2 hours, before randomly allocating them to home or hospital treatment. There was no significant difference in the 6-week mortality between the home group (13 per cent) and the hospital group (11 per cent). The article concluded that 'for the majority of patients to whom a general practitioner is called because of suspected infarction, hospital admission confers no clear advantage'.

Avoidance of transportation risks

By looking after patients at home the risks of an ambulance journey to hospital can be avoided. This factor takes on added significance in rural practices where some patients may live a considerable distance from a hospital and roads are often rough and winding.

Mulholland and Pantridge (1974) found that a heart-rate which was inappropriately rapid and likely to adversely affect the magnitude of the infarct occurred during movement of one-third of patients with acute myocardial infarction. Pain relief prior to movement did not significantly reduce the incidence of a rapid heart-rate.

Two other studies have shown that deaths during transportation account for 18–22 per cent of prehospital deaths (McNeilly and Pemberton, 1968; Nixon, 1968).

Several French studies of transportation between hospitals of selected groups of ill patients have shown that serious collapse, arrhythmias, cardiac arrest, acute respiratory insufficiency or fits occurred in 5 per cent of cases, and 15–30 per cent developed mild hypotension (Cara *et al.*, 1957; Cardoso, 1964; Hurtaud, 1965; Pichard, Poisvert and Hurtaud, 1970; Poisvert, 1962; Radiguet and Pichard, 1967).

A study of in-hospital transportation of 50 cardiac patients revealed that 90 per cent had an increase in heart-rate, 84 per cent showed arrhythmias, and 44 per cent had arrhythmias which constituted indications for emergency therapy (Taylor *et al.*, 1970).

Waddell *et al.* (1975) found a significant incidence of hypotension (28 per cent) in critically ill patients being transported by ambulance. Other studies have described isolated instances of collapse which seem to have been related to sudden jolting of the ambulance (Cullen, Douglas and Danziger, 1967; Pichard, Poisvert and Hurtaud, 1970; Snook, 1972).

There would seem to be no logical reason to inflict an ambulance journey on a patient with a struggling myocardium, and there is considerable evidence that it is harmful (Colling, Carson and Hampton, 1978).

Continuity of care

One of the strengths of the British National Health Service is the principle that each individual is registered with a general practitioner who provides 'personal, primary and continuing medical care' (Royal College of General Practitioners, 1972). Over the years individuals and families can build a relationship of mutual trust and respect with their doctor, perhaps best reflected in the term 'family doctor'.

An acute myocardial infarction is one of the most major medical events which can occur in an individual's life. The combination of severe pain, enforced bedrest and connotations of sudden death can be extremely frightening. The patient can derive much comfort from knowing the doctor who is looking after him, and realizing that the same doctor and nurse will be in attendance each day, managing the acute stages of his illness, his mobilization and rehabilitation.

Complaints of lack of information are prominent in items of dissatisfaction expressed by hospital patients in several studies (Cartwright, 1964; Congalton, 1969; Dunkelman, 1979; Hawkins, 1979; Ley, 1977; Parkin, 1976; Reynolds, 1978). One reason for this may well be the fact that several different doctors and nurses are usually involved in the hospital care of a patient. This can allow dilution of responsibility and increases the likelihood of conflicting information being given. In one survey of hospitalized myocardial infarction patients and their relatives, communication was seen as often being inadequate, vague and conflicting (Mayou, Williamson and Foster, 1977).

The continuity of care provided by the general practitioner and nurse at home reduces the possibility of such confusion and encourages the patient and his relatives to seek information about his condition. Evidence from general practitioner studies reveals much higher levels of patient satisfaction regarding communication than in hospital studies (Kaim-Caudle and Marsh, 1975; Kincey, Bradshaw and Ley, 1975; Varlaam, Dragoumis and Jeffreys, 1972).

Improved rehabilitation and compliance

It has been suggested that hospitals are unsuccessful in conveying their beliefs about the need for an active convalescence after myocardial infarction to patients and their relatives (Mayou, Williamson and Foster, 1977). The general practitioner can play a key role in coordinating and supervising rehabilitation and it is probable that he will be more effective than hospital services in establishing a graded rehabilitation programme and in avoiding the dissatisfaction and difficulties which commonly arise from conflicting, inadequate or inappropriate advice (Mayou, Foster and Williamson, 1976).

Much research has now shown that the dissatisfaction patients feel with communication, and their subsequent failure to follow advice, are in part due to their failure to understand and remember what they are told (Ley et al., 1976). If the continuity of care described above allows a better exchange of information than in hospital, this should lead to improved compliance from the patient. Several studies have shown a strong relationship between patients' satisfaction with the consultation and their following the advice they are given (Francis, Korsch and

Morris, 1969; Korsch, Crozzi and Francis, 1968; Korsch, Freemon and Negrete, 1971).

SOCIAL/PSYCHOLOGICAL

Comfort and familiarity of home

It is well recognized that the first few hours after a myocardial infarction are the most dangerous; the risk of life-threatening arrhythmias and sudden death is at its highest. It is therefore essential to minimize anxiety and allow the patient complete rest after relieving pain adequately. The familiarity and comfort of the patient's own home can provide the ideal environment for nursing. Bearing in mind that many patients are genuinely afraid of hospitals it is thought that a continuing peaceful and secure home atmosphere might well prevent the development of some complications of myocardial infarction (Mather *et al.*, 1976).

Conversely, interaction with hospitals and staff can significantly affect a patient's heart-rate and rhythm (Järvinen, 1955; Lynch, 1977; Thomas, Lynch and Mills, 1975). Indeed a disproportionate number of patients dying in hospital after acute myocardial infarction do so shortly after ward rounds (Järvinen, 1955). In the case of the older patient, management in his own home with known attendants may prevent the disturbing disorientation which can occur after hospital admission (Sleet, 1976).

Reduced stress for spouse

The wives of men who have had a myocardial infarction suffer major psychological effects (Adsett and Bruhn, 1968; Skelton and Dominian, 1973; Wynn, 1967). Skelton and Dominian (1973) studied 65 wives whose husbands had been admitted to a coronary care unit. Feelings of loss, depression and guilt were common at the time of the infarction. The authors concluded that 'possibly the illness is a less traumatic experience for the wife if the patient is treated at home'.

In addition to reducing psychological stress, keeping a husband at home avoids the domestic upheaval of admission to hospital, and the disruption to life caused by travelling to and from hospital.

Home care enables the general practitioner to involve the spouse actively in the care and subsequent rehabilitation of her husband right from the start of his illness. This can be satisfying and rewarding for the wife and provides the general practitioner with an excellent opportunity to allay fears and instil positive attitudes in both husband and wife, hopefully reducing the chances of overprotection which can occur following discharge from hospital.

OTHER

Cost-effectiveness

The estimated cost of the National Health Service in 1980 was £11 500 million (Office of Health Economics, 1979). General medical services (primary care) account for 6 per cent of this total (£690 million) whereas the hospital service consumes a massive 82 per cent (£9430 million). Stringent cash limits now apply to the hospital service and therefore expansion of current coronary care facilities and extension of mobile coronary care units must be at the expense of developments in other hospital-based specialties. The cost of caring for a patient with a myocardial infarction in the community is a fraction of the hospital costs, especially if a coronary care unit has been involved.

With the current interest in audit, doctors are beginning to examine their behaviour and decision-making more critically, especially in the area of cost-effectiveness. There is a growing realization that the gathering of objective evidence of performance and outcome must be a central feature of audit (Fraser, 1981).

If the present economic trends continue it will become increasingly difficult to justify indiscriminate use of such expensive resources as coronary care units for all myocardial infarction patients. Ultimately the combination of professional scrutiny and economic restrictions may result in doctors using the facilities of coronary care units more rationally.

Enhanced job satisfaction for general practitioner and nurses

A final argument for home care is that it can provide a most rewarding experience for the general practitioners and nurses involved. With the establishment of vocational training for general practice in the United Kingdom more and more general practitioners have had experience of working in coronary care units and are familiar with using and reading electrocardiograms. Managing myocardial infarction patients at home enables the general practitioner to practise and maintain these skills.

Nursing such patients at home is challenging and requires close liaison between the general practitioner and his community nurse. However, being involved right from the start, and helping a patient proceed from the absolute bedrest associated with a major medical emergency, through mobilization to rehabilitation and return to work, can provide intense professional and personal satisfaction for doctor and nurse.

CONCLUSION

In any one year the average British general practitioner will encounter nine patients with acute myocardial infarction. Depending on his decision these patients will be cared for in hospital or at home. This decision may well have far-reaching implications for the individual patient and his family, as well as significant effects on the costs to the National Health Service, and his own professional satisfaction.

There are sound medical, social, psychological, professional and economic reasons for deciding to treat the majority of myocardial infarction patients at home.

References

Adgey, A. A. J. (1977). Pre-hospital Coronary Care with a Mobile Unit. In Colling, A. (ed.). *Coronary Care in the Community*. p. 97. (Edinburgh: Croom Helm)

Adgey, A. A. J., Allen, J. D. and Geddes, J. S. (1971). Acute phase of myocardial infarction. *Lancet*, **2,** 501

Adsett, C. A. and Bruhn, J. G. (1968). Short-term group psychotherapy for post-myocardial infarction patients and their wives. *Can. Med. Assoc. J.*, **99,** 577

Cara, M. *et al.* (1957). Le transport d'urgence des asphyxiques par les médicines du laboratoire expérimental de physique de l'assistance publique à Paris. *Anesthés., Analgés. Réanimation*, **14,** 942

Cardoso, P. (1964). Physio-pathologie du transport en ambulance. *Ann. Anesthésiol. Franç.*, **5,** 645

Cartwright, A. (1964). *Human Relations and Hospital Care*. p. 73. (London: Routledge and Kegan Paul)

Cochrane, A. M. G., Ghosh, P. and Evans, D. W. (1976). Analysis of time intervals involved in admission to a coronary care unit. *J. R. Coll. Gen. Practit.*, **26,** 648

Colling, A., Carson, P. and Hampton, J. (1978). Home or hospital care for coronary thrombosis? *Br. Med. J.*, **1,** 1254

Colling, A., Dellipiani, A. W., Donaldson, R. J. and MacCormack, P. (1976). Teeside coronary survey: an epidemiological study of acute attacks of myocardial infarction. *Br. Med. J.*, **2,** 1169

Congalton, A. A. (1969). Public evaluation of medical care. *Med. J. Aust.*, **2,** 1165

Crampton, R. S., Aldrich, R. F., Gascho, J. A., Miles, J. R. and Sillerman, R. (1975). Reduction of prehospital, ambulance and community care death rates by the community-wide emergency cardiac care system. *Am. J. Med.*, **58,** 151

Cullen, C. H., Douglas, W. I. C. and Danziger, A. M. (1967). Mortality of the ambulance ride. *Br. Med. J.*, **3,** 438

Dunkelman, H. (1979). Patients' knowledge of their condition and how it might be improved. *Br. Med. J.*, **2,** 311

Francis, V., Korsch, B. M. and Morris, M. J. (1969). Gaps in doctor-patient communication. Patients' responses to medical advice. *N. Engl. J. Med.*, **280,** 535

Fraser, R. C. (1981). Audit at work. The future. *Br. Med. J.*, **282,** 1199

Gilchrist, I. C. (1971). Factors affecting admission to a coronary care unit. *Br. Med. J.*, **4,** 153

Hackett, T P. and Cassem, N. H. (1969). Factors contributing to delay in responding to the signs and symptoms of acute myocardial infarction. *Am. J. Cardiol.*, **24,** 651

Hawkins, C. (1979). Patients' reactions to their investigations: a study of 504 patients. *Br. Med. J.*, **2,** 638

Hill, J. D., Hampton, J. R., Mitchell, J. R. A. (1978). A randomised trial of home-versus-hospital management for patients with suspected myocardial infarction. *Lancet*, **1,** 837

Hill, J. D., Holdstock, G. and Hampton, J. R. (1977). Comparison of mortality of patients with heart attacks admitted to a coronary-care unit and an ordinary medical ward. *Br. Med. J.*, **2,** 81

Hurtaud, J. P. (1965). Reflexions sur le transport des traumatisés craniens. *Ann. Anesthésiol. Franç.*, **6,** 281

Järvinen, K. A. (1955). Can ward rounds be a danger to patients with myocardial infarction? *Br. Med. J.*, **1,** 318

Kaim-Caudle, P. R. and Marsh, G. N. (1975). Patient-satisfaction survey in general practice. *Br. Med. J.*, **1,** 262

Kincey, J., Bradshaw, P. and Ley, P. (1965). Patients' satisfaction and reported acceptance of advice in general practice. *J. R. Coll. Gen. Practit.*, **25,** 558

Korsch, B. M., Crozzi, E. and Francis, V. (1968). Gaps in doctor-patient communication. I. Doctor-patient interaction and patient satisfaction. *Paediatrics*, **42,** 855

Korsch, B. M., Freemon, B. and Negrete, V. F. (1971). Practical implications of doctor-patient interaction analysis for paediatric practice. *Am. J. Dis. Child.*, **121,** 110

Lancet (1979). Coronary-Care Units – Whcre Now? (Editorial). **1,** 649

Ley, P. (1977). In Rachman, S. (ed.) *Contributions to Medical Psychology.* p. 9. (Oxford: Pergamon Press)

Ley, P. *et al.*, (1976). In *Communications in Medicine.* (London: Oxford University Press for the Nuffield Provincial Hospitals Trust)

Lynch, J. J., Paskewitz, D. A., Gimbel, K. S. and Thomas, S. A. (1977). Psychological aspects of cardiac arrythmia. *Am. Heart J.*, **93,** 645

Mather, H. G., Morgan, D. C., Pearson, N. G., Read, K. L. Q., Shaw, D. B., Steed, G. R., Thorne, M. G., Lawrence, C. J. and Riley, I. S. (1976). Myocardial infarction: a comparison between home and hospital care for patients. *Br. Med. J.*, **1,** 925

Mather, H. G., Pearson, N. G., Read, K. L. Q., Shaw, D. B., Steed, G. R., Thorne, M. G., Jones, S., Guerrier, C. J., Eraut, C. D., McHugh, P. M., Chowdhury, N. R., Jafary, M. H. and Wallace, T. J. (1971). Acute myocardial infarction: home and hospital treatment. *Br. Med. J.*, **3,** 334

Mayou, R., Foster, A. and Williamson, B. (1976). Hospital-treated myocardial infarction and the general practitioner. *J. R. Coll. Gen. Practit.*, **26,** 654

Mayou, R., Williamson, B. and Foster, A. (1976). Attitudes and advice after myocardial infarction. *Br. Med. J.*, **1,** 1577

McCormick, J. S. and Fry, J. (1972). Myocardial infarction: the case for home care. *Update,* **4,** 473

McKenzie, G. J., Ogilvie, B. C., Turner, T. L., Fulton, M. and Lutz, W. (1971). Coronary-care unit in a district general hospital. *Lancet,* **2,** 200

McNeilly, R. H. and Pemberton, J. (1968). Duration of last attack in 998 fatal cases of coronary artery disease and its relation to possible cardiac resuscitation. *Br. Med. J.*, **3,** 139

Moss, A. J. and Goldstein, S. (1970). The pre-hospital phase of acute myocardial infarction. *Circulation,* **41,** 737

Mulholland, H. C. and Pantridge, J. F. (1974). Heart-rate changes during movement of patients with acute myocardial infarction. *Lancet,* **1,** 1244

Nixon, P. G. F. (1968). In Julian, D. G. and Oliver, M. F. (eds.) *Acute Myocardial Infarction: Proceedings of a Symposium.* p. 29 (Edinburgh: Livingstone)

Office of Health Economics (1979). *Compendium of Health Statistics, Third Edition.* London: Office of Health Economics

Office of Population Censuses and Surveys (1979). *Mortality Statistics: Cause (series DH 2).* (London: HMSO)

Parkin, D. M. (1976). Survey of the success of communications between hospital staff and patients. *Public Health,* **90,** 203

Pichard, E., Poisvert, M. and Hurtaud, J. P. (1970). Les accélérations et les vibrations dans la pathologie liée au transport sanitaire. *Rév. Corps Santé,* **11,** 611

Poisvert, M. (1962). Transports des tétaniques graves. *Agressologie,* **3,** 592

Radiguet, P. and Picard, P. (1967). Mise en condition et transport des comateux par la route. *Rév. Corps Santé,* **8,** 65

Reynolds, M. (1978). No news is bad news: patients' views about communication in hospital. *Br. Med. J.*, **1,** 1673

Royal College of General Practitioners (1972). *The Future General Practitioner – Learning and Teaching,* p. 1. (London: British Medical Journal)

Royal College of General Practitioners, Office of Population Censuses and Surveys, and Department of Health and Social Security (1974). *Morbidity Statistics from General Practice. Second National Study, 1970–71* (London: HMSO)

Shaw, G., Groden, B. and Hastings, E. (1971). Coronary care in a general hospital. Results and observations on the first year's work in the unit in the Southern General Hospital, Glasgow. *Scot. Med. J.*, **16,** 173

Sherman, M. A. (1979). Mobile intensive care units. An evaluation of effectiveness. *J. Am. Med. Assoc.*, **241,** 1899

Skelton, M. and Dominian, J. (1973). Psychological stress in wives of patients with myocardial infarction. *Br. Med. J.*, **2,** 101

Sleet, R. A. (1976). Case for the home treatment of myocardial infarction. *Update,* **12,** 33

Smyllie, H. C., Taylor, M. P. and Cunningham-Green, R. A. (1972). Acute myocardial infarction in Doncaster. I. Estimating size of coronary-care unit. *Br. Med. J.*, **1,** 32

Snook, R. (1973). Medical aspects of ambulance design. *Br. Med. J.*, **3,** 574

Taylor, J. O., Landers, C. F., Chulay, J. D., Hood, W. B. and Abelmann, W. H. (1970). Monitoring high-risk cardiac patients during transportation. *Lancet,* **2,** 1205

Thomas, S. A., Lynch, J. J. and Mills, M. E. (1975). Psychosocial influences on heart rhythm in the coronary-care unit. *Heart Lung,* **4,** 746

Varlaam, A., Dragoumis, M. and Jeffreys, M. (1972). Patients' opinions of their doctors – a comparative study of patients in a central London Borough registered with single-handed and partnership practices in 1969. *J. R. Coll. Gen. Practit.*, **22,** 811

Waddell, G., Scott, P. D. R., Lees, N. W. and Ledingham, I. McA. (1975). Effects of ambulance transport on critically ill patients. *Br. Med. J.*, **1,** 386

Walsh, M. J., Shivalingappa, G., Scaria, K., Morrison, C., Kumar, B., Farnan, C., Chaturvedi, N. C., McC. Boyle, D. and Barber, J. M. (1972). Mobile Coronary Care. *Br. Heart J.*, **34,** 701

Wynn, A. (1967). Unwarranted emotional stress in men with ischaemic heart disease. *Med. J. Aust.*, **2,** 847

The case for hospital care

Joseph H. Levenstein

In being asked to argue in favour of hospital care versus home care in acute myocardial infarction (AMI), it must be appreciated that this is a debate in absolutes. We are not debating whether some patients managed at home will do as well as a similar group in hospital (Levenstein, 1982). Rather, we are discussing which choice we would make if only one could be chosen for *all* our patients.

TWO PHASES OF ACUTE MYOCARDIAL INFARCTION

The first point to appreciate is that the management of acute myocardial infarction is divided into two phases: the *early prehospital phase* (usually between 0–4 hours after onset of symptoms) and a *later phase* (usually 4 hours after onset of symptoms). In the early prehospital phase management is usually effected by the general practitioner or a mobile intensive coronary care unit (MICCU). It has been shown that a prompt and effective management by the general practitioner in the early phase can be as effective as that of mobile intensive coronary care unit (Levenstein, 1976a). The patient is stabilized, pain is relieved and anti-arrhythmic prophylaxis given. The greatest risk of sudden arrhythmic death is in the early phase.

The question now is where do we manage the patient in the later phase – at home or at hospital? On a temporal scale the immediate prehospital phase is short and the later phase is long. However, there is still a strong possibility of the patient succumbing from a sudden, 'electrical', arrhythmic death. This risk will decrease exponentially over the next 48 hours to 7 days but nevertheless it is still there. In fact 10 per cent of acute myocardial infarction patients will suffer a ventricular fibrillation during this period (Levenstein, 1976a).

CORONARY CARE UNITS

The intensive coronary care units (ICCU) evolved in the hospital setting because of this risk of sudden arrhythmic death in acute myocardial infarction (Levenstein, 1976b). Beck coined the phrase 'hearts too good to die'; by this he meant that patients, who could have had even a small infarction, could suddenly succumb because of electrical derangement. Thus initially all patients with acute myocardial infarction were placed together and if they suffered a ventricular fibrillation they were defibrillated. Lown added another dimension to intensive coronary care unit management in the mid-1960s when he proclaimed, 'sudden arrhythmic death in AMI did not come unannounced'. There were premonitory warning arrhythmias which, if treated, prevented the advent of terminal arrhythmias. These could be detected by continuous cardiac monitoring.

The effect of the intensive coronary care unit on hospital mortality was dramatic. In most instances the death rate decreased by 50 per cent (Levenstein, 1976a). This was attributed solely to the prevention of arrhythmic death.

Thus there is irresistible logic in placing those with electrically unstable hearts, who can die at any minute, under constant surveillance. Arrhythmias occur in 80 per cent of patients with acute myocardial infarction. Several of these are either lethal or forerunners of lethal arrhythmias. Others are haemodynamically compromising, and if not reversed can result in further extension of the infarction.

There have been some strides forward in the management of gross pump failure (congestive cardiac failure, pulmonary oedema and cardiogenic shock). In fact, such patients could not survive in the home environment – the supportive machinery and nursing care involved in ventilation and tracheostomy for severe pulmonary oedema, or the insertion of a Swan–Gantz catheter in a patient with cardiogenic shock are but a few examples.

Thus both for pump failure and 'electrical instability' the intensive coronary care unit would appear to be the best place for a patient following an infarction.

HOME CARE STUDIES – DEFECTS OF METHODOLOGY

The arguments for home management in acute myocardial infarction must obviously hinge around the Bristol (Mather et al., 1976) and Nottingham (Hill et al., 1978) studies. These studies suffer from essential defects and they certainly could not provide the answer as to whether all patients with acute myocardial infarction should be treated at home or hospital. A key defect in the studies is they do not separate the two phases of acute myocardial infarction. Moreover *all* patients were not randomized. Patients who required hospitalization as a result of complications were excluded, for example.

The Bristol study was attacked by the Joint Working Party of the Royal College of Physicians and the British Cardiac Society (1975), for 'randomizing only a small ill-defined minority of their patients'. Pantridge's group (Belfast) highlighted the failure of the Bristol study to appreciate the importance of which phase the patient was treated in (Boyle, Adgey and Geddes, 1976). Of the 47 patients (out of 450) treated within 1 hour after onset of symptoms (early phase) there was a death rate of 26 per cent within 1 month. This compares very favourably with the 1-month mortality of patients seen in the first hour after onset of symptoms of the Cape general practitioners (South Africa) (7.0 per cent) and the Belfast group (8.6 per cent).

The Nottingham study indirectly appreciated the importance of the early phase. Each patient had the presence of a trained and equipped team in the patient's home for 2 hours. Thereafter, randomization took place. However, 24 per cent of 349 patients were excluded from randomization because of various factors. These included successful resuscitation, complications of acute myocardial infarction, coincidental diseases requiring hospital admission or those socially unsuitable for home treatment.

Another important criticism of home-care studies is the failure to give details of the mechanism of death of patients dying at home. If some of these were sudden arrhythmic deaths obviously they could have been prevented or treated in the intensive coronary care unit.

HOSPITAL IS BEST

Implicit in the patient selection for these studies is the belief that certain patients must be excluded as they require hospitalization. Other criteria that have been suggested for hospitalization include the time after onset that patients were seen, the age of the patient, where the incident occurred (for example, in a street or at work) and whether an intensive coronary care unit is available or not.

Thus if one had to choose *one* management strategy for all cases of acute myocardial infarction, home or hospital, there could be little doubt that the hospital intensive coronary care unit management would be the most effective.

References

Beck, C.S. Pritchard, W.S. and Feil, H.S. (1947). *J. Am. Med. Assoc.*, **135,** 985

Boyle, McC., Adgey, A. A. J. and Geddes, J. S. (1976). Treatment of myocardial infarction. *Br. Med. J.* **3,** 581

Hill, J. O. *et al.* (1978). *Lancet*, **2,** 838

Joint Working Party of the Royal College of Physicians and the British Cardiac Society (1975). The care of the patient with coronary heart disease. *J. R. Coll. Phys. Lond.*, **10,** 5

Levenstein, J. H. (1976a). Emergency management of acute myocardial infarction by the GP. *S. Afr. Med. J.* **50,** 531

Levenstein, J. H. (1976b). Myocardial infarction and the evolution of the intensive coronary care unit. *S. Afr. Med. J.*, **50,** 918

Levenstein, J. H. (1982). Home versus hospital care. *Update.* In Press

Lown, B. (1967). *Br. Heart J.*, **29,** 469

Mather, H. G., Morgan, D. C., Pearson, N. G., Read, K. I. Q., Shaw, D. B., Steed, G. R., Thorne, M. G., Lawrence, C. J. and Riley, J. S. (1976). Myocardial infarction: a comparison between home and hospital care. *Br. Med. J.*, **1,** 925

Commentary

The numbers of likely acute myocardial infarctions occurring in 1 year in a population of 2500 will be approximately nine, but of these two to three will be 'instant deaths' within 30 minutes of the onset of attack; two to three will occur in places or circumstances where the victim is taken by emergency ambulance to hospital; three to five will be seen by the family physician in the first instance – of these perhaps two to three may be considered suitable for home care, on the criteria stated.

One question which has to be asked is whether the two or three cases of acute myocardial infarction managed at home each year provide enough experience for the home care team?

If the expected mortality is 10–20 per cent then if only two to three cases are managed each year a death should occur less often than once every 3–5 years – not a great impact on the family physician.

The question must also be asked whether any of the home deaths may have been avoided if the patient had been in a hospital tensive coronary care unit; the answer to this is 'possibly'. It may also be argued that transporting the patient, plus the stresses of being in an intensive coronary care unit, could also cause avoidable deaths.

To this particular dilemma there are no crystal-clear 'all-or-none' answers. It is likely that some low-risk situations may warrant home care. However, as in obstetric care home deliveries should be the exception and shared care between hospital delivery and home

maternity supervision may be the ideal – so the care of acute myocardial infarctions should be a compromise between hospital intensive coronary care unit supervision for the first week, followed
by home supervision and rehabilitation.

5 Is obesity worth treating?

The issues

What exactly is obesity? Although it is easy to imagine that fat people are those who overeat it is certainly not the whole story. For reasons unknown some individuals tend to obesity, yet apparently their food intake is no greater, or even less, than many of their fellows who are thin. There are many aspects of the nature and causes of obesity on which we are very uncertain.

Why should obesity be treated? Statistics are produced (usually from life insurance organizations) to show the increased risks to life of obesity; other reports suggest excess morbidity from obesity. These conclusions have been challenged.

Obesity is considered as a lifestyle bad habit that should be amenable to correction and lead to prevention of – what? Personal cosmetic dissatisfaction is a common reason for seeking weight reduction – success depends on motivation. How much should the family physician be involved in such efforts? Long-term results of attempts at slimming and weight control are uncertain and generally have low rates of success – so how worthwhile are the tremendous efforts?

The case for treating obesity
Robert B. Taylor

Weight control as an actual or potential medical problem is faced daily by the busy family practitioner. The following is a representative case history.

Mrs M J, age 37, was found upon routine examination to weigh 77 kg (169 lb), 40 per cent above the ideal weight for her height of 162 cm (64 in). Her blood pressure was slightly elevated at 154/94 and she had venous varicosities of the lower extremities. Her 10-year-old son, seated in the waiting room, was noted to appear overweight. Also, at the time of his routine examination 1 month ago, Mrs M J's husband had been found to have a serum triglyceride level of 236 mg/dl.

The clinical situation briefly described presents a constellation of issues for the physician: Should weight control be stressed in the management of Mrs M J's mild hypertension? Should Mr M J be encouraged to lose weight to reduce his serum triglyceride level (and, by implication, reduce his risk of cardiovascular disease)? Should the physician request an examination of the apparently overweight 10-year-old son? And should dietary advice be offered for the 14-year-old normal-weight daughter who shares the family diet? Should weight control be advocated for any individual who has no risk factor or disease other than excessive body weight?

The attainment of ideal body weight is accepted as a worthwhile goal by most primary physicians. The vigour with which this goal is pursued varies widely among clinicians, and there is no universal agreement as to when weight control programmes should be advised, which programmes should be selected for which patients, and how vigorously such measures should be advocated.

Controversy regarding the physician's role in weight control has broad implications. Weight control is but one of several lifestyle interventions which have the potential to affect health (Taylor, 1982). Nevertheless, the outcome of such interventions is not readily predictable and is confounded by a host of variables including genetic heritage, individual motivation, and family influence. Further, efforts to control weight or otherwise influence lifestyle are, for physician and patient alike, time-consuming, often frustrating, and frequently unsuccessful. Hence it is appropriate to ask: What are the health implications of obesity that might make weight control a justifiable use of medical resources? Is advocacy of weight control an appropriate role for the family physician? What clinical interventions are appropriate for use in family practice? What are the outcomes by which success or failure could be measured?

HEALTH IMPLICATIONS OF OBESITY

The database concerning any medical disorder involves three dependent variables: mortality, morbidity, and the quality of life.

Mortality

Mortality data related to obesity is not as clear-cut as might be presumed. With the possible exception of instances involving the Pickwickian syndrome, mortality can seldom be attributed directly to obesity. Over-weight individuals die of other causes which may or may not be related to excessive body weight. Hence data on mortality and body weight, in both retrospective and prospective studies, become inexorably intertwined with multiple factors. One study of 200 morbidly obese men revealed a 12-fold excess mortality from ages 25–35 and a 6-fold excess mortality from ages 35–44, with the ratio decreasing with advancing age (Drenick *et al.*, 1980). A large number of epidemiological studies have suggested that body weight may be involved in early death, notably from coronary heart disease (Kannel and Gordon, 1973; Kannel and Thom, 1979; Multiple Risk Factor Intervention Trial Group, 1978). Par-ticularly striking evidence has evolved from the ongoing Alameda County (California) study (Wiley and Camacho, 1980), which has shown that those persons who utilize healthful lifestyle practices, including weight control, have a greater life-expectancy than those who do not. For example, a 45-year-old male who practises six or seven of the health habits listed in Table 5.1 has an 11-year greater life-expectancy than the

Table 5.1 Physical health status and health practices: a study of 6928 adults. Source: Belloc and Breslow (1972)

Health practices associated with positive health status

1	Maintaining weight - (−5% to +19.9% of ideal weight for men, +5% to +9.9% for women)
2	Eating breakfast daily
3	Not eating between meals
4	Sleeping 7–8 hours per night
5	Exercising regularly
6	Using alcohol moderately or not at all
7	Never smoking cigarettes

individual who practises three or less (Belloc, 1973). This life gain is particularly noteworthy when compared with Breslow's (1979) assertion that from 1900–70, a period of dramatic advances in medical technology, the life-expectancy of a 45-year-old male increased by only 4 years.

Morbidity

Morbidity related to obesity includes not only the cosmetic defect of excessive adipose tissue, but a wide variety of other disorders. The associ-ation of obesity with cardiovascular disease is well documented in the previously cited studies (Kannel and Gordon, 1973; Kannel and Thom, 1979; Multiple Risk Factor Intervention Trial Group, 1978). That overweight is a risk factor for coronary heart disease is not universally accepted, and Keys (1979) has asserted, 'At this time in our society, obesity is felt to be a cosmetic defect and thereby can cause emotional disturbances, but unless it is extreme or associated with high blood pressure it is not a risk factor for coronary heart disease for men of middle age or older'. Nevertheless, the association of overweight with increased coronary heart disease risk factors – hypertension, hyperlipidaemia, and diabetes mellitus – is too well documented to be ignored, and physicians continue to consider excess body weight as increasing the risk of coronary heart disease.

Less well known is the relationship of overweight to cancer. A 20-year study by the American Cancer Society (1979) involving more than 1 million persons found that excessive body weight (more than 40 per cent overweight) was associated with higher rates of cancer of the uterus, ovary, breast, and gallbladder in women. Men who were 40 per cent or more overweight had higher rates of colon–rectum and prostate cancer.

Quality of life

More difficult to quantitate is the *quality of life*. However, as part of the Alameda County study researchers (Wiley and Camacho, 1980) have developed an index of 'positive health' as determined by RIDIT (relative to an identified distribution) value. In their study of 6928 adults, they found that 'positive health' as determined by RIDIT value was positively correlated with good health habits, including weight control (see Table 5.1) (Belloc and Breslow, 1972). A follow-up study of 3892 adult survivors published in 1980 continued to show a positive correlation between health habits and 'overall health outcomes nine years later, controlling for initial level of health' (Wiley and Camacho, 1980). Evidence that the impact of weight control on physical health can influence the quality of life can be inferred from the study of Vaillant (1979), who followed 185 men for four decades, from adolescence to mid-life, and compared mental and physical health; he found a strong statistical correlation between physical health status and mental health as measured by an adult adjustment score.

THE FAMILY PHYSICIAN'S ROLE

How the individual family physician approaches weight control in day-to-day practice will be determined by sociocultural, individual, and medical issues. Involved in these issues are economics, value systems, and various perceptions of the physician's mission.

Is weight control a cost-effective use of the physician's time?

The physician, an important resource of society, should, some say, focus on those activities most likely to augment the health of the greatest number. And he should do so at the lowest possible cost. Is weight control counselling an appropriate use of valuable physician time, or should his efforts be directed more toward disease prevention and therapy?

What about the individual's own value system?

Does the individual have the right to be overweight? Morbidly obese? Similar questions must concern tobacco use, alcohol abuse, and other behaviours likely to cause disease, and hence the use of expensive health care resources? If the physician believes that the individual 'should' strive for weight control, does the physician have the right to advocate weight reduction? To use coercive tactics? In short, does the physician have the right to impose *his* value system – in this instance the meritorious attainment of ideal weight – on the patient?

Factors influencing the physician's role in weight control and other health promotion efforts

There are three factors (Taylor, 1981): The first is the traditional problem-oriented approach to health care. The physician is trained to find the problem and then seek a remedy, or perhaps a means to prevent the problem. Such an approach may suffice when a problem of obesity is identified, but what is the physician's role when no 'problem' exists, and the only need is for weight *control* rather than cure of a morbid condition? Linked to problem-oriented practice is the physician's medical value system, which accords maximal prestige and financial awards upon curative behaviour; the highest fees go to the surgeon who excises a diseased organ. Somewhat less value is ascribed to preventive care, and even less merit and financial reward to time-consuming counselling regarding weight control, whose only outcome may be the enhancement of health.

CLINICAL INTERVENTIONS

Clinical interventions in weight control must begin with motivation. In some instances the impetus to control weight will originate with the physician, prompted by a family history of obesity, incipient hypertension, increased coronary heart disease risk, or some other identifiable health problem. In most instances, however, the motivation to control weight will arise with the patient, either offered during the consultation or discovered upon physician questioning. The urge to lose weight is widespread in western society. In a report on lifestyles and personal health care of 4473 individuals in six different occupations by the American Academy of Family Physicians (1979), almost two-thirds of respondents in each group reported a desire to lose weight, and almost half wanted to lose 4.5 kg (10 lb) or more. Dissatisfaction with personal body weight was considerably higher among women than among men for all groups except executives. Nevertheless, no more than 10 per cent of any sample group had followed a weight control diet during the prior 6 months, and of those who tried to lose weight, half or less succeeded.

A number of weight control strategies are used in clinical practice, often employed in combination (Table 5.2) (Ureda and Taylor, 1982).

Table 5.2 Weight control strategies. Source: Ureda and Taylor (1982)

1	Behavioural techniques	6	Hypnosis
2	Diet prescription	7	Drug therapy
3	Exercise	8	Fasting
4	Individual psychotherapy	9	Surgery
5	Group support		

Williams and Riser (1978) describe the use of hypnotically induced visual imagery for weight control: 'I picture myself becoming more and more slender every day. I visualize how I'll look when I've lost 5 more pounds and ....' Diet prescriptions, whether self or physician-prescribed, are often used but long-term results have been disappointing (American Academy of Family Physicians, 1979). The risk of major surgery must be considered with all operative interventions such as jaw wiring, gastric plication, or intestinal bypass. A 1978 study (Dahms, Molitch and Bray, 1978) compared drug therapy, placebo, and behavioural therapy in an outpatient obesity clinic; no difference in weight loss was found among the treatment groups, and the researchers concluded that behavioural therapy is the preferred approach, involving little physician time, modest cost, and no drug side-effects.

The behavioural approach to weight control, perhaps supplemented by other techniques including exercise, group support, or occasional brief fast, is currently used by many family physicians. Based upon the early work of Pavlov (1927) and Skinner (1938), behavioural techniques to control weight utilize seven steps in behaviour modification listed in Table 5.3 (Tapp *et al.*, 1978). Behavioural techniques in family practice

Table 5.3 Behavioural modification techniques in weight control

1	Define behaviour: eating
2	Obtain baseline record: eating diary
3	Establish long-range goals and rewards: target weight
4	Determine behaviour necessary to attain goal: guidelines for healthy eating
5	Share responsibility for ongoing care: patient, physician, spouse–family involvement
6	Record programme as a contract: behaviour modification agreement, individual or family
7	Provide behavioural reinforcement: appropriate feedback for healthful eating behaviour

are likely to be most effective when other family members are involved (Taylor, 1979); for example, Brownell *et al.* (1978) studied the effect of couples training and partner cooperativeness in the behavioural treatment of obesity, finding that subjects in a spouse training group lost significantly more weight than subjects whose spouses did not share in the weight control training programme. In all behavioural techniques, feedback about performance is important, and is described by Ferguson (1975) as the key feature in any behavioural modification programme.

OUTCOMES

The outcomes of any medical intervention will involve three areas: therapy, disease prevention, and health promotion.

Weight control is important in the treatment of high blood pressure, hypertriglyceridaemia, diabetes mellitus, and a number of other disorders (Johnson, Katunas and Epstein, 1973; Reisin *et al.*, 1978). By reducing weight, the individual may help prevent coronary heart disease, cancer, diabetes mellitus, and other disorders whose onset may depend, in part, upon the prior weight status of the individual (Stamler *et al.*, 1980). Weight control in the context of health promotion – the enhancement of physical and emotional wellbeing – will depend upon the motivation of both patient and physician to achieve optimum physical and emotional wellbeing. Weight control as part of a self-improvement programme also involving other health practices (see Table 5.1) will also pay dividends of decreased morbidity and mortality.

The short-term outcomes of any behavioural intervention involve changes in the target behaviour itself, the true measurement of success or failure in behaviour modification efforts. That is, is the patient eating the correct food, at the correct time, using the correct technique? Intermediate outcomes involve physiological consequences, such as blood lipid and sugar levels, blood pressure, and body weight. The long-term changes in morbidity and mortality that may derive from weight control involve a variety of diseases; because these benefits are realized only in the distant future, they provide scant reinforcement for day-by-day behavioural change, and hence merit frequent mention to the patient during continuing care.

As the effects of lifestyle on health become increasingly apparent, there is, according to Mahoney and Arnkoff (1979), a growing conviction that 'disease is less a matter of random misfortune than the result of a failure to develop health enhancing behaviour'. Such behaviours are subject to a wide variety of environmental influences – social and ideological environments involving the home, work, mass media, and health care providers (Jenkins, 1979). As the provider of primary health care services for all members of the family, the family physician is potentially able to influence family mortality, morbidity, and quality of life, as concerns weight control and other health-related behaviours. Such interventions may have implications regarding disease therapy and prevention as well as health promotion. The potential outcome of clinical intervention regarding body weight may be profound. Whether or not the family physician and the individual patient will achieve their joint potential in weight control will be determined by sociocultural, individual, and medical value systems. There is a growing body of evidence that weight control is a worthwhile activity for the family physician. The integration of weight control and other health-promoting activities into clinical practice will be a continuing challenge to the family physician.

References

American Academy of Family Physicians (1979). *A Report on Lifestyles/Personal Health Care in Different Occupations*. (Kansas City: American Academy of Family Physicians)

American Cancer Society (1979). *Cancer Prevention Study 1959–1979*. (New York: American Cancer Society)

Belloc, N. B. (1973). Relationship of health practices and mortality. *Prev. Med.*, **2,** 67–81

Belloc, N. B. and Breslow, L. (1972). Relationship of physical health status and health practices. *Prev. Med.*, **1,** 409–21

Breslow, L. (1979). A positive strategy for the nation's health. *J. Am. Med. Assoc.*, **242,** 2093–5

Brownell, K. D., Heckerman, C. L., Westlake, R. J., Hayes, S. C. and Monti, P. M. (1978). The effect of couples training and partner cooperativeness in the behavioral treatment of obesity. *Behav. Res. Ther.*, **16,** 323–33

Dahms, W. T., Molitch, M. E., Bray, G. A., *et al.* (1978). Treatment of obesity: cost-benefit assessment of behavioral therapy, placebo, and two anorectic drugs. *Am. J. Clin. Nutr.*, **31,** 744–8

Drenick, E. J., Bale, G. S., Seltzer, F. and Johnson, D. G. (1980). Excessive mortality and causes of death in morbidly obese men. *J. Am. Med. Assoc.*, **243**, 443–5

Ferguson, J. M. (1975). *Learning to Eat: Behavior Modification for Weight Control* (leader manual). (Palo Alto: Bull Publications)

Jenkins, C. D. (1979). An approach to the diagnosis and treatment of problems of health related behavior. *Int. J. Health Educ.*, **22**, 1–24

Johnson, B. C., Katunas, T. M. and Epstein, F. H. (1973). Longitudinal change in blood pressure in individuals, families and social groups. *Clin. Sci. Molec. Med.* **45** (Suppl), 35s–45s

Kannel, W. B. and Gordon, T. (eds) (1973). *The Framingham Study: An Epidemiological Investigation of Cardiovascular Disease.* DHEW Publ No (NIH) 74–618. Washington: US Department of HEW, Public Health Service, National Institutes of Health

Kannel, W. B. and Thom, T. J. (1979). Implications of the recent decline in cardiovascular mortality. *Cardiovasc. Med.*, **4**, 983–8

Keys, A. (1979). Is overweight a risk factor for coronary heart disease? *Cardiovasc. Med.*, **4**, 1233–43

Mahoney, M. J. and Arnkoff, D. B. (1979). Self-management. In Pomerleau, O. E., Brady, J. P. (eds) *Behavioral Medicine: Theory and Practice.* p. 75. (Baltimore: Williams and Wilkins)

Multiple Risk Factor Intervention Trial Group (1978). The multiple risk factor intervention trial. *Ann. NY Acad. Sci.*, **304**, 293–308

Pavlov, I. P. (1927). *Conditioned reflexes* (New York: Dover Publications)

Reisin, E., Abel, R., Modan, M., *et al.* (1978). Effect of weight loss without salt restriction on the reduction of blood pressure in overweight hypertensive patients. *N. Engl. J. Med.*, **298**, 1–6

Skinner, B. F. (1938). *The Behavior of Organisms.* (New York: Appleton-Century-Crofts)

Stamler, J., Farinaro, E., Mojonnier, L. M., Hall, Y., Moss, D. and Stamler, R. (1980). Prevention and control of hypertension by nutritional hygenic means. *J. Am. Med. Assoc.*, **243**, 1819–23

Tapp, J. T., Krull, R. S., Tapp, M. and Seller, R. H. (1978). The application of behavior modification to behavior management: guidelines for the family physician. *J. Fam. Pract.*, **6**, 293–9

Taylor, R. B. (1979). Family behavior modification. *Am. Fam. Phys.*, **19(3)**, 176–81

Taylor, R. B. (1981). Health promotion: can it succeed in the office? *Prev. Med.*, **10**, 258–62

Taylor, R. B. (1982). *Health Promotion: Principles and Clinical Applications.* (New York: Appleton-Century-Crofts)

Ureda, J. R. and Taylor, R. B. (1982). Weight control. In Taylor, R. B. (ed.). *Health Promotion: Principles and Clinical Applications.* (New York: Appleton-Century-Crofts)

Vaillant, G. E. (1979). National history of male psychologic health: effects of mental health on physical health. *N. Engl. J. Med.*, **301**, 1249–53

Wiley, J. A. and Camacho, T. C. (1980). Lifestyle and future health: evidence from the Alameda County Study. *Prev. Med.*, **9**, 1–21

Williams, M. W. and Riser, E. A. (1978). Teaching the obese to act and think thin. *Behav. Med.*, **5(8)**, 26–7

The case against treating obesity
Denis Craddock

If obesity is considered to be abnormal then it must be about the most common abnormality affecting adults in western civilization. Depending on how obesity is defined, different observers estimate the prevalence of obesity in adults as lying between 20 and 50 per cent.

To define obesity, one must first of all define normal weight, and then decide what deviation from this is to be considered abnormal. Weight tables provide a useful guideline for comparisons between groups of people but are of little assistance when dealing with individuals.

The tables most commonly used are still those prepared by the New York Metropolitan Life Assurance Society (1959), which give desirable weights in indoor clothing for men and women of small, medium, and large frames. Frame size is difficult to evaluate in the obese except for research purposes, and the current tendency is to accept that the limits of normal weight should be from the lower limit of the small frame at each height to the upper limit of the large frame. Many observers classify as overweight those who are 10 per cent above the upper limit of these tables, and as obese those who are 20 per cent above. The difference between the two limits however, varies from 12 kg (27 lb) in small women to 18 kg (40 lb) in large men so that many individuals of slender build can carry 9 or 13 kg (20 or 30 lb) of extra fat and still be classified as normal. Even applying these strict standards, between 10 and 30 per cent of adults over 30 years are obese.

As far as the individual patient is concerned, the best or ideal weight approximates to what he or she weighed at the age of 20–25 if fit and lean at this time. (Most men and women seem to remember their weights when they married!). For those who have no certain knowledge of their early adult weight or who were overweight at that time the estimation of skin-fold thickness in the triceps and subscabular areas will suffice. A skin-fold 2.5 cm (1 in) thick or more in women, or 2 cm ($\frac{3}{4}$ in) or more in men gives a good correlation with total body fat and indicates obesity. The Ten State Nutrition Survey (US Department of Health, 1972), using these criteria, found that 20–25 per cent of adult white males and 35–40 per cent of white females were obese. In black males it was 15–20 per cent, but in black females 40–50 per cent.

Obesity thus affects a large proportion of all patients in western civilization who consult their family physicians. How important is it medically?

MORTALITY AND MORBIDITY OF OBESITY

Recent research and further evaluation of earlier work have shown that obesity *per se* is nothing like so serious a health risk as was previously thought. The mortality statistics of the New York Metropolitan Life Assurance Society (1959) were based on deviations from *average* weight rather than from ideal or 'best' weight, that is, the weight resulting in least mortality, so that the increased mortality resulting from a weight of 25 per cent above *average* is equivalent to that arising from 35–40 per cent above 'best' weight even using the old figures (Hutchinson, 1961).

Similar results were shown by the recent American Cancer study (Lew and Garfinkel, 1979) in which mortality only increased for weights in excess of 20 per cent above average weight (30–35 per cent above ideal). The updated Framingham Study (Sorlie, Gordon and Kannel, 1980) also showed that moderately overweight was associated with the lowest mortality rates.

The recent Dusseldorf mortality study (Klesse *et al.*, 1980) on 36 050 patients who attended clinics from 1960–77 even went so far as to show that only grossly obese patients (90 per cent above ideal weight) had higher mortality rates than the regional population of 17 million, while the moderately obese patients (less than 35 per cent above ideal weight) had a lower mortality rate.

Nevertheless, particularly in young men, the length of time that obesity exists makes them increasingly at risk, and young men weighing more than 35 per cent over best weight showed on 30 years follow-up to have mortality rates 50 per cent above those of national controls (Sørensen and Sonne-Holm, 1977).

OBESITY AS AN INDEPENDENT CORONARY RISK FACTOR

Coronary artery disease occurs more frequently in obese individuals but only if there are additional risk factors of hypertension, impaired glucose tolerance and low HDL cholesterol levels. The evidence is well summarized by Berger *et al.* (1980). Even when extra risk factors are associated with obesity and patients might be expected to be highly motivated to lose weight, initial weight loss is rarely sustained. A 3-year follow-up of patients with a personal or family history of heart disease in Dundee, Scotland (Bateson, 1979) showed that the average loss was only 2 kg ($4\frac{1}{2}$ lb) in men and 4 kg ($8\frac{1}{2}$ lb) in women.

LONG-TERM RESULTS OF TREATMENT

The treatment of obesity often is successful for a few months, but the tendency to relapse is great and very few individuals treated by physicians attain their ideal weight; in my own series only seven out of 150 maintained their ideal weight after 10–18 years (Craddock, 1977). Most series followed up after some years show that the majority of patients have not maintained any weight loss at all (for a fuller discussion see Craddock, 1978, Chapter 11.) Published reports are from individual physicians or clinics with special interest in the subject. The long-term results of those normal physicians who regard treatment of the obese as a chore are likely to be much worse.

SMOKING AS A HEALTH RISK COMPARED WITH THAT OF OBESITY

Smoking is a much greater risk to health than obesity as has been shown by the American Cancer Society follow-up of 750 000 men and women (Lew and Garfinkel, 1979), which excluded about 10 per cent who had recently lost weight, were ill, or had a history of serious illness. This is the first large-scale survey which separates obese smokers from obese non-smokers. The risk to life of moderate obesity in a non-smoker is less than that of the average overweight person who smokes 20 or more cigarettes each day. Even if stopping smoking is associated with a 20 per cent increase in weight, a substantial fall in mortality is likely to result. It follows that the time physicians spend in persuading patients to give up smoking produces far more important and lasting effects on the patient's health than the ongoing care of moderate obesity.

Those smokers who are dependent upon the effects of nicotine for their wellbeing (and this has been estimated at around 70 per cent of all smokers) can avoid putting on weight on giving up smoking by obtaining their nicotine from special chewing gum (Russell, Raw and Jarvis, 1980).

OBESITY AND HYPERTENSION

Diagnosis and control of hypertension produce a far greater effect in protecting the patient's health than the treatment of obesity, and life-expectancy may be increased by 5–30 years as a consequence. If obesity is associated with hypertension compliance is usually good. Stamler *et al.* (1978) found that over 60 per cent of 519 middle-aged men maintained a 5 kg (11 lb) weight loss for 10 years as a result of which blood pressure fell 7–16 mmHg systolic and 4–10 mmHg diastolic.

WHO SHOULD RECEIVE TREATMENT FROM DOCTORS?

Obesity should be treated if it is causing symptoms which can be relieved by weight loss or if it is associated with hypertension. Gross obesity, and obesity in young men should be treated, but treatment of uncomplicated moderate obesity in the general population is a mammoth task with which physicians cannot cope unless they have a strong personal interest in the condition. The treatment of this type of obesity is not cost-effective in terms of time, and most individuals of this type can be dealt with adequately by other means.

WHO SHOULD TREAT THE MODERATELY OBESE?

I believe that all the listed agencies could expand the range of their activities with advantage:

Commercial slimming groups

In the commercial slimming groups overweight women receive sympathetic attention from group leaders who have also experienced the stress of trying to reduce their calorie intake below what they need to satisfy their hunger while lean members of their families eat all they wish with impunity. Moral support from other group members is a potent factor in the success of these groups whose results are comparable to any from physicians. (Stunkard, Levin and Fox, 1970.)

Groups run by health departments

In Britain and the United States an increasing number of health authorities are funding obesity clinics. These are staffed by nutritionists and nurses trained in health education with general supervision by medical staff. In the majority of overweight people the results are as good as those of individually supervised weight reduction (James and Christakis, 1966).

Groups run by members of a practice team

In Britain, group practice is becoming the norm for family doctors. Ancillary workers employed by the group or seconded from the local health authority are increasingly being asked to run slimming clubs on practice premises. This enables those obese patients who are too shy to join a commercial group to obtain treatment for a condition which many of them feel is wasting the doctor's time.

Behavioural therapy by psychologists

The altering or modification of eating behaviour involving the place and manner in which food is eaten as well as the type of food yields good long-term results providing increased exercise is included in the behavioural programme (Stalonas, Johnson and Christ, 1978; Miller and Sims, 1981).

THE DANGERS OF TREATING THE UNCOMPLAINING OBESE

These dangers vary considerably in the six age-groups with which I shall deal.

Babies

A certain amount of fat is physiological for a babe in arms and the majority of plump babies achieve normal weight by school entry (Poskitt and Cole, 1977). Perhaps 10 per cent of overweight babies become fat children and they are likely to be found amongst those who gained weight rapidly in the first 6 months of life.

Children

In my own experience and from a survey of the literature many overweight children are from broken or unhappy homes (Craddock, 1978). Many of them are also emotionally immature and tend to turn to food for comfort. Most of them are brought along unwillingly by their mothers, and it can make them more unhappy if they are put on a strict diet without going into their background and also the family's eating habits.

Treatment can only be successful if an obese child really wishes to lose weight and cooperates with the treatment. If the child is being deprived of enjoyable food while other members of the family are eating more or less what they want, it is asking too much of the child to expect full cooperation. The whole family's eating habits should be assessed and modified towards a healthier one so that calorie control can be avoided and a free type of diet substituted. The health of the whole family is indeed likely to benefit by their sacrifices on behalf of the overweight member.

Teenagers

The treatment of overweight teenagers is fraught with difficulty and possible danger unless a careful assessment is made of the individual's attitude to food, to her parents and to her own body and personality. I use the feminine gender because it is in young teenage girls that the main risk of anorexia nervosa arises. Crisp, Palmer and Kalucy (1976) report that it may occur in as many as 1 in 100 schoolgirls in their mid-teens. These girls have an eating problem which usually starts with a loss of food control and obesity. They are usually immature and may have been pressurized by one or both parents to attempt to achieve academic or other success which may be beyond their potential. They rarely have a good relationship with their parents and their change from a rounded plumpness to a lean and almost masculine configuration usually signifies that they are subconsciously afraid of the challenge of their developing sexuality.

Growing teenagers should be encouraged to take a minimum of 1000 calories daily of protective foods with an additional rationed amount of junk foods if they cannot live without them.

Dieting can be potentially dangerous in other teenagers and young women who are emotionally stable but need to keep slim for their chosen careers. Dancing and modelling students, for instance, may be excessively concerned about their diet in order to be slim and achieve higher success in their careers. They need assurance that a small subcutaneous layer of fat is physiological for young women, and indeed is necessary to provide their rounded contours.

Adults with emotional needs to eat

Obesity may be protective against anxiety and depression as was found in a survey in a London suburb (Crisp and McGuiness, 1976), and as I have often noticed amongst my own patients. The majority of my long-term dietary failures have had an obvious need to eat for comfort because they have unfulfilled emotional needs. These should be advised that moderate obesity is a reasonable compromise with their life situation and they need encouragement to accept the situation with equanimity. Frequent attempts at dieting followed by relapse tend to lead to frustration and unhappiness.

Some people have a need to be large in body to compensate for deep-seated feelings of inadequacy. This applies to many middle-aged men and some single women in a position of authority. The portly bank official and the matronly senior nursing officer are prime examples.

Middle-aged women

Moderately obese middle-aged women who do not seek weight control are usually satisfied with the way they look. Many of them have put on weight during pregnancy and their husbands and children are used to their image and do not wish them to change. Other women would prefer to be slimmer but enjoy their food too much to be willing to give up the pleasures of eating what they like.

The aged

Many old people are lonely and eating is one of the few pleasures in life left to them. Those obese individuals who have associated risk factors for cardiac health have already been eliminated and we are left with a hard core of overweight old people whose obesity is unlikely to be detrimental to their health. In fact, Andres (1980) even goes so far as to say that mild or moderate obesity in this age group may have a protective effect against certain diseases. Physicians should therefore be aware of the possible dangers of trying to persuade fat old people to lose weight.

HEALTH EDUCATION

The word doctor comes from the Latin word for 'teacher', but many physicians forget that their role today should primarily be preventive.

Obesity would cease to be a problem if everyone ate natural unrefined foods and stopped eating when their hunger was satisfied.

I believe that the best way to create a healthy nation and to avoid obesity is to teach healthy eating habits to mothers of families, and that the time when women are most amenable to health education is in the antenatal period. I have shown that health education at this time works in practice by reducing amongst my own patients the average amount of fat laid down in pregnancy from the 4.0 kg (8.8 lb) shown in British series to about 0.8 kg (1.7 lb) (Craddock, 1970).

Out of a consecutive series of 100 women under my personal antenatal care, 60 were either overweight at the start of the pregnancy or laid down excessive fat during the first 5 months. After dietary advice 58 of these women either lost weight or gained less weight. With 33 of them the advice to eliminate from their diet sugar, white flour or items containing them was all that was necessary. The remainder needed more detailed advice in addition particularly as to the reduction of animal fat or foods containing it.

These women who have been taught to eat natural foods at the expense of refined products have passed on the knowledge to their children; only three out of 167 children born to these women and remaining under my care are overweight. In contrast, out of 165 children in my practice whose mothers were not cared for by me during pregnancy, no less than fourteen were brought to me for advice concerning obesity (Craddock, 1978).

SUMMARY

The following conclusions can be drawn

(1) Obesity as a health hazard is not as great as was previously supposed.

(2) Concentrating on treating patients who are slightly or moderately obese can distract attention from the more important health measures of controlling smoking and hypertension, both of which are more dangerous to life and health and are more amenable to control.

(3) Attempting to coerce or discipline patients into losing weight when they have a need to eat for compensation may do positive harm to some of them, particularly children.

(4) Weight control by group therapy, as in the major commercial groups or groups run by public health authorities or medical ancillaries, produces at least as good results as those of doctors in hospitals or general practice, and is therefore the method of choice for most moderately obese individuals who want to lose weight.

(5) Time spent in educating patients in healthy eating habits particularly during pregnancy will produce greater benefit than the same amount of time spent in treating the already moderately obese.

References

Andres, R. (1980). Effect of obesity on total mortality. *Int. J. Obesity*, **4**, 381

Berger, M., Berchtold, T., Gries, F. A. *et al.* (1980). Indications for the treatment of obesity. In: *Recent Advances in Obesity Research III*, p. 1 (London: John Libby)

Bateson, M. (1979). Dietary advice and obesity. *Br. Med. J.*, **2**, 1585

Craddock, D. (1970). The normal weight gain in pregnancy: a series from general practice. *J. Obstet. Gynaecol. Br. Emp.*, **77**, 728

Craddock, D. (1977). The free diet: 150 cases personally followed up for 10 to 18 years. *Int. J. Obesity*, **1**, 127

Craddock, D. (1978) *Obesity and its Management, 3rd edn.* (Edinburgh, London and New York: Churchill Livingstone)

Crisp, A. H. and McGuiness, B. (1976) Jolly fat: relationship between obesity and psychoneurosis in the general population. *Br. Med. J.*, **1**, 79

Crisp, A. H., Palmer, R. L. and Kalucy, R. S. (1976). How common is anorexia nervosa? *Br. J. Psychiatr.*, **128**, 549

Hutchinson, J. J. (1961). Clinical impressions of an extensive acturarial study of build and blood pressure. *Ann. Intern. Med.*, **54**, 90

James, G. and Christakis, G. (1966). Current progress and research: New York City Bureau of Nutrition. *J. Am. Diet. Assoc.*, **48**, 303

Klesse, R., Berchtold, P., Dannehl, K. *et al.* (1980). The Dusseldorf mortality study. *Alim. Nutr. Metab.*, **1**, 4, 291

Lew, E. A. and Garfinkel, L. (1979). Variations in mortality by weight among 750 000 men and women. *J. Chron. Dis.*, **32**, 563–576

Metropolitan Life Assurance Society. (1959). *Statistical Bulletin No. 40.* (New York: Metropolitan Life Assurance Society)

Miller, P. M. and Sims, K. L. (1981). Evaluation and component analysis of a comprehensive weight-control program. *Int. J. Obesity*, **5**, 57–65

Poskitt, E. M. F. and Cole, T. J. (1977). Do fat babies stay fat? *Br. Med. J.*, **1**, 7

Russell, M. A. H., Raw, M. and Jarvis, M. J. (1980). Clinical use of nicotine chewing gum. *Br. Med. J.*, **1**, 1599–1602

Sørensen, T. I. A. and Sonne-Holm, S. (1977). Mortality in extremely overweight young men. *J. Chron. Dis.*, **30**, 359–367.

Sorlie, P., Gordon, T. and Kannel, W. B. (1980). Body build and mortality. The Framingham Study. *J. Am. Med. Assoc.*, **243**, 1826

Stalonas, P. M., Johnson, W. G. and Christ, M. (1978). Behaviour modification for obesity: the evaluation of exercise, contingency management and program adherence. *J. Consult. Clin. Psychol.*, **46**, 463–469

Stamler, R., Stamler, J., Riedlinger, W. F. *et al.* (1978). Weight and blood pressure. Findings in hypertension screening of 1 million Americans. *J. Am. Med. Assoc.*, **240**, 1607–1610

Stunkard, A., Levine, H. and Fox, S. (1970). The management of obesity. *Arch. Intern. Med.*, **125**, 1067

US Department of Health. (1972). *Ten State Nutrition Survey 1968–70.* (Washington DC: US Department of Health)

Commentary

There is no universal acceptance of definitions of objective criteria for obesity – subjectively 'obesity' is any excessive weight considered so by patient, physician or both. On balance a strong case has been made out that obesity is a health hazard and should be treated actively.

The following are bases for effective weight reduction

(1) personal support and supervision
(2) frequent and regular attendance at slimming groups
(3) clear and easy directions and plans
(4) good motivation
(5) group stimulus
(6) visible incentives
(7) commercial organizations are as effective and often *more* effective than physicians in achieving weight reduction.

6 Diabetes: strict control or flexibility in management?

The issues

The aims of diabetic treatment are: correction of hyperglycaemia; control of symptoms; prevention of complications; normal life and good health; and avoidance of any side-effects of treatment.

In asking how possible and how realistic are these aims in practice the following questions can be asked: To what lengths should rigidity go in treatment? What degrees of control can be achieved in normal practice? Are serious complications really preventable by strict control? How can a balance be struck between a normal lifestyle and good control?

The case for strict control
Robert G. Russell

Prior to the discovery of insulin in 1921 and its introduction into general use in 1922 the life-expectancy of an insulin-dependent diabetic (IDD) varied from a few weeks to a few years following diagnosis. The most frequent cause of death was ketoacidosis often precipitated by infection.

Following the introduction of insulin, ketoacidosis became increasingly less common, and the later introduction of antibiotics further reduced its incidence so ketoacidosis became an infrequent cause of death in diabetes.

A decade or more after insulin came into general use it became increasingly apparent that the longer survival of insulin-dependent diabetics allowed time for other problems to arise and that the prevention of ketoacidosis was not the definitive answer to the problem of diabetes. Certain patients who had suffered from diabetes for 10 or 15 years developed lesions of the small blood vessels, particularly of the kidney and the retina, leading sometimes to renal failure and blindness. The individual vascular lesions of the small vessels are unique to diabetes, both insulin-dependent and maturity-onset types. Peripheral neurological lesions, both motor and sensory, also occurred in some patients. Diabetics were also noted to be more at risk from cardiovascular and peripheral vascular disease than non-diabetics, diabetic females losing the protection from atheroma that their sex normally enjoys.

AETIOLOGY

The tendency to develop diabetes is an inherited trait precipitated to actual disease by environmental factors.

We may argue that the aetiology of the microangiopathy of diabetes arises in one of two possible ways. Either the microangiopathy and its sequelae are a direct result of the metabolic defect, or the tendency to develop microangiopathy is a separate inherited trait occurring in individuals with an inherited diabetic trait.

If the first of our possibilities is true then it follows without doubt that correction of this metabolic defect, and therefore strict control of the blood glucose level, would at best prevent or at worst postpone or reduce the onset of the microvascular complications of diabetes. However, if the second possibility is true the position is less secure.

Support for the second possibility may be claimed from animal experiments in non-hereditary diabetes. Fifteen dogs were made severely diabetic either by alloxan or by pituitary growth hormone and were maintained in a poorly controlled state for from 1–5 years (Engerman and Bloodworth, 1965). All the dogs developed glomerulosclerosis and seven of them developed Kimmelstiel–Wilson nodules identical to those found in the glomeruli of human diabetics. Characteristic retinopathy developed in three dogs who had been diabetic for more than 4 years. This demonstrates that the complete syndrome of diabetic microangiopathy can be developed in animals with non-hereditary diabetes.

Diabetes in man following severe pancreatic disease or removal of the pancreas may be complicated by the development of characteristic lesions in the eye, kidney or both (Duncan, MacFarlane and Robson, 1958).

WHAT STRICT CONTROL?

Strict control means the maintenance of blood glucose at levels as near physiological as possible. It is possible to achieve normal postprandial blood glucose levels in non-insulin-dependent diabetics (NIDD) either by control of diet only or by diet plus oral hypoglycaemic agents. The serum glucose level in health seldom varies outside the range 3.3 to 6.2 mmol/l, and it is against this variation that levels of control must be assessed.

To achieve normoglycaemia at all times in a patient suffering from insulin-dependent diabetes over a prolonged period is impossible. Control must be a compromise between that degree of normoglycaemia during the 24 hours that it is possible to achieve without the occurrence of unacceptable levels of hypoglycaemia. Insulin dosages and dietary regimes should be adjusted to achieve preprandial normoglycaemia and a high-fibre diet to avoid spikes of postprandial hyperglycaemia. It must be accepted that strict control cannot be achieved without occasional attacks of mild hypoglycaemia. To achieve strict control of insulin-dependent diabetics the worst possible regime is a single dose of long-acting insulin assessed by urinalysis and symptoms only.

ASSESSMENT OF CONTROL

The assessment of control of diabetes by body weight, measurement of glucose in urine and infrequent blood glucose levels is inadequate to achieve good control. Even if there is no glycosuria and a normal renal threshold the blood sugar may vary from hypoglycaemic levels to 10 mmol/l. Frequent measurement of blood glucose enables much stricter assessment of control to be made and better control is therefore possible.

Recent developments of reflectance meters based on the enzyme strip principle are now available, and these make direct reading of blood glucose levels possible. Even simpler are the BM 20–80 test strips which give a reasonable estimate of blood glucose over a wide range. Both these methods may be used either in the consulting room or by the patient in his own home. They may be done both fasting and postprandially at frequent intervals in patients with sufficient motivation. Estimations several times daily for a few days will give a more accurate assessment of the overall level of control than will less frequent single measurements taken at a clinic attendance. A high level of acceptability to self-monitoring of blood glucose has been found among young patients (Sönksen, Judd and Lowy, 1978).

Methods of assessing glycosylated haemoglobin (HbA_{1c}) are now becoming available. The proportion of this haemoglobin and its intermediates provide an index of mean blood glucose over the previous month (Gonen and Rubenstein, 1978). This could become an important method of assessing control, albeit retrospectively.

BENEFITS OF STRICT CONTROL

It is important to decide whether strict control of blood glucose is related to the incidence and progression of diabetic complications.

Short-term benefits

Acute diabetic symptoms and ketoacidosis are quickly relieved by prompt and adequate treatment with insulin and all patients are sufficiently motivated to avoid a recurrence of these symptoms. Such a level of control, however, may be inadequate to prevent the occurrence of other complications.

There is no doubt that excellent control of the level of blood glucose in the diabetic mother throughout her pregnancy has a very significant effect on the outcome of that pregnancy (Essex, 1976). Strict control of diabetes and low neonatal mortality demands high levels of motivation. The reduced incidence of neonatal hypoglycaemia and the reduction in fetal mortality are certainly due to strict control of blood glucose levels. There is some evidence that good regulation of diabetes reduced the number of malformed fetuses (Leslie *et al.*, 1978; Pedersen and Molsted-Pedersen, 1978).

Clinicians who have wide experience of the treatment of diabetes have noted the importance of the maintenance of near normal blood glucose levels in the treatment of soft tissue infections and the fact that these infections occur very much more frequently in patients with excessive hyperglycaemia.

Long-term benefits

Poor control of diabetes in the young is often associated with poor growth and development, and often with amenorrhoea in the female. With good control these faults are corrected.

It is, however, the vascular disease of diabetes that gives rise to most controversy and responsible for most of the more distressing long-term diabetic complications. This presents as either small blood vessel disease or microangiopathy, or large blood vessel disease, principally atheroma and arteriosclerosis.

Microangiopathy with the Kimmelstiel–Wilson nodule in the kidney and characteristic retinopathy is exclusive to diabetes.

Although disease of the large blood vessels is common in diabetes and tends to occur at an earlier age it is also common in the non-diabetic population and obviously has other aetiological factors than hyperglycaemia, although it is tempting to argue that the hyperglycaemia and abnormal lipid profile of uncontrolled diabetes are significant contributory factors to its development.

Because of other factors such as age, hypertension and smoking habits, involved in large vessel disease, and because of the later onset of maturity diabetes and frequent difficulty in establishing the date of onset of the disease even at the time of diagnosis, it would be better to confine our main arguments to microangiopathy in juvenile onset diabetics with the onset of disease fairly early in life.

Diabetic retinopathy is the commonest cause of blindness under the age of 65. The cause of one-half of deaths of patients who develop diabetes before the age of 20 is chronic renal failure due to diabetic nephropathy.

It cannot be proved that maintaining a normal or near normal blood glucose in diabetic patients will prevent or delay the onset of retinopathy or nephropathy. The clinical studies which are available have been retrospective because of the difficulty in carrying out a prospective study due to the unjustifiability of dividing patients into well-treated and badly treated groups, and the length of time – 10–20 years or more – that would be required to carry out the study.

A study of 140 patients with diabetes of 10–29 years' duration and onset during childhood concluded that the only identifiable factor bearing a constantly significant relationship to the incidence and severity of retinopathy was the degree of control of the diabetes (Hardin *et al.*, 1976).

A study at the Joslin Clinic involving 451 patients with onset of diabetes under 30 years and duration of diabetes from 10–36 years collected data on complications and factors including sex, age at onset of diabetes, duration of the disease, insulin dosage and degree of control over the duration of the disease. The latter was graded as excellent, good, fair or poor. Analysis of this study at all stages indicated that the incidence of retinopathy, arterial calcification, and nephropathy was less in patients who had maintained excellent or good control (Keiding, Root and Marble, 1952).

A study in Belgium (Pirart, 1977) has suggested that poor control was associated with the more severe forms of small blood vessel disease. In this study involving 4398 diabetics followed over 25 years the duration and severity of hyperglycaemia was the only factor which correlated with the development of microangiopathy and that increasing hyperglycaemia was associated with a high frequency of severe diabetic retinopathy.

PRACTICE EXPERIENCE

In the limited number of patients in general practice it would be wrong to relate isolated episodes occurring in that group to the whole. One does tend, however, to be influenced more by personal experience than by any other single factor and my impression is similar to that of the vast majority of physicians who take a particular interest in diabetes, that patients who take care to maintain good control of their diabetes tend to have less severe problems from diabetic complications than those who do not. In general practice I have experience of only two cases of ocular palsy complicating diabetes.

The *first case* was a patient whose palsy was his presenting symptom. He had a long history of diabetic symptoms and his blood sugar was in excess of 20 mmol/l. The *second patient* was insulin-dependent and had been so for 25 years. He was a fastidious man whose diabetic control had been excellent and who had no detectable evidence of small blood vessel disease. He suffered a severe back injury and his diabetes became poorly controlled during his immobility. During this period of poor control he developed an ocular palsy.

The palsies of both patients recovered totally after a few weeks of good control, but I have yet to see a similar occurrence during a period of strict control.

THE CASE

Those who detract from the benefits of strict control of blood glucose levels base their opposition on the premise that diabetic microangiopathy is a trait occurring in diabetics but with a course independent of the metabolic defect and therefore of levels of hyperglycaemia. They further argue the risks of hypoglycaemia and the disruption of normal social life by the efforts necessary to monitor strict biochemical control.

Although it is impossible to provide definitive evidence that maintenance of normal blood glucose levels prevents microangiopathy in diabetes, the evidence presented in clinical reports strongly indicating hyperglycaemia as the dominant factor in the occurrence of severe blood vessel disease, together with experimental evidence of typical microangiopathy in non-hereditary diabetes, and the widespread impression of clinicians that strict control of blood glucose is beneficial, is in my opinion very strong evidence in its favour.

Attacks of profound hypoglycaemia, sufficient to cause neurone damage in well-controlled, conscientious diabetics are extremely rare. With increasing patient self-monitoring of glycaemic levels and therefore increasing awareness of control the frequency of these attacks will diminish. The social disruption involved in adherence to a simple diet, injections two or more times daily, and occasional finger-pricks are not very much in excess of the efforts required to attain only poor control; the ultimate benefits are worth the increased effort.

The next decade will see more convincing evidence of the benefits of strict control as a result of increased biochemical monitoring, particularly in the home.

References

Duncan, L. J. P., Macfarlane, A. and Robson, J. S. (1958). Diabetic retinopathy and nephropathy in pancreatic diabetes. *Lancet*, **1**, 822

Engerman, R. L. and Bloodworth, J. M. B. Jr. (1965). Experimental retinopathy in dogs. *Arch. Ophthalmol.*, **73**, 205

Essex, N. (1976) Diabetes and pregnancy. *Br. J. Hosp. Med.*, **15**, 333

Gonen, B. and Rubenstein, A. H. (1978). Haemoglobin A_{1c} and diabetes mellitus. *Diabetologia*, **15**, 1

Hardin, R. C., Jackson, R. L., Johnson, T. L. and Kelly, H. G. (1956). The development of diabetic retinopathy. Effects of duration and control of diabetes. *Diabetes*, **5**, 397

Keiding, N. R., Root, F. H. and Marble, A. (1952). Importance of control of diabetes in prevention of vascular complications. *J. Am. Med. Assoc.*, **150**, 964

Leslie, R. D. G., Pyke, D. A., John, P. N. and White, J. M. (1978). Haemoglobin A_c in diabetic pregnancy. *Lancet*, **3**, 958

Pedersen, J., Molsted-Pedersen, L. M. (1978). Congenital malformations: the possible role of diabetes care outside pregnancy. *CIBA Found. Symp. No. 63*, 65671

Pirart, J. (1977) Diabetes mellitus and its degenerative complications: a prospective study of 4400 patients observed between 1947 and 1973 (in three parts). *Diabète et Métab.*, **3**, 97, 173 and 245

Sönksen, P. H., Judd, S. L. and Lowy, C. (1978). Home monitoring of blood glucose. *Lancet*, **1**, 729

The case for realistic control

Douglas G. Garvie

When discussing the management of diabetes most general practitioners will be able to recall patients whose clinical progress seems to have been little influenced by the degree of their control.

For example I can recall a female nursing auxiliary who developed diabetes at the age of 19, shortly after being found to have pulmonary tuberculosis. She was always a very irregular attender at the hospital diabetic clinic, never varied her insulin dosage, never checked her urine and paid little if any attention to dietary advice. Now, 30 years later, she copes normally with a demanding full-time job. She now attends a general practice-based diabetic clinic, is of ideal weight, her blood sugars are always within normal limits and she has no evidence of any diabetic complications.

At the other end of the spectrum is a dentist whose diabetes was diagnosed when he was aged 57, after he developed a paronychia; he was found only 2 months later to have extensive diabetic retinopathy requiring frequent photocoagulation, and bilateral cataracts developed 2 years after that. He attends the practice diabetic clinic regularly, his blood glucose remains within normal limits, his urine is free of sugar, he sticks closely to his diet and he takes his oral antidiabetic agent regularly. Despite this careful attention to detail he has had to retire prematurely because of failing vision and now, 5 years after diagnosis, he has severe retinopathy, peripheral neuropathy and absent peripheral pulses.

Had the nursing auxiliary been more cooperative, her present freedom from complications might well have been attributed to the tightness of her control. But would the dentist have fared much worse if he had just forgotten about his diabetes?

In his book *Clinical Diabetes Mellitus* Malins (1968) outlines the aims of treatment in diabetes as:

(1) The elimination of symptoms
(2) The avoidance of side-effects of treatment, notably hypoglycaemia
(3) A normal life in society
(4) The maintenance of good health for a reasonable span
(5) The amelioration of complications.

He goes on to counsel against 'rigid and unimaginative care'. These aims are at the root of good general practice, and I believe that they are compatible with the maintenance of adequate, if not strict control of diabetes.

WHAT IS 'STRICT CONTROL'?

What do we mean by 'control' of diabetes? Do we believe that it means freedom from symptoms? We are indeed of the estimation that there are equally as many undiagnosed asymptomatic diabetics in the population as are known. What happens to them? Do we mean normoglycaemia? If so we should remember that the blood glucose level in a normal person fluctuates continuously and a single measurement taken at an instant of time cannot do more than give a very rough estimate of the degree of control of the metabolic disorder. We should also remember that hyperglycaemia is only one of the metabolic consequences of diabetes and there are other measures of control now available, such as glycolisated haemoglobin. Those who have recently provided evidence that very tight control of blood sugar levels reduces the risk of microvascular retinal changes used a regime of multiple insulin injections, and in some cases a continuous infusion of insulin by a subcutaneous pump. Is this sort of regime practical on a wide scale and is it justified? Diabetes is a lifelong disease. Is it not likely that this type of management will create a population of diabetic neurotics obsessed by the precise level of their self-monitored blood glucose, and continually anxious about the proper functioning of the increasingly technical equipment required for its measurement and the administration of their precisely regulated insulin requirements?

WHAT IS 'EARLY DIAGNOSIS'?

I have previously referred to the considerable number of undiagnosed diabetics in the population. We do not know for how long their blood sugar levels have been above normal before diagnosis. The incidence of diabetes rises sharply with increasing age, and about half the cases will not be diagnosed until an age when life-expectation is comparatively short and when, as in my second example, much damage may already have been done. By this time diabetes may be one of a number of problems of a degenerative nature and it is likely that many will die with, and not because of, their diabetes.

More than 10 per cent of diabetics first diagnosed over the age of 60 already have retinopathy at the time of diagnosis, while a third of those who have been diabetic for over 30 years have normal fundi. In any consideration of retinopathy, as Lundbaek (1953) showed many years ago, we must distinguish between the presence of retinopathy and the resultant disability which is frequently much less.

Similarly when discussing the long-term consequences of diabetes we have to consider both morbidity and mortality. So far as morbidity is concerned, although there is some recent evidence, based on a small number of cases, that very strict control of the blood sugar level slows down or even reverses the progression of the microvascular changes of retinopathy, evidence that such control affects the development or progression of peripheral vascular disease, atheromatous degeneration, peripheral neuropathy or nephropathy, is lacking. On the contrary the development of nephropathy and neuropathy seem to depend more on the duration of the diabetes than its severity. Further, although atherosclerosis of the coronary and peripheral vessels is common in diabetes, the precise contribution of the diabetic state in its pathogenesis is not known and the roles of hyperglycaemia, lipid abnormalities and increased platelet adhesiveness and aggregation are not clear. Approximately half of the diabetic population of the western world (although not of Japan) die of atherosclerotic heart disease, and at least another 10 per cent of cerebrovascular episodes.

While atheroma may be more common in diabetics than non-diabetics, nevertheless it is highly likely than an improvement in morbidity and mortality is more likely to result from the prevention of obesity, the control of hypertension and the elimination of cigarette smoking than from an attempt to maintain blood sugar levels within strict limits. The changes in the blood vessels may be associated with, rather than caused by, the biochemical abnormalities.

An examination of a large series of diabetics from Birmingham (Hayward and Lucena, 1965) showed that in men over the age of 50, who had been diabetic for less than 15 years, and who had otherwise a first-class quality of life, there was no excess mortality. Similarly, a study from the United States of America many years ago (Dolger, 1947) showed that the duration of diabetes when retinopathy was first seen, was the same, irrespective of whether control had been good or bad.

GENETIC FACTORS

The role of genetic factors in the development of complications has recently been examined. For example it is known that chlorpropamide/alcohol 'flushers' are less likely to develop retinopathy than 'non-flushers' – the tendency to flushing being genetically determined. It has also been shown that genetically determined fast acetylators are less prone to neuropathy than slow acetylators. Clearly, further work has to be done but at present these findings offer further evidence that the development of at least some complications is likely to be genetically determined and not solely due to the blood glucose level.

EFFECTS OF DRUG THERAPY

What about the effects of drug therapy? The first requirement in the control of diabetes is the imposition of some degree of carbohydrate restriction with the object of achieving a more satisfactory weight as well as leading to a reduction in the blood sugar level. However, there is no universal agreement on precise dietary requirements. In many cases dietary controls alone are adequate, but in some there will be a need for either insulin or an oral hypoglycaemic agent. In the young person there will be almost a universal requirement for insulin, but in the middle-aged and elderly only a small number will require insulin and less than 50 per cent need an oral agent.

It seems that many physicians administer oral hypoglycaemic drugs to patients in the pursuit of some predetermined optimum level of blood glucose concentration without always considering the possible harmful effects. Many patients will experience mild side-effects in the form of skin rashes, headaches, digestive disorders and bowel disturbances, while a few will develop blood dyscrasias or toxic hepatitis. Even mild side-effects may cause problems of non-compliance thereby lessening the degree of control. The biguanides have been reported to lead to troublesome side-effects in up to 25 per cent of patients. Occasionally side-effects are extremely serious; it was reported from the United States of America some years ago that phenformin was associated with an increased risk of death from myocardial infarction (University Group Diabetes Program, 1975). It was also found that the same drug, usually when administered to patients in adverse circumstances (for example, with renal or hepatic impairment), was prone to cause potentially fatal lactic acidosis.

Insulin and oral agents result in a lowering of the blood glucose level and almost all diabetic patients on insulin, and a proportion treated with an oral agent, will experience hypoglycaemic episodes. The more strict is the control, the more likely that hypoglycaemia will occur. While in a mild degree it is probably no more than an inconvenience, occasionally severe hypoglycaemia may result in a prolonged period of unconsciousness with a consequent loss of memory and a varying degree of dementia. A severe price to pay for the pursuit of therapeutic excellence!

ART OF THE POSSIBLE

By the nature of their scientific training, physicians are accustomed to believe that good medical practice must mean a precise correction of any underlying abnormality and an attempt to continually strive for normality, whether this be in respect of levels of blood pressure, haemo-globin or biochemistry. Too great a preoccupation with scientific accuracy can lead to a neglect of other less easily measured aspects of patient care. The aim should always be to achieve as near normality as possible consistent with the comfort and wellbeing of the patient. This is particularly true in the diabetic in view of the scarcity of evidence that slavish attention to the maintenance of a 'normal' blood sugar level significantly affects the long-term results. What is possible may not be ideal, but it should at least be practical.

References

Dolger, H. (1947). Clinical evaluation of vascular damage in diabetes mellitus. *J. Am. Med. Assoc.*, **134,** 1289–91

Hayward, R. E. and Lucena, B. C. (1965). An investigation into the mortality of diabetes. *J. Inst. Actuaries*, **91,** part 3, 390, 286–336

Lundback, K. (1953). *Long-term Diabetes.* (Copenhagen: Munksgaard)

Malins, J. M. (1968). *Clinical Diabetes Mellitus.* (London: Eyre and Spottiswoode)

University Group Diabetes Program (1975). *Diabetes*, **24,** Suppl. No. 1, 65

The case for flexibility below 11.0 mmol/l
A. I. M. Bartelds

The topic for discussion is whether general practitioners should try to achieve strict control in patients suffering from diabetes mellitus. By strict control we mean the maintenance of such metabolic balance as will prevent the diabetic patient's blood sugar levels from exceeding the desired upper and lower tolerance limits.

The principal aim of strict control is to prevent the long-term compli-cations of the disease, namely, vascular and neural disorders and the development of cataract. The means for achieving this aim are adjust-ment of lifestyle, diet, oral hypoglycaemic agents and insulin. Adjustment in lifestyle and diet are invariably prescribed, whereas insulin or oral hypoglycaemic agents are dependent on the type of diabetes as well as on blood sugar levels. The underlying assumption is that the long-term complications of diabetes mellitus are, or may be, due in considerable measure to the reversible metabolic abnormalities which accompany the disease; and, moreover, that the degree of metabolic disorder is related to blood sugar levels, the latter being the determining factor in the physi-cian's decision to control the patient.

DIABETES MELLITUS: A CHRONIC DISEASE

With a few exceptions, secondary types of diabetes mellitus are incurable and chronic. The change in the patient's metabolism is permanent, manifesting itself in insulin deficiency or imbalance. Although the life-expectancy of patients suffering from the disease has increased since the discovery of insulin and its metabolic function, this irreversible condition is a common cause of premature death and diminished fitness.

The immediate dangers inherent in the disease, although reduced, still exist. Moreover, long-term risks remain. Diabetics, therefore, require regular care and supervision.

The chronic nature of diabetes, however, does not only affect the relation between the patient and the health care system – it is a way of life. A booklet published in the Netherlands is aptly titled *Living with Diabetes*. One of its views is that 'a diabetic can, to all intents and purposes, lead a normal and healthy life in spite of his metabolic disorder'. It goes on to describe the conditions under which this can be achieved: a great number of 'do's' and 'dont's' as well as the kind of moderation necessary in very many areas of life if metabolic balance is to be maintained. In actual fact and contrary to the above quotation, life and work patterns have to change once diabetes has been diagnosed. A person who is found to have diabetes mellitus will have to learn to live with the changes that carry certain threats – if only because of the numerous beliefs which are about. Every diabetic patient can recall the anxious questions which came to mind during the first hours, days and weeks following 'the verdict'. One wonders whether physicians are ever sufficiently aware of such fears when they are preoccupied with abnormal blood sugar levels and other possible consequences of metabolic disturbances. Diabetics have to learn to live with their diabetes and one has to ask: what can patients themselves do?

WHAT CAN PATIENTS DO FOR THEMSELVES?

When diabetes mellitus has been diagnosed the doctor and his patient face the task of deciding how they can both contribute to keeping the situation under permanent control. A necessary first condition is an appointment to discuss how this can best be arranged. Such a discussion is not unusual in itself. There have always been discussions of this kind between doctor and patient. However, many discussions could be criticized as being a form of one-way traffic. The patient is told to collect urine samples four times daily and to hand them in when he comes for the usual check-up, or he is told to report to the laboratory several times on a given day to have blood samples taken. The doctor receives the results of the tests and informs the patient whether they are satisfactory or not. It is accepted without too much concern that patients will see to it that they are 'all right' by the time they are to be checked, with a slight relaxation in the application of the rules at other times. This is seen as a minor and acceptable expression of protest against the uninspiring and condescending attitude of some doctors.

This situation has begun to change. In long-term care of conditions such as diabetes, chronic obstructive lung diseases and hypertension, there is an increasing encouragement of self-help, self-control and, where necessary, self-treatment.

Self-help

The question of self-help is a topical one and accords with the wishes of most, if perhaps not all, patients. It constitutes a development, partly initiated by doctors, which may, in various ways, lead to lesser dependence of the patient on the health care system. It seems proper that doctors and other health care workers should listen carefully when patients attempt to answer the question 'what can you yourself do about your problem?' The mere fact that a patient should comply with his doctor's wishes by taking care that his blood sugar level is compatible at the time of check-up with the doctor's expressed aim suggests that the patient's views might be very instructive.

A DIABETIC'S ANSWER

In 1979 and 1980 the Netherlands Institute for General Practice organized a number of symposia on the care of diabetic patients under the title 'From specialized control to self-care'. Apart from pathologists and diabetic specialists, the participants in these symposia consisted of general practitioners, district nurses, dieticians, and last but not least diabetics. The programme, which contained lectures and discussions, concluded with a personal answer by a female diabetic patient to the question of what patients themselves can contribute. The patient answered that the question consisted of three parts, namely, (1) what do patients wish to do, (2) what must they do, and (3) what can they do themselves? This particular patient, an active member of the Dutch Association of Diabetics, knows from her own experience in counselling a considerable number of diabetics who have consciously chosen to ignore their condition. In addition, the degrees of involvement of those diabetics who do wish to participate may differ. A diabetic's burden is often heavy enough as it is, so that he may lack the energy not only to acquire more knowledge about his condition but also to act upon such knowledge either voluntarily or as a matter of necessity. Living with a chronic illness is a continuous process of psychological adjustment which shows similarities to a state of bereavement (Moors, 1978). Not everyone will always be in a balanced state of mind under such conditions, with the result that the responsibility for action is often gladly left to those who make the rules.

Self-monitoring

The possible contribution that the patient himself can make, after a period of accurate information gathering on the course of his own diabetes and on diabetes in general, lies in the stabilization of the condition. Self-monitoring is the first step. The next step, taken in consultation with the patient's own doctor, consists in the ability and permission to interpret and act upon the results of this monitoring.

The view has been expressed that 'The physician provides the theory and the patient its application; both can be of equal importance' (Velde-Veening, 1979).

WHAT IS THE DOCTOR OBLIGED, ABLE OR WILLING TO DO?

When doctors ask patients who suffer from chronic diseases to answer the question of what they themselves can do, an interesting thing happens, at least in our experience: the question is thrown back at the doctor. Not only in discussions with patients at symposia but also during their own consultations can doctors expect to be asked to what extent they are willing, able and obliged to give diabetic patients material and moral support. It is precisely in the area of chronic diseases that the general practitioner is thought to have an important role to play. The general practitioner is expected to treat the patient near his or her domestic environment. This provides the greatest chance that enough attention is paid to the implications of the disease for the functioning of patient and family alike – in other words, a form of treatment which does not overemphasize the medical technicalities, but which concentrates on all the practical implications of learning to live with the disease. Moreover, this kind of treatment can take into account the way in which diabetics are affected by everyday family life and, conversely, how families, relationships with marriage partners or child-rearing may be affected by diabetes.

According to this view, then, the general practitioner is regarded as a technical adviser and counsellor, somebody to provide clarification and solutions to problems not only in emergencies but as a kind of permanent force behind the scenes. It should be clear from this that the general practitioner can do a great deal if he is willing; and this partly determines what he has to do.

In short, the general practitioner must choose from three areas of obligation: (1) to know, (2) to know-how-to, and (3) to act. One of the choices concerns the degree of patient participation that should be aimed for. This has to be weighed against many other possible choices.

Below 11.0 mmol/l again?

In accordance with what we set out to do, the discussion has narrowed down to the degree of patient involvement that should be aimed for. We shall, therefore, from now on confine ourselves to this issue. It should be stressed, however, that this is by no means the only choice to be made in the guidance of patients with diabetes mellitus.

First, in view of the rather discursive nature of our discussion, we owe a brief explanation for the appearance of the precise figure 11.0 mmol/l in the title of this paper. This figure refers to the blood sugar level which Pirart (1977) defines as the upper limit for strict good control. It represents a blood sugar level of 200 mg. Pirart's study involves the monitoring of 4400 patients from 1947–73 in the first stage and concerns the incidence of the dreaded degenerative complications caused by diabetes. That is, a causal link is assumed. The study was prospective in nature and, therefore, inherently more reliable than a retrospective study. A randomized double-blind study, in which causal links between degrees of control and prevalence (and incidence) of complications could be measured, has never been undertaken for medico-ethical reasons.

One of the results of the researches of Pirart and his colleagues is that 'The only two factors with which the frequency of specific complications clearly correlates for all groups and sub-groups have been the duration and intensity of hyperglycaemia'. As regards blood sugar levels Pirart observes the following: 'The determinant lower level of glycaemia appears to settle around 200 mg/dl in the course of the day'.

Great value is attached to Pirart's study since he had personally subjected all the previously published studies to sharp methodological scrutiny and, in the majority of cases, had discovered a number of weaknesses which made their results less convincing. His own research, being prospective and methodologically sound, did in the long run provide strong indications with pleas for strict control; that is, for an approximation to the physiological norm. The question whether this norm should serve as guideline in a fundamentally changed metabolic situation is a purely theoretical one. Less speculative, however, are the new insights gained from diabetes studies in the last few years, which cast some doubt on Pirart's answer to the question whether strict control prevents complications in diabetic patients. There is, for example, evidence to suggest that the incidence and seriousness of diabetic retinopathy is partly genetically determined (Pyke and Tattersall, 1973) and, furthermore, that the absence or presence of certain HLA antigens as well as the association with other genetic markers points to the existence of a defence mechanism which reduces the likelihood of complications. At present it is assumed that the clinical picture of diabetes mellitus is genetically heterogeneous. This view is supported by clinical evidence which indicates that a number of diabetics show no complications even after years of moderate or poor control. On the basis of these recent insights an unequivocal answer cannot be given to the question of whether strict control should be the practitioner's aim in the prevention of complications. This does not imply, of course, that the positive correlation, established by Pirart, between the incidence of complication and the degree and duration of hyperglycaemia is of no significance. There remains, particularly for patients who depend on insulin, the risk of hypoglycaemia and its consequences, which are also somewhat unclear.

DIABETES MELLITUS AND GENERAL PRACTICE

As far as the general practitioner is concerned, the debate about the necessary measure of involvement by the diabetic patient covers only part of his professional territory with regard to diabetes mellitus. General practice studies (Van Weel and Tielmans, 1981) show that it is only in exceptional circumstances that general practitioners treat insulin-dependent diabetics and certainly not if such patients are difficult to control. The general practitioner's specific domain is more likely to involve the treatment of diabetics who are not dependent on insulin, the mature-onset type of patient. This group of older patients is male or female in approximately equal proportion and, in the majority of cases, receives only dietary treatment. It is particularly with reference to this group that the question has to be asked whether a blood sugar level below

11.0 mmol/l should be strictly aimed at, in view of the often advanced stages of arteriosclerosis. The general practice studies already referred to show that slightly more than 90 per cent of patients had, at their latest check-up, a glucose level below 15 mmol/l, which was considered satisfactory. Less satisfactory, particularly for this group of patients, is the lack of information about the complications characteristic of diabetes. Optimal treatment is, therefore, difficult to define.

What does seem desirable, with regard to this group, is that general practitioners should take note of symptoms which may lead to diminished mobility. It is essential, particularly in the case of elderly patients, that foot problems should be closely watched. The aim here is prevention or, failing that, prompt enough treatment to leave the patient at least with a leg to stand on, in the figurative as well as the literal sense. It would also seem desirable that patients should be able to expect more of their legs than just the ability to carry them to the local health centre for the next test.

SUMMARY

Diabetes mellitus is a chronic disease. This means, in essence, that a patient in whom diabetes mellitus has been diagnosed must be made to embark on a course of instruction in order to enable him to accept his condition and to live with it.

The general practitioner will primarily treat and advise patients who are not insulin-dependent, particularly those older patients whose symptoms may be due to a change in glucose tolerance rather than diabetes mellitus. Little is known with any certainty about this group of diabetics, especially of the rates of degenerative complications. Research into the relationship between control (= blood glucose levels) and the onset of degenerative complications has been confined largely to insulin-dependent diabetics. In fact, findings in this area are controversial in view of the results obtained from genetic research into diabetes (Pyke, 1979).

The general practitioner, therefore, should not aim at strict control, attempting to achieve physiological normality, rather at lightening the burdens of diabetes, particularly in elderly diabetics.

References

Moors, J. P. C. (1978). Mensen met hoge bloeddruk en hun huisarts. *Huisarts en Wetenschap*, **21,** 221
Pirart, J. (1977). Diabetes mellitus and its degenerative complications: a prospective study of 4400 patients observed between 1947 and 1973 (in 3 parts).

Diabète et Métab, **3,** 97, 173 and 245. (Full translation in two parts published in *Diabetes Care*, **1,** 168, 252 (1978)

Pyke, D. A. (1979). Diabetes: the genetic connections. *Diabetologia*, **17,** 333

Pyke, D. A. and Tattersall, R. B. (1973). Diabetic retinopathy in identical twins. *Diabetes*, **22,** 613

Van Weel, C. and Tielemans, C. (1981). Diabetes mellitus in een huisartsen-praktijk. *Huisarts en Wetenschap*, **24,** 13

Velde-Veening, M. v. d. (1979–1980). What can the patient do for himself? NHI-symposium

Commentary

Diabetes is a disease of family practice. A practitioner with 2500 patients may expect 25–30 known diabetics plus a number of undiagnosed diabetics in the community; of these some 40 per cent will be on insulin, 40 per cent on hypoglycaemic drugs, and 20 per cent on diet regimes only.

While one of the major aims in treatment is restoration of hyperglycaemia to normal (at least below 10 mmol/l) often this is very difficult, perhaps impossible, to achieve in actual practice, without serious hypoglycaemic attacks. Even with the most enthusiastic endeavours of family practitioners and specialists it is not possible to achieve normal levels of blood sugar.

Fry (1981), in an audit of diabetics in his practice, found good control (blood sugar below 10 mmol/l) in only 43 per cent and poor control (above 20 mmol/l in 18 per cent – this was in spite of intensive efforts between practitioners and specialists.

It is difficult to relate the extent and frequency of complications to the control of hyperglycaemia achieved – there are reports supporting both sides, for both strict and flexible control.

A compromise, therefore, is necessary: The diabetic has to be informed of the importance of the principles of diabetic control – diets, adherence to correct dosage of drugs, regular checks and supervision and general attention to health including non-smoking, and on his/her own responsibilities. The family practitioner has to follow a planned regime for the care of his diabetic patients with regular objective assessments. Difficulties in control of the diabetic state will require the help of specialists – but often they are no more successful in controlling stubborn hyperglycaemia.

The life of a diabetic is hard enough, so it should not be made harder by excessive rigidity and attempts to control a hyperglycaemia that it is not possible to achieve.

Reference

Fry, J. (1981). Self-check: Diabetes. *Update*, **23,** 1105

7 Antibiotics for acute otitis media and sore throat?

The issues

Acute otitis media and tonsillitis are among the most frequent conditions of children and young adults. They have always been prevalent,with no decrease in prevalence over the past 25 years.

The causes of these common infections are uncertain – specific organisms have been isolated in less than one-half of attacks. Antibiotic-sensitive bacteria are found in a minority of attacks.

The questions to be answered here are as follows: Should antibiotics be used for *all* attacks and if so on what grounds? Should antibiotics be used for *some* attacks and if so on what criteria? What are the risks and dangers of not treating acute otitis media and tonsillitis with antibiotics? What are the benefits of treating *all* cases with antibiotics?

The case for antibiotics
Niels Nørrelund

Now 40 years old I have for 8 years worked in a practice in partnership with two colleagues of the same age. We care for some 5000 patients in a Danish rural district. They live within 10 km of our clinic, and we are on duty day and night throughout the year.

SOME CASES

Acute otitis media

The other night I was called by family F living on a small farm about 10 km from my practice, to attend to a 4-year-old feverish child complaining of headache. She had been bedridden with fever for a couple of days, and her mother had given her aspirin. The parents were afraid that she might have meningitis.

Apart from the usual children's diseases the girl had never been ill. Her general condition was good, she was well hydrated with a temperature of 39.7 °C, and one of the eardrums was burning red with the light reflex gone. There was no stiff neck or any other signs of meningitis.

I know this home very well. The parents are sensible, good observers whenever their children fall ill. The mother was relieved when told that it was only a question of otitis media, and I instructed her in the use of a powdered, broad-spectrum penicillin preparation.

On my way home I called in on the family J, whom I was seeing frequently. Only that morning Mrs J had consulted me about her 3-year-old boy, who is always ill: nasal catarrh, bronchitis, eczema, diarrhoea, recurrent otitis, eating problems. These have been some of the main talking-points at our recent consultation meetings.

That day the child had again become catarrhal, had a little fever, and kept touching one of his ears. Chest examination was normal, the pharynx inflamed, both eardrums red, and the light reflex was gone on the left side.

The child's nose had been running for a couple of days, but now she was afraid that the child had earache. It should be mentioned that the boy had undergone adenoidectomy a year ago. At the same time both of his ears had been sucked out, and a great deal of viscous secretion had been recovered from the middle ears. Grommets were inserted but within a month they fell out. The little boy has had antibiotics prescribed at least a dozen times in his short life, and last time he was given erythromycin. Following a previous treatment a fine spotted rash developed, which I reckoned was due to penicillin allergy. I prescribed erythromycin mixture again.

Sore throats

Here I can cite the case of BA, a 13-year-old boy, who consulted me about an inflamed throat. He had pain on swallowing and was sweating. His temperature had not been taken. He is a big, strong boy who is usually healthy. But at the time he was warm and perspiring, and both tonsils were enlarged with coverings, almost meeting when he put out his tongue. Otoscopy and pulmonary stethoscopy was normal. I prescribed penicillin V and ordered him to go home to bed.

During my afternoon visits I saw a 7-year-old girl VM, who has been kept indoors for a couple of days owing to mild fever and pain on swallowing. She is an only child, and her mother, being very solicitous with her, had been hoping that the sore throat would pass off with much hot tea and by keeping the child indoors. Apparently, it had not cleared.

In the case of a lady PP with a fever of 38.3 °C the pharynx was red, there was no hypertrophy of tonsils and no oxudate, nor other abnormal findings. She was given penicillin V for 7 days.

GOOD OLD PENICILLIN

Haemolytic streptococci are killed off by penicillin. A substantial proportion of throat infections are caused by these bacteria. Clinically we are unable to distinguish between those infections caused by haemolytic streptococci and viral infections. An apparently minor pharyngitis may be due to streptococci, while an apparently just as 'typical' streptococcal throat may be caused by viruses. Accordingly, the aetiology cannot be predicted on the basis of the clinical picture.

In my opinion, every patient with a sore throat should be treated with penicillin V.

I do not take swabs routinely from my sore throat patients. Geographically my access to bacteriological facilities is difficult. It is, of course, with the complicating conditions, such as rheumatic fever and glomerulonephritis that I am concerned about. They have become exceedingly rare in Denmark, but is that not just because we have been so liberal in prescribing penicillin? Is it not an obvious thought that those two diseases would recur, if we returned to observe the haemolytic streptococcus instead of killing it? Has the haemolytic streptococcus not been tamed by the atoxic penicillin?

In the old days before the penicillin became available, otitis media was a feared illness, which even could be lethal. Many patients developed complications, and mastoidectomies were common. Chronic ear discharge frequently produced partially or completely deaf ears.

Nowadays it is quite different. Complications are unusual, but earaches are still frequent among children, most of whom have earache at some time or other, and many consult a doctor at least once because of otitis.

My standard treatment for otitis media is a broad-spectrum penicillin preparation as *Haemophilus influenzae* and pneumococcus frequently cause these infections. If a patient has had earache for 24 hours, and I find a bulging, red eardrum with the landmarks obliterated, I prescribe broad-spectrum penicillin.

I am convinced that because of penicillin therapy, otitis media has changed from being an aggressive extremely unpleasant illness into a still painful, but on the whole fairly peaceful condition, seldom leaving serious sequelae.

I do not perform myringtomy to collect specimens and I never take swabs from the ear.

I do not have serious scruples about my liberal application of penicillin. It is a cheap safe drug. It has been suggested that over-liberal use of penicillin prevents children from forming antibodies against other organisms, such treatment contributing to the possible recurrence of the condition. This has never been substantiated.

PENICILLIN ALLERGY?

Many children have been labelled as allergic to penicillin on far too loose a foundation. Often the events are as follows: penicillin therapy has been commenced, and 1 or 2 days later the mother calls to say that the child has developed a fine spotty rash. It is decided over the telephone that the rash is probably due to penicillin allergy and, accordingly, this is recorded in the patient's notes.

One may safely continue the oral penicillin treatment, since often the rash disappears, so it cannot have been due to allergy. If, however, the rash is aggravated it is advisable to discontinue the penicillin and record the child as allergic to the drug. In my experience it is very rarely a question of penicillin allergy, but of an uncharacteristic rash in connection with a viral disease for which antibiotics should not have been prescribed. If the patient should turn out to be allergic to penicillin it is no problem as other drugs are available.

Until the opposite has been proved, I shall assume that the control of otitis media is due to a liberal policy of antibiotics.

EXPECTATIONS OF THE PATIENT

As a general practitioner one sees numerous patients with complaints which do not at all tally with what one has learned at medical school. It is an everyday occurrence for me to disappoint patients, because I cannot give an explanation for their symptoms. I may say that a specific symptom is at any rate quite harmless and not a manifestation of a serious illness, and that it will wear off on its own. Unfortunately, I am unable to offer any effective medicine.

These consultations are tedious, as I do not meet the patient's expectations. I only give negative information: 'You do not suffer from cancer! You have no thrombus!' The patient might rightly counter, 'But what is it, then?' I do not know! I was never taught anything about this particular set of symptoms. For example, a patient has tonsillitis. My academic knowledge tells me that the infection is probably due to a virus. Accordingly, my penicillin V is ineffective, but it may well be that it is due to haemolytic streptococcus, and in that case nobody can blame me for my prescription. I may also have to say reluctantly that I am going to take a specimen from the throat to be examined at a laboratory in a neighbouring town, with the result expected after 3 days. Until then the patient must stay in bed and take aspirins. When the result is known I may prescribe penicillin.

The patient population is accustomed to expect that a child with fever and earache should be treated with penicillin. I cannot deny that my prescriptions are influenced by what I think is expected by the patient population. I see so many patients for whom I feel I cannot do anything, that I should find it difficult to survive as general practitioner if I did not seize opportunities to offer something useful when it is available.

THE HOLISTIC CONCEPT OF ILLNESS

Most patients with otitis and sore throat hardly ever consult their practitioners. On the other hand, a few with the same conditions constantly consult their general practitioner. What characterizes these latter patients?

Rarely do they try to help themselves. They think their children are less robust than other children, so they do not find it difficult to consult their doctors. Why is earache an illness in one home and an inconvenience in another? What does it mean to a home when a child is ill? Why are the same children repeatedly attacked by infectious diseases, and by other diseases as well?

Sociological interest in studying illnesses originates partly from the observation that a human being's inclination to regard himself or others as ill cannot be explained satisfactorily by referring to medical standards. Some children experience the bulge of a red eardrum as extremely painful, while others hardly notice. Some children feel terribly sick with tonsillitis, others find it trifling.

As a general practitioner I ought to be able to compare a number of different approaches to the treatment of even comparatively banal infectious diseases. How does the family live? How does the family react mutually and in relation to the surroundings? Have the children got many friends? How do they get on at school? What do the parents know about illnesses? Which disease model do the parents believe in? I think that Illich (1976) is right in stating that an analysis of the disease pattern over the last hundred years shows that the environmental conditions are of vital importance to the general state of health in any population.

In his treatment of otitis the otologist often seems to manage only by looking into the ear, while we general practitioners, ideally, should try to utilize some of the many factors mentioned above. We are not experts on otitis or sore throats, but we ought to be experts on the groups of people who have chosen to consult us, and our acquaintance over several years teaches us a great deal about them, about their fears and anxieties among other factors.

CONCLUSION

Otitis media still is a substantial clinical problem, a frequent disease causing much suffering. It must be up to general practitioners to treat the illness promptly and efficiently in an attempt to prevent the condition from becoming recurrent or chronic. If possible, they should prescribe cheap safe drugs – both these conditions are fulfilled by penicillin.

As the portal of entry of haemolytic streptococcus is often the throat, the introduction of penicillin has virtually caused the disappearance of diseases associated with streptococcal infections, such as rheumatic fever and glomerulonephritis. I am convinced that if penicillin treatment of streptococcal tonsillitis is discontinued in a few years we shall again experience rheumatic heart diseases and nephritic uraemia. Who would dare try this experiment, when we possess a safe cheap drug which always kills haemolytic streptococci?

Reference

Illich, I. (1976). *Limits to Medicine*. (London: Marian Boyars)

The case against antibiotics

Michael J. Whitfield

ACUTE OTITIS MEDIA

Traditional views

I was taught that otitis media needs treating with antibiotics, and that the use of penicillin over the last few decades has been the main reason behind the reduction in mastoid infections and complications resulting from it. This still is the traditional teaching in medical schools. *Pneumococcus* is the most common infecting agent accounting for nearly one-half of the cases of all series regardless of age. Most studies show *Haemophilus influenzae* to be the second most frequent agent in preschool-aged children and some have shown this organism to be a significant cause of infection in older children as well. *Lancefield Group A beta-haemolytic streptococci* are found in all age-groups but less commonly in infants than in older children.

Personal experience

Having worked as a general practitioner for over 15 years this traditional approach has had to be questioned. The first time I questioned it was with the numerous complaints of earache experienced by my elder child. Examination sometimes revealed a bright red eardrum with no light reflex, sometimes just an injected tympanic membrane with or without deafness. Initially he was given courses of antibiotics on each occasion, but it became so frequent one year that a more conservative approach was adopted, using analgesics alone. To my surprise the results were identical, the pain lessened quickly, the deafness responded within a day or so and his tympanic membrane did not rupture as it had done on one occasion after starting antibiotics. I still occasionally use antibiotics for otitis media but usually only if after 2 or so days' conservative treatment there has been no improvement.

It is very easy to slip into the way of prescribing antibiotics for all earaches forgetting that before antibiotics became available traditional methods of treatment with analgesics proved perfectly adequate. The mildly injected, or wax-obscured, tympanic membrane, the fractious child who will not permit examination – how easy it is to prescribe an antibiotic, but is this what doctors should be doing?

Reports from studies

What evidence have we that antibiotics have any effect on otitis media? Fry (1958) was the first to question the routine prescribing of antibiotics in acute otitis media. He reported his observations on 552 episodes of otitis media and had complete resolution in 85 per cent of his study group without the use of antibiotics. Follow-up revealed no differences in number of recurrences or degree of hearing loss between this group and those receiving antibiotics.

Despite this, Bass *et al.* (1973) stated that 'controlled clinical trials have shown antimicrobials to be of definite benefit in the treatment of acute otitis media.' They quote three trials.

The first, by Rudberg (1954), had a number of methodological problems: patients were able to opt for antibiotic treatment, 'patients treated conservatively *usually* received placebos', and the measurement of response was the duration of aural discharge. The penicillin-treated group of these hospital patients certainly improved more than those treated conservatively.

Halstead *et al.* (1968) reported a well-controlled study of 89 children. Oral ampicillin, oral penicillin/sulpha mixture and placebo were compared and no superiority was demonstrated for either antibiotic group when compared with placebo.

Laxdal *et al.* (1970) conducted a controlled study of 142 children. This again was not a double-blind study and they found that for children under 3 years of age ampicillin had a distinct advantage over placebo, but this did not apply to those children over 9 years.

In a recent study, Meistrup-Larsen *et al.* (1980), using a double-blind method, compared 149 children aged 1–10 years treated with oral penicillin V against placebo. They found that penicillin had a significant effect on pain relief on the second day of treatment, but no differences were found on otoscopy or tympanometry after 1 week, 1 month or 3 months in placebo and the penicillin group.

Van Buchem, Dunk and Van't Hof (1981) found no differences in a well-designed double-blind trial of 239 ears (117 children) between those treated with antibiotics, myringotomy and placebo.

My contention is that antibiotic prescribing is *only indicated* if simple measures such as analgesics are not relieving symptoms and signs within 48 hours.

SORE THROATS

A sore throat is a common complaint in general practice, but most people complaining of a sore throat do not consult a general practitioner. The reason for consultation may as well be a concomitant emotional disorder as the severity of the symptom.

What causes and effects?

Throat cultures grow *beta-haemolytic streptococci* in approximately one-third of cases of acute tonsillitis, various viruses are grown in a further third and in about one-third no organisms are isolated.

Non-suppurative complications such as rheumatic fever and acute glomerulonephritis have been associated with beta-haemolytic streptococci Lancefield Group A infections of the pharynx and tonsils, and in order to prevent the onset of these diseases and to reduce the likelihood of suppurative complications the traditional teaching has been to prescribe penicillin to those cases from which the beta-haemolytic streptococcus has been isolated.

There is considerable variation in the frequency with which general practitioners in different countries routinely perform throat swabs; in the United Kingdom they are rarely performed; in the United States frequently.

The eradication of the beta-haemolytic streptococcus required a 10-day course of oral or injectable penicillin. Most patients stop taking penicillin when the sore throat is better – usually long before eradication of the beta-haemolytic streptococcus is achieved.

Why antibiotics?

Two reasons are traditionally put forward for prescribing antibiotics for sore throats: firstly it will eradicate beta-haemolytic streptococci (if present) and prevent suppurative and non-suppurative complications; and secondly it may shorten the illness.

To give an example of the first reason: although Rammelkamp *et al.* (1952) showed that prescribing penicillin to young men in army camps during the last war eradicated the beta-haemolytic streptococci and prevented acute rheumatic fever the natural history of sore throats nowadays is not so straightforward. Haverkorn *et al.* (1971) in community studies in Holland have shown that beta-haemolytic streptococcal throat infections frequently occurred with no symptom of sore throat, that ASO titre rises occurred with no evidence of symptoms or even positive cultures on throat swabs, and that most sore throats were not associated with ASO titre increases. They concluded that there was no need to search out beta-haemolytic streptococcal throat infections in order to prevent acute rheumatic fever.

The incidence of acute rheumatic fever has fallen dramatically over the last few decades in most European countries and when it does occur there is little evidence of preceding sore throat. This has occurred despite persistence of the streptococci in the community, and therefore the conclusion must be that either the streptococci have changed in some subtle way or, more likely, that the hosts have changed and that they are more resistant. There is therefore little point in trying to eradicate beta-haemolytic streptococci in patients complaining of a sore throat.

To give an example of the second reason: studies by Chapple *et al.* (1956) and Brumfitt and Slater (1957) demonstrated that penicillin therapy shortens the illness of patients with a sore throat by up to 24 hours. Whitfield and Hughes (1981) in a recent double-blind study of penicillin V versus placebo showed that no clinical type of sore throat responded significantly better to penicillin than to placebo even when there was fever, purulent tonsils and lymphadenitis present. It is difficult to justify, by any reason other than habit, that doctors keep on prescribing penicillin for sore throats.

Why not antibiotics?

What further arguments are used to justify the use of penicillin?

(1) '*It is safe.*' Is it? Idsøe and colleagues (1968) examined all reports of penicillin allergy and concluded 'penicillin allergy is common and can be fatal' but anaphylactic death appears very uncommon with oral penicillin. As Howie (1975) has stated 'the probability is that nephritis and rheumatic fever on the one hand and penicillin anaphylaxis on the other, are too uncommon to allow any individual doctor to make an appropriate assessment of comparative risk in patients with possible streptococcal illness on the basis of his clinical experience'. Complications of penicillin therapy apart from allergic response exist. These include vaginal candidiasis and gastrointestinal upsets.

(2) '*It is cheap.*' Penicillin V is certainly cheap, but many doctors are persuaded to prescribe more expensive antibiotics for upper respiratory tract infections which are certainly not cheap. The encouragement of

patients to return for further treatment for similar symptoms is likely to increase the cost of medicines needlessly.

(3) '*I must prescribe something and penicillin is a reasonably safe drug.*' This need of the doctor to prescribe has recently been examined. Do patients, in fact, expect a prescription? Cartwright and Anderson (1981) have shown that nowadays fewer patients in the United Kingdom (41 per cent, as opposed to 52 per cent in 1964) said they expected or hoped for a prescription at their last consultation but were given one in two-thirds of cases both times. Illich (1975) in *Medical Nemesis* claims that we are 'medicalizing society'. From Cartwright's study it would appear that he has some justification for this claim. Surely it would be better to advise patients with sore throats to use an aspirin gargle, to explain how to use it effectively and to leave the patient free to contact the doctor again if resolution of symptoms does not occur within 3–4 days – the usual length of the illness. Stott and Davis (1979) in examining the content of any consultation felt that one part of each consultation should be the doctor examining whether he is likely to modify the future health-seeking behaviour of the patient. They claimed that prescribing antibiotics for a cold could lead the patient to expect a similar medicine on each subsequent episode of cold. Prescribing antibiotics for each otitis media and sore throat is likely to modify patients' expectations of future treatment. That this behaviour occurs can be seen by examining the American experience with sore throat management – most patients expecting and demanding a throat swab and if streptococci are present a course of penicillin.

(4) '*Why should we change our treatment habits?*' Because they make no difference to the outcome of the illness. We no longer bleed our patients, we no longer subject them to uvulectomies or operate on their tongue tie, so why persist with medicalizing them when in most cases they get better by themselves?

References

Bass, J. W., Frostad, A. L. and Schooler, R. A. (1973). Antimicrobials in the treatment of acute otitis media. *Am. J. Dis. Child.*, **125,** 397

Brumfitt, W. and Slater, J. H. D. (1957). Treatment of acute sore throat with penicillin. *Lancet*, **1,** 8

Cartwright, A. and Anderson, R. (1981). *General Practice Revisited.* (London: Tavistock Publications)

Chapple, P. A., Franklin, L. M., Paulett, J. D., Tuckman, E., Woodall, J. T., Tomlinson, A. J. H. and McDonald, J. C. (1956). Treatment of acute sore throat in general practice. *Br. Med. J.*, **2,** 705

Fry, J. (1958). Antibiotics in acute tonsillitis and acute otitis media. *Br. Med. J.*, **2,** 883

Halstead, C., Lepow, M. L., Balassanian, N., Emmerick, J. and Wolinsky, E. (1968). Otitis media. *Am. J. Dis. Child.*, **115,** 542

Haverkorn, M. J., Valkenburg, H. A. and Goslings, W. R. O. (1971). Streptococcal pharyngitis in the general population. A controlled study of streptococcal pharyngitis and its complications in The Netherlands. *J. Infect. Dis.*, **124,** 339

Howie, J. G. R. (1975). The case against use of antibiotics in upper respiratory tract illness. *Update*, **10,** 1351

Idsøe, O., Guthe, T., Willcox, R. R. and de Weck, A. L. (1968). Nature and extent of penicillin side-reactions with particular reference to fatalaties from anaphylactic shock. *Bull. WHO*, **38,**159

Illich, I. (1975). *Medical Nemesis.* (London: Calder and Boyars)

Laxdal, O. E., Merida, J. and Trefor Jones, R. H. (1970). Treatment of acute otitis media. *Can. Med. Assoc. J.*, **102,** 263

Meistrup-Larsen, K. J., Mygind, N., Thomsen, M. *et al.* (1981). Penicillin in acute otitis media: A double-blind, placebo-controlled trial. *Clin. Otolaryngol.*, **6,** 5

Rammelkamp, C. H. *et al.* (1952). Studies on the epidemiology of rheumatic fever in the armed services. In Thomas, L. (ed.) *Rheumatic Fever.* (Minneapolis: University of Minnesota Press)

Rudberg, R. D. (1954). Acute otitis media. *Acta Otolaryngol.* (Stockholm), *Suppl.* **113,** 1

Stott, N. C. H. and Davis, R. H. (1979). The exceptional potential in each primary care consultation. *J. R. Coll. Gen. Practit.*, **29,** 201

Van Buchem, F. L., Dunk, J. H. M. and van't Hof, M. A. (1981). Therapy of acute otitis media: myringotomy, antibiotics, or neither? *Lancet*, **2,** 883.

Whitfield, M. J. and Hughes, A. O. (1981). Penicillin in sore throat. *Practitioner*, **225,** 234

Commentary

The dilemma here is whether family practitioners are to base their management of acute otitis media and tonsillitis on accepted scientific principles or on subjective impressions from personal experiences?

The case for a scientific approach is that there is no certainty of exact causes of the infections. Some may not be caused by antibiotic-sensitive organisms and some may not be infectious at all but have some other immunological reactions. There also are trials quoted showing that there are no great measurable benefits from antibiotics.

The case for using antibiotics in all attacks is that since we cannot decide clinically or even bacteriologically which are caused by which organisms it is best to assume that all require specific therapy. Antibiotics are safe, cheap and effective and the public do expect them – but one wonders whether the medical profession should follow or lead?

Diseases are not static, they change with time. Acute otitis media is no less prevalent but it is a much less serious condition now than 25 years ago. Acute throat infections likewise are less severe but no less prevalent. Rheumatic fever has become rare in developed countries. These changes are most likely to have occurred because of improved social conditions and better general health, and decreased virulence of streptococci and other causal bacteria. The contributions of antibiotics here are uncertain.

8 Premenstrual tension and the menopausal syndrome – specific treatment?

The issues

Can premenstrual tension and the menopause be considered as normal physiological states or must they to be looked on as pathological disorders with psychosocial overtones?

We have to discover: What are the causes of the symptoms – hormonal imbalances, psychoemotional disturbances or personal, family or social upsets? And if they are to be treated, by what treatments, and how effective are they?

The case for specific therapy (1)
Gillian Strube

Although unpleasant premenstrual and menopausal symptoms have been recognized for hundreds of years, it has only recently become possible to treat them effectively. Like all new ideas in medicine, the concept has been subjected to the wild swings of the pendulum of fashion and suffered from the protestations of both supporters and antagonists. In this case too, as when chloroform was first used to ease the pains of labour, the arguments have been moral and ethical as much as clinical. Should women be offered relief from symptoms which are part of their natural burden?

Now that the battlecries are beginning to fade and the smoke to blow away, it is possible to see the issues more clearly.

123

The facts are important and should be separated from the emotions which surround the subject and which emanate as much from the male chauvinist 'it's all hysterical female nonsense' side as from the feminist corner.

PREMENSTRUAL SYNDROME (PMS)

The facts are as follows:

(1) Unpleasant symptoms affect large numbers of women during the premenstruum and beginning of menstruation.

(2) These symptoms include headache, oedema, increase in weight, depression, anxiety, muddled thinking, indecision, irritability and lethargy. There may be exacerbation of other diseases such as asthma, epilepsy and rheumatoid arthritis.

(3) Secondary to, or associated with, these symptoms there is an increase in the incidence of violent crime, suicide, alcoholic excess, baby battering and marital discord during the premenstruum.

(4) Similar symptoms may occur at other times and in other women and have nothing to do with the menstrual cycle.

(5) Not all symptoms experienced by women between 15 and 50 are associated with the menstrual cycle.

(6) The symptoms and signs are difficult to measure although there is a remarkable consistency in the findings of successive workers studying the subject.

(7) No clear aetiology has been demonstrated.

(8) All studies of the results of treatment have demonstrated a powerful placebo effect.

(9) The intensity of the symptoms varies from time to time and is clearly stress-related in many women.

The case against specific treatment for PMS usually rests on the high rate of placebo response, the clear stress-linked nature of many of the symptoms, the fact that it 'is not a disease', and on the difficulty in identifying the aetiology. I will deal with these points in turn.

Placebo response is high in many conditions from asthma to the pain of bone metastases. Since the aetiology of PMS, obscure as it is, clearly involves the hypothalamus at least, it is not surprising that the placebo response is especially marked. It has to be considered, in assessing the relative merits of the various treatments available, but it is no excuse for neglecting to treat the condition altogether.

Many symptoms and diseases in modern western society are stress-related. If doctors denied treatment to patients suffering from them, then migraine, eczema, hypertension and asthma, amongst many others, would go unrelieved.

Deciding what is a disease is a pointless exercise. If only diseases should be treated, and if 'natural' or physiological processes are not diseases, then what happens to patients with the degenerative processes associated with ageing, including prostatic problems? In very few conditions which doctors treat, be they diseases or unpleasant physiological processes, is the outcome significantly altered by the treatment. Most medical treatment is used for self-limiting, non-fatal conditions and is symptomatic or palliative, designed less to cure than to make life more comfortable.

Regarding aetiology, medical practice has grown out of empirical treatment applied to conditions, the cause of which was unknown. If doctors had waited to understand clinical conditions fully before applying treatment, Withering would never have used extract of foxglove or Jenner the cowpox.

The successful treatment of PMS depends on accurate diagnosis. Many women are unaware of the cyclical nature of their symptoms, others attribute everything to the premenstrual syndrome. Doctors are unlikely to think of the diagnosis, if the patient does not mention the link, or may fall into the trap of using it to cover a wide variety of unrelated problems. A menstrual chart, with the main symptoms written in as they occur, is essential for accurate diagnosis and should be kept for at least 3 months before starting treatment.

Choice of treatment

Many of the studies so far conducted have been badly designed, some have given conflicting results, while in others the results have been unclear. To be convincing, a study has to involve large numbers of women over many months. The diagnosis in each case must be accurate and the trial must be double-blind. Such trials are now under way, but in the meantime we have to make do with the most reliable results available. These appear to show that dydrogesterone, taken by mouth during the second half of the cycle, is superior to placebo; thiazide diuretics are probably effective in some women, and pyridoxine may also be.

Progesterone, by injection or suppository, and oral progestogens clearly work well for many women but they have not been subjected to sufficiently prolonged and well-controlled trials for their efficacy to be held to be proven.

MENOPAUSE

In many ways the problems of the menopause present doctors with a dilemma similar to that of the PMS. The symptoms are stress-related, difficult to measure, variable from one woman to another and in the same woman at different times, and the precise aetiology is unclear. However, the case for specific treatment is much stronger.

The facts are as follows:

(1) Many women, perhaps 30 per cent, suffer unpleasant symptoms related to the menopause. A smaller proportion, perhaps 10 per cent, are seriously distressed or incapacitated by them.

(2) The symptoms include hot flushes or sweats, insomnia, depression, headache, dyspareunia, loss of libido, aches and pains, poor concentration and irritability.

(3) Apart from flushes and sweats, these symptoms may occur apart from the menopause.

(4) Not all symptoms in women aged between 35 and 65 can be attributed to the menopause.

(5) The symptoms are difficult to measure.

(6) Trials of treatment show a strong placebo response.

The case for treating severe menopausal symptoms, especially when hot flushes predominate, is now well established. There have been many well-constructed, long-term trials, and there is no doubt that hot flushes are dramatically improved by oral oestrogens, as is the insomnia which accompanies them. With reasonable care, hormone therapy is safe and without serious side-effects. Normal safeguards include a careful history, measurement of blood pressure, breast and pelvic examination and cervical cytology. There is good evidence that endometrial hyperplasia can be avoided by giving oral oestrogen for 3 weeks at a time, with progestogen added to the second half of the course, followed by a week's break. This usually produces withdrawal bleeding during the pill-free week, but it is light and for most women a small price to pay for the relief of their symptoms. A woman who has had a hysterectomy may take continuous oestrogen alone. Hormones should not be given to a woman with a history of mammary, uterine or ovarian carcinoma, thromboembolism or liver disease. Care is needed in the hypertensive, grossly obese, diabetic, smokers and those with severe varicose veins.

As well as producing a dramatic improvement in the flushes, oestrogen has been shown to be significantly better than placebo in a number of other symptoms including vaginal dryness, irritability, anxiety, urinary frequency and headaches. Depression is frequently improved. For women of menopausal age without hot flushes, pyridoxine may be helpful. Whether this is simply a placebo effect is not clear but even if it is, no-one should be denied it, if it helps. At least it is safe, unlike the tranquillizers and hypnotics which have been used in the past and which often exacerbate the symptoms.

Post-menopausal osteoporosis and degenerative arthritis form a problem of a different kind to that posed by the symptoms of the menopause. They are costly conditions in terms both of misery to the patients concerned, and in cost to the health services in treatment of fractures and painful symptoms. There is no doubt that they occur and are severe in some women, particularly those who have had a premature menopause caused by bilateral oophorectomy or irradiation. Routine treatment with prophylactic oestrogens appears to reduce the incidence of these conditions, although not to reverse them once they have developed. It seems logical to treat all women, who have had a hysterectomy and bilateral oophorectomy, for benign conditions before the menopause with oestrogens for a prolonged period. How long this should be is difficult to say but many women make the decision for themselves and stop after a few years.

The problems of PMS and of the menopause are responsible for a large amount of human misery in modern western society. The misery affects not only the women themselves but also their husbands, children, friends and colleagues. When PMS is linked with crime and road accidents, the rest of the community is affected. It is a subject which doctors cannot dismiss lightly.

With safe, effective treatment available, there is no longer any excuse for neglect, however benign.

The case for specific therapy (2)
K. Gill

> To women, biology is most important;
> to men, intelligence
> *after Osofsky*

INTRODUCTION

'Menopause indicates the final menstrual period and occurs during climacteric.' This definition, accepted at the First International Congress on Menopause in 1976, suggests that this article had best discuss the climacteric, which is 'that phase in the ageing process of women marking the transition from the reproductive stage of life to the non-reproductive stage' (Utian, 1978).

During this phase, 30–40 per cent of all women have symptoms and complaints which can be summarized as 'climacteric syndrome'. In this respect, distinction should be made between the surgical and the natural menopause.

EPISTEMIC ASPECTS

For an understanding of the rich diversity of symptoms and complaints of this period, a description of the climacteric syndrome should be preceded by a discourse on the nature and existence of women. I shall confine myself to some statements found in the works of Simone de Beauvoir: 'that woman has an uncertain perception of her own physicality in herself, as a means to do someting ... and that woman has an uncertain grip on the world' (Buytendijk, 1966).

Depending on the kind of civilization in which they live, some women may be relieved that the reproductive stage of life is over, and consequently adopt a positive attitude. Other women, who still desire children, may experience this phase of life as 'partial death' (Deutsch, cited in Van Keep, 1973). Their complaints may be ascribed largely to the undesired ageing process.

The average menopausal age in our western civilization is estimated to be 51 years, with a standard deviation of 3.8 years. Oestrogen production diminishes from age 40 on, and some 25 per cent of women over 40 notice irregularities in the menstrual cycle.

For a good understanding it is useful to distinguish between symptoms and complaints in this phase. The non-specific symptoms include amenorrhoea, vasomotor instability, weight gain, osteoporosis, atrophic skin lesions, sometimes facial hirsutism, atrophic vaginitis with dyspareunia, pruritus vulvae, urinary incontinence, insomnia, headache, backache, nervousness, fatigue, depression and anxiety. Specific complaints are flushes and acute bouts of perspiration.

The above list of non-specific symptoms – which could easily be extended – shows what women may have to cope with in the climacteric, in somatic as well as in psychological, psychosocial and social terms. We know from a study by Aakster and Jaszmann (1979) that, of 22 climacteric complaints that were related to a large number of independent variables, ageing was the most conspicuous.

THE OECOLOGY OF THE FEMALE CLIMACTERIC

In our youth-centred society with its emphasis on attractive appearance, sex and clothes, the climacteric assumes extra dimensions when the children leave the parental home, the woman's own parents become infirm and dependent, or die, and the partner's sexual interest wanes. Whereas the male partner usually reaches the peak of his professional/ social achievement in this period, the woman faces a change of role and a functional vacuum. Her principal task has been completed.

At that time it largely depends on her coping behaviour whether she can adequately assimilate and integrate these stressful life events and learn to accept herself in the new phase of life. Other factors of evident importance in this respect are phenomena accompanying the climacteric, possible organic disturbances (arthrosis) and circumstances which may present themselves.

Since we know that most symptoms and complaints of the climacteric are not exclusively of a medical nature, it is the above aspects that should largely determine the general practitioner's strategy.

THE FAMILY DOCTOR'S STRATEGY

Four out of ten women with climacteric complaints in The Netherlands seek medical advice, and most regard the family doctor as the most suitable adviser.

The oestrogen deficiency has prompted several investigators to regard the perimenopause as a deficiency disease, and to prescribe oestrogens for life (Wilson, 1966). Others, however, caution against this therapy in view of uterine carcinoma, hypertension, thromboembolic processes or cholelithiasis observed in many of the patients so treated.

It has been demonstrated, moreover, that there is no absolute correlation between the degree of oestrogen deficiency and the severity of symptoms. In view of this, the family doctor is well advised to focus primarily on the psychosocial complaints. This is not an easy task, because there are still numerous misconceptions both in the world of science and among the women concerned.

In nearly all western countries, general practitioners are seeing increasing numbers of women from a wide variety of ethnic groups in their surgeries; consequently they cannot ignore cultural aspects in their strategy. And further differentiation of strategy is required for married and unmarried women, women with and without a profession or occupation, and women with both a natural and a surgical menopause. A detailed discussion of all these aspects would exceed the scope of this article.

Women in the climacteric are bound to have more complaints than women of any other age group; and these complaints may mask a depression. After careful history-taking it is of primary importance to gain an impression of the premenopausal woman (if the family doctor does not already have this impression). The following questions may be broached in the interview: How does the woman experience the empty-nest phase? Does she want more children? Is she still employed or at work, or does she want to be? How is her sex life? Are there changes in the household or in the family? Has she experienced physical changes?

Once a diagnosis is established, the patient should be given insight into this physiological process by transfer of knowledge in the therapeutic interview. An empathic interest in her problems – her flushes and bouts of perspiration as well as her insomnia, fatigue, loneliness and nervousness – can produce a therapeutic result.

The individual therapy can be supported, if necessary, by prescribing anxiolytics of the benzodiazepine group of tricyclic antidepressants to combat sleep disorders, anxiety, depression and somatic complaints without organic cause.

If after this the patient asks for treatment with oestrogens, and if there are no contraindications such as history of mammary or uterine carcinoma, diabetes mellitus, myoma, endometriosis or thromboembolic processes, then oestrogens may be prescribed at the lowest effective dosage for no more than 6 weeks. Coope (1981) has demonstrated in a random double-blind crossover trial that oestrogens have no effect on depressions in the climacteric.

SUMMARY

Four out of ten women seek the family doctor's advice for the climacteric as a biosocial phenomenon. He is regarded as the expert *par excellence* to provide information and guidance on complaints of which the aetiology still remains to be defined in detail.

The general practitioner should bear in mind the biological as well as the psychosocial and sociocultural aspects of the climacteric, and by means of the history he should gain an impression of the woman's views, attitude and available knowledge.

References

Aakster, C. W. and Jaszmann, L. J. B. (1979). Bestaat er een patroon in de klachten? In: Jaszmann, L. J. B. and Haspels, A. A. (eds.) *De Middelbare Leeftijd van de Vrouw.* (Utrecht: Bunge)

Buytendijk, F. J. J. (1966). *De Vrouw. Een Existentieel-Psychologische Studie.* (Utrecht/Antwerp: Aula Books)

Coope, J. (1981). Is oestrogen therapy effective in the treatment of menopausal depression? *J. R. Coll. Gen. Practit.,* **31,** 134–140

Utian, W. H. (1978). *The Menopause Manual. A Woman's Guide to the Menopause.* (Lancaster: MTP Press)

Van Keep, P. A. (1973). The Aging Woman. In: Keep, P. A. van and Lauritzen, C. (eds.) *Ageing and Estrogens.* (Basle/Paris/London/New York: S. Karger)

Wilson, R. A. (1966). *Feminine Forever.* (New York: M. Evans)

The case against specific treatment
Alistair Moulds

It seems nowadays that the only significant hormonal event in a woman's life that is accepted by everyone as being physiological is the menarche. The menopause has become increasingly regarded as an ovarian deficiency disease and the premenstrual syndrome (PMS) is now so established as a *bona fide* illness that crimes alleged to have been committed under its influence can *a priori* be successfully defended.

One natural process which will affect every woman and another which affects the majority of menstruating women (30 per cent seriously) have become viewed by a significant section of public and medical opinion as abnormal. The large variety of distressing symptoms with which both conditions may be associated or coincide with are now held, without proof, to be the result of a causal relationship. Widespread social, psychiatric and physical problems are now happily explained purely in terms of non-threatening, socially acceptable hormonal changes. Uneasy thoughts of psychosomatic components, which may need to be coped with primarily by the sufferer, can be ignored as the responsibility for the cure of physical disease is firmly in the hands of doctors.

In a society much occupied in trying to eliminate sex differences it is understandable that distress apparently attributable to biological disadvantage should evoke strong feelings, resulting in pressure on sufferers to demand specific treatment to abolish their symptoms and on doctors to prescribe it. As a result male doctors, particularly, have been publicly castigated for ignoring, ridiculing or ineffectually treating literally hordes of suffering females.

Perhaps this would be acceptable if there was evidence that women actually were biologically inferior or disadvantaged compared to men and that hormone patterns therefore required 'correcting'. This is patently not the case. Women have a lower mortality rate than men in every age-group and have a greater expectation of life. All men, except those in social class I, have a lower life expectancy than even social class V woman. Women, it appears, are healthier than men though their perceptions of what constitutes health may well be different. It seems fair to assume that lifelong hormone patterns must be responsible for much of this feminine advantage and it seems strange that, with so little understanding of the underlying mechanisms, some doctors and patients should be so keen to interfere with and upset natural balances.

PREMENSTRUAL SYNDROME (PMS)

The term PMS covers a wide range of psychic and somatic symptoms occurring in the 10–14 days prior to menstruation. Those most often described are irritability, depression, exhaustion, panic, painful or tender breasts, oedema, stomachache, nausea and headache. Virtually all other known symptoms have also been embraced by PMS, the only criterion for their inclusion being that some woman at some time has suffered from them premenstrually. Accidents, suicide attempts and child-battering are more frequent than at other times.

There is no doubt that premenstrual changes exist but their existence does not imply that they are due to disease or that they need treatment. Normality for a woman is cyclical, being determined by powerful hormone changes. The irritability, anger and emotional lability of the premenstrual phase is no more an illness than the euphoria, placidity, tolerance and 'womanliness' of the postmenstrual phase. The increased sensitivity that makes women less tolerant of unpleasantness and minor difficulties premenstrually may also make them more creative, more enterprising, more productive and more appreciative of art, music and the world in general. Why then should we try to abolish or modify this when we have only measured a few easily observed disadvantages and have made no attempt to see any of the advantages that undoubtedly exist?

No-one knows the basic cause(s) of PMS. Psychological factors certainly play an important role in the majority of cases and as the syndrome only occurs in the second half of cycles it seems fair to infer that some direct or indirect hormonal influence must be at work. Despite many theories the research evidence is not sufficient or consistent enough to allow anyone to venture beyond generalizations.

The most often quoted hormonal 'cause' is progesterone deficiency which some studies have shown to be present in about 20 per cent of women with PMS. Recent work has strongly challenged this theory, finding no relationship with progesterone levels and also showing that there is no direct relationship between progesterone levels and levels of symptoms.

Neither knowing nor understanding the causes of a perceived problem has ever stopped doctors from producing 'cures' for it. So it is for PMS where in uncontrolled studies the claims for success for nearly all types of treatment are impressive. Everything and anything (natural progesterone; progestogens; vitamin B$_6$; lithium carbonate; methyltestosterone; oestrogens; the pill; tranquillizers; relaxation classes; regular meals; salt restriction; aspirin; orgasm; bromocriptine; calcium alone or with magnesium; hypnosis; acupuncture; diuretics; emotional support; special diets; ibuprofen; amphetamines) applied with sufficient therapeutic enthusiasm will be effective in relieving certain symptoms in 50–70 per cent of patients. Almost all the proposed treatments are largely or completely ineffective in more severe forms of the syndrome and the response to treatment often defies explanation.

No *one* treatment has been proved effective in a properly controlled study, and not surprisingly the studies that have bothered to include a placebo have shown a consistently high response to it. This placebo response is in fact most striking and few studies have continued long enough to allow for its abatement.

What then of the supposedly specific treatments currently being most vociferously promoted?

Thiazide diuretics

These will relieve symptoms of fluid retention whatever its origin. However, their injudicious use has in fact been cited as a possible cause of PMS!

Synthetic progestogens

Much promoted by the drug industry, these may worsen symptoms, as they actually *lower* plasma progesterone levels.

Progesterone (injection or suppository)

This has also been much promoted by some authorities on the basis of anecdotal and uncontrolled studies. In a recent double-blind crossover controlled trial comparing with placebo it was found that in the majority of cases placebo was more effective than progesterone, though never significantly so.

The pill

As PMS may occur in both ovulatory and anovulatory cycles there seems little advantage to be gained by suppressing ovulation.

Pyridoxine (B₆)

Used in PMS on the basis of unproved claims that it relieved depression in pill users, there is no evidence that it is effective.

Summing up, therefore: physiological changes have been redefined as pathological and despite a lack of understanding of the underlying mechanisms involved are being enthusiastically treated by a large variety of remedies, none of which is any more or less effective or specific than a placebo. It seems strange that when we have a superfluity of real diseases to treat and a paucity of real resources with which to do it we should spend so much time, energy and money in pursuit of a chimera.

MENOPAUSAL SYNDROME

Human females are the only female animals to live to any significant extent beyond their reproductive years. Round about the age of 50 when women may already be experiencing anxieties about future functioning, doubts about their attractiveness and sexuality, and fears of approaching old age, sudden hormone changes can be associated with unpleasant symptoms which act as a potent, emotive and inescapable reminder that one phase of life has ended. The power that this change has to act as a focus for all manner of sexual, emotional, social and even political discontents cannot be underestimated.

As with PMS a huge variety of symptoms have been ascribed to the fall in circulating oestrogen levels that accompanies the menopause for no better reason than that these symptoms happen to have been experienced coincidentally with it. No doubt endocrine changes do act directly to cause some symptoms though it seems a bit too easy to assume that falling oestrogen is the only significant change when various other hormone levels are also altering.

Be that as it may symptoms of vasomotor instability (sweats, hot flushes) and atrophic vaginitis are plausibly claimed to be helped by hormone (oestrogen) replacement therapy or HRT. For all the other possible symptoms, including a large number which at other times of life – except premenstrually – would be assumed to be psychogenic in origin, it is clear that HRT offers no advantage over placebo.

What then are the supposed advantages gained by giving HRT to menopausal women, in other words by treating them as if they are now suffering from a lifelong oestrogen deficiency disease?

Relief of symptoms of vasomotor instability

Oestrogen is highly effective in treating flushes and sweats. Unfortunately for its protagonists so is placebo and as far back as 1937 a double-blind trial comparing oestrogen, placebo and phenobarbitone showed that the highest proportion of cures (85 per cent) was achieved by placebo injections. Other well-conducted trials have also shown that there is a considerable placebo response with flushes.

In most women flushes are very variable and clear up spontaneously for long periods. Placebo improvement may be continued whereas improvement after oestrogen is not only not long-lasting but also subject to a marked rebound effect such that withdrawal provokes severe flushing prompting requests for a return to HRT. Thus patients may quickly become dependent on oestrogen, and flushing which would have resolved with the passage of time will now need treatment for the rest of the patient's life – a self-defeating process if ever there was one!

Reversal of atrophic vaginal changes

Vaginal dryness or atrophy will be greatly helped by oral HRT or oestrogen creams. Even the creams may provoke postmenopausal bleeding which would then need investigation.

I cannot understand why vaginal age changes are so significant that long-term hormone treatment should be considered necessary to reverse them. KY jelly will provide any lubrication necessary for sexual activity without any risk of adverse effect.

Prevention of atherosclerosis

There is a considerable weight of evidence to suggest that this is not the case. It could even be plausibly argued that long-term HRT increases the incidence of cardiovascular disorders.

Without going into great detail the most important factor to consider is that while oestrogen administration reduces serum cholesterol levels and low density lipoprotein levels it increases the concentrations of very low density lipoproteins (VLDL), which are thought to be of paramount importance in the development of atherosclerosis.

Prevention and alleviation of osteoporosis

More evidence is needed before any valid conclusions can be made on this topic. Ageing seems to be the most important determinant of bone loss and HRT seems to delay, for a limited period only, the accelerated bone resorption found in postmenopausal osteoporotic women.

Whether this is of practical value or not is open to question. Even if it were it is doubtful if that value would outweigh the massive expense and considerable long-term risks of giving HRT to all postmenopausal women.

On the debit side HRT may be associated with side-effects such as breast tenderness, fluid retention, uterine bleeding and gastrointestinal upset. It may also increase the risk of endometrial cancer (a risk estimated at being six times that of non-oestrogen users) and gallbladder disease (by 2.5 times).

Summing up, therefore: like PMS a physiological process has been redefined as pathological. A large variety of advantages have been claimed for an apparently specific treatment which in fact is often no more effective than a placebo. Even for those symptoms where it may be more effective than placebo it can be argued that the already known serious long-term risks appear to be greater than the less tangible benefits claimed.

Commentary

Most family practitioners are male and it is suggested that they may be less than sympathetic towards these female disorders.

With increasing media information the expectations of women have altered and many demand and expect treatment of unpleasant premenstrual tension and menopausal symptoms. The fact that there are so many recommended forms of treatment implies that no one is completely satisfactory for all situations. It is likely also that there may be more than one single cause of the symptoms – that not all are caused by hormonal imbalances.

Good care of premenstrual tension and menopausal symptoms requires truly a holistic approach. Attention must be paid to and time allowed for discussion of the patient's personal fears and problems and of family situations and difficulties.

Because of significant placebo effects the likely benefits of many of the drugs recommended have to be viewed with much critical scepticism. Probably sympathetic support over the stressful periods is more important than polypharmacy.

9 Acute backache – active or passive treatment?

The issues

Rarely does a week go by without an acute backache being seen by a family practitioner. The causes of most 'acute backs' are undetermined, and whatever is done, the majority of them will get better within a short while.

Therefore, accepting that we do not know the causes and that most acute backs will recover – should we embark on *active therapies* or be satisfied with more (or less) masterly *conservative* care?

The case for active treatment
Peter B. Martin

WHAT IS ACUTE BACKACHE?

Acute backache is a painful and frustrating symptom which affects a large proportion of the population at some time or other in their lives. Pain in the back may be due to any disease of the vertebral column and the associated muscles, ligaments and nerves. Referred pain from diseases of other organs, for example a duodenal ulcer, may also be felt in the back.

For the purposes of this discussion acute backache refers to pain due to some mechanical derangement of the vertebral column and its associated structures. Symptoms due to other diseases such as neoplasms, infections or inflammatory arthritis are quite a different management problem. Having considered and excluded other significant diseases it is reasonable to use the working hypothesis that the symptoms are mechanical in

139

origin. During the examination of the patient one should be able to demonstrate an alteration in the mobility of one or more vertebrae which may be associated with muscle spasm, tenderness in the muscles or ligaments or nerve root irritation.

WHO GETS ACUTE BACKACHE?

The patient with acute backache is normally a well person who is suddenly disabled by pain and muscular spasm. Once he or she realizes that there is no serious underlying disease, anxiety is often replaced by a feeling of frustration. Impatient to get better unless they have other reasons for adopting the sick role, such as a compensation claim, they may be irritated by what they see as a negativistic approach if conservative methods are used exclusively. 'How is it,' the patient may ask himself 'that this learned physician is so impotent when faced with such a simple problem?' Not surprisingly, patients who are slow to get better often vote with their feet and their chequebooks for the ministrations of fringe medicine practitioners like osteopaths and acupuncturists.

No respector of age or profession, acute backache can strike down just about anybody at any time. The peak incidence is in the third and fourth decades and then there is a slow decline in incidence in the 50s and 60s. Surprisingly surveys have not shown any marked association with any particular occupation, though there is some increased incidence in people who sit down to do their jobs. The doctor who bends over to pick a pencil up is just as likely to be afflicted as the building site labourer who heaves tonnes of material about every day.

WHAT HAPPENS TO ACUTE BACKACHE?

The natural history of an acute attack of backache is that 80 per cent get better in 3–4 weeks. The immediate prognosis is therefore quite good and whatever treatment you use it will appear to have a good success rate. However, backache is common and though most attacks are not prolonged the total number of working days lost is enormous and this is damaging to the economy, both the patient's and the nation's.

Each general practitioner in the United Kingdom sees about 25–35 new incidents of backache per 1000 patients per year. This adds up to 1 000 000 new incidents and the loss of 10 000 000 to 15 000 000 working days per year in the United Kingdom. Any treatment that can shorten the length of the illness, even by only a few days, will be received with gratitude by the patient and nationally it would have considerable economic benefits.

WHAT TO DO WITH ACUTE BACKACHE?

Though we are discussing a problem that is very common, the pathological processes that produce the pain are poorly understood. The specialist or even the superspecialist is hard put to it to make a precise diagnosis in most cases. The vertebral column is a complex structure and the aetiology of the pain is often multifactorial. It is not surprising, therefore, that yet another patient with backache tends to produce a feeling of gloom in the family practitioner and a retreat into the safety of conservative treatment is the usual result. After all, if you know that the patient will get better quite soon there is no incentive for great therapeutic efforts. I would suggest, however, that if one had acute backache, and particularly if there were recurrent episodes, one would search very hard for ways and means of shortening the disability. A 1 or 2-week illness is immensely preferable to a 3 or a 4-week one.

Though conservative treatment may not be ideal for all patients it is just as important not to be too optimistic about what one can do. One must be quite clear about management objectives, which in the acute situation should be the relief of pain, mobilization and an early return to work. Permanent cure is an unrealistic goal because a mechanical derangement that has occurred once can occur twice, or for that matter any number of times.

What can the family doctor do, apart from offering sympathy and analgesics? In selected cases manipulation, local injections of anaesthetics and steroids and mobilizing exercises may all be helpful. The techniques and indications are easy to learn. The key to success is the correct selection of suitable cases because in some patients active treatment may be contraindicated. Many of the clinical trials of manipulation in the treatment of backache have been quite useless because no serious effort was made to select cases appropriately. One might just as well carry out a trial of appendicectomy in the treatment of unselected cases of abdominal pain. Such a trial might well conclude that appendicectomy was not a good treatment for abdominal pain.

MANIPULATION

Manipulation has been practised in one form or another in virtually every culture. Practitioners vary from the highly educated graduates of osteopathic or chiropractic colleges to the folk healers of rural areas who practise an art, the secrets of which have been handed down through generations of the same family. It is reasonable to suppose that a form of treatment that has been so popular in so many cultures has some real efficacy. Perhaps the best recommendation is the number of patients who suffer from recurrent backache who dash off to their favourite osteopath every time they get 'stuck'. More objective evidence has emerged from some clinical trials that patients do improve more quickly with manipulation than with placebo treatment. There is general agreement however that there is no long-term benefit from manipulation. Quicker relief – yes, but no cure!

There are many techniques of manipulation and the family physician is advised to become familiar with one or two simple procedures. Osteopathic physicians often run courses for their orthodox colleagues and it is well worth while attending one of these.

The simplest technique is to lay the patient prone and to identify the dysfunctional vertebra by pressure on the vertebral spines. A sharp vertical thrust is then given to the vertebra with the heel of the palm and with the arm locked straight.

The other commonly used manipulation is to give a firm rotational thrust to the spine using the thigh as a lever or by fixing the upper girdle and then rolling the pelvis with the other hand. This latter manœuvre is known in the United States as the 'million-dollar roll' – an allusion to the fact that it has earned vast sums of money for its practitioners.

If manipulation is going to be helpful then this is apparent quite quickly. There is no virtue in continuing to manipulate day after day if there is no progress. Sometimes it is worth referring the patient to a specialist manipulator like an osteopath or a physiotherapist if you feel that the patient should respond to manipulation, but where you have not had any success with your own efforts.

Possible risks

Before manipulating anybody it is important to exclude those cases where it may be dangerous. The possibilities of secondary neoplastic deposits, osteoporosis, rheumatoid arthritis or fracture must be considered. In the older or the chronically ill patient it is wise to have an X-ray done first. In the younger patient a good history and examination should virtually exclude these conditions and then I do not think that an X-ray is mandatory. If the patient is in severe pain, the associated muscle spasm may make manipulation impossible and then conservative treatment must be used, at least to begin with. The other contraindication is any evidence of nerve root pressure, with loss of power, reflexes or sensation.

LOCAL INJECTIONS

One of the features of the acute backache syndrome is that there are often areas of acute tenderness in the muscles or the associated tendons in the paravertebral, sacral or gluteal regions. These appear to be secondary to the dysfunction in the vertebral joints and they usually manifest themselves some time after the onset of the backache. Once established, these tender areas may cause considerable disability due to the associated pain and muscle spasm. They may also persist for some time after the original problem in the vertebral joints has resolved.

Injections of a mixture of a local anaesthetic solution and a parenteral steroid preparation into the lesion will often relieve the pain and tenderness dramatically. Personally, I use 0.5 per cent lignocaine and prednisolone but any similar preparations will suffice. There is not very much in the literature about the effectiveness of local anaesthetic and steroid injections. One difficulty is the fact that it is virtually impossible to produce an adequately controlled trial on these preparations. I continue to use them because I get consistently good results though I am not at all sure how they work. One recent trial showed that water was just as good as steroids when injected intra-articularly. Is this just a placebo effect or does the action of sticking the needle into the joint and altering its hydrodynamics produce a therapeutic effect?

Some acupuncturists say that simply inserting a needle over the tender spot and then leaving it there for a while is just as effective. I have tried this and it does seem to work, though the number of cases that I have treated is too small for me to draw any conclusions. Physiologists are now producing some reasonable explanations for the effects of acupuncture techniques, so we ought to take them seriously and some trials ought to be done. In the meantime I am convinced that I can give some of my patients relief from pain using injections.

EXERCISES

There is no clear evidence that exercises improve the rate of recovery of acute backache. Only a few trials have been reported and these have been inconclusive. However, though pain relief may not be achieved there may be other objectives for the use of exercises.

One feature of patients with backache is that they tend to become rather depressed and passive if the pain is at all prolonged. Recovery is then delayed by the fear of movement and a positive approach to their problem motivates them to mobilize more quickly.

A programme of exercises gives the patient something definite to do and makes them realize that limited activity is quite safe. Psychologically this is important because it replaces fear and apprehension with some confidence. There may also be some physical benefits. Immobility produces muscle wasting, and isometric exercises to the back, leg and abdominal muscles counteract this process. Muscle power must be maintained and if possible improved in the recovery phase. Strong abdominal muscles do have some supportive effect on the back, and strong leg muscles are needed if the patient is to learn to lift by using the legs rather than by flexing and extending the back.

There are therefore some good psychological and physical reasons for asking the patient with acute backache to do some exercises in the recovery phase. However, it is important to prescribe appropriate exercises. In the very acute situation where there is a lot of pain and spasm, exercises are simply impossible, except for isometric ones applied to the legs and abdomen. In particular, it is important to avoid flexion exercises if you suspect a disc lesion because flexing the spine greatly increases the intradisc pressure. In practice, it is best to begin with simple extension exercises and then to proceed to rotations carried out by swinging the arms round from side to side while standing up. This is particularly useful for promoting mobilization. If done smoothly and in a relaxed manner so that as the arms swing round they produce a torsional effect on the spine, the patient effectively does a gentle manipulation on himself.

Exercises therefore can be helpful but must be used carefully and with proper instruction. The doctor must make sure the patient knows exactly what to do and when.

CONCLUSIONS

Ideally, the family doctor should be able to make decisions about which therapeutic approach is best for any particular illness by looking up the literature and reading the definitive papers on the subject. Sometimes a carefully executed trial of treatment produces results which leave no doubt about which is or is not the best method. In many instances however the type of illness or the complicated nature of the treatment makes a definitive trial virtually impossible. Acute backache is one of these conditions. The aetiology is multifactorial and the treatments I have been discussing make it difficult to have proper controls. Many of the trials that have been done have been invalidated by the fact that no serious effort was made to select appropriate patients for the treatment under investigation and I think that it is fair to say that the trials to date have proved nothing – either for or against the treatments under discussion. For the moment we will have to rely on experience, clinical judgement and the opinions of our patients. Certainly, patients who are offered active treatments usually jump at the chance and even more significantly they come back for more if they have another attack.

I am convinced that I am able to have a significant effect on the course of acute backache in many patients, though I am realistic enough to know that I have no panaceas and no permanent cures.

Further reading

Arthritis and Rheumatism Council, Industrial Survey Unit. Report on Rheumatism in Industry. (1969)

Bartelink, D. (1969). The role of abdominal pressure in relation to the pressure on the lumbar intervertebral disc. *J. Bone Jt. Surg.*, **39B,** 718

Burns, C. (1975). The low back pain syndrome in general practice. *Update*, **10,** 753

Curtis, P. (1975). Osteopathic methods in family practice. *Update*, **10,** 753

Hult, L. (1954). Cervical, dorsal and lumbar spinal syndromes. A field investigation. *Acta. Orth. Scand., Suppl. 17*

Iller-Paine, O. (1977). The back pain campaigners. *Gen. Practit.*, December 2

Kay, R. (1977). *Update*, **15,** 1093

Morley, T. (1977). Remedies for back trouble. *Gen. Practit.*, December 16

Richards, A. (1974). The management of disc lesions in the surgery. *Gen. Practit.*, June

Royal College of General Practitioners. (1974). *Morbidity Statistics from General Practice. Second National Study.* (London: HMSO)

Sims-Williams, H. *et al.* (1978). Controlled trial of mobilisation and manipulation for patients with low back pain in general practice. *Br. Med. J.*, **2,** 1338–1340

Ward, I. *et al.* (1968). Low back pain. *J. R. Coll. Gen. Practit.*, **15,** 128

The case for conservative management
Jack Froom

Approximately 2 billion people in the world will suffer from attacks of back pain in the next decade (Nachemson, 1976). The costs in terms of discomfort and disability are incalculable. Yet, the aetiology, mechanisms of pain production, and most effective therapy for these attacks are either unknown or matters of controversy. The entity is poorly understood and the attacks are unwelcome both to patient and therapist.

Reference to recent literature, however, may point to areas of reasonable agreement and facilitate formulation of a rational approach to the care of patients with this problem. The practitioner treats patients with back pain daily. Lack of precise information does not relieve him of the responsibility to provide the *best possible* advice to the ailing patient, even if the suggestion given is that no intervention is appropriate.

INCIDENCE

Among principal reasons for visits to physicians in the United States back symptoms rank fourth after throat symptoms, cough and upper respiratory infections. In 1977, 10.7 million office visits, or 1.9 per cent of all visits, were made for back pain (National Ambulatory Medical Care Survey, 1980). A similar high frequency is noted in Great Britain, where 1.8 million adults consult their general practitioners annually because of back pain (Wood and Bradley, 1980). These data underestimate the extent of the problem, because many persons with back pain do not seek medical care. One population survey of 1410 adults reported that 21 per cent had experienced back pain in the preceding two weeks (Dunnell and Cartwright, 1972), while another noted that 18 per cent of 1135 adults reported 'being often bothered with a pain in the back' (Nagi, Riley and Newby, 1973). Among employees in several occupations that included both sedentary and heavy work, 12.9 per cent suffered from back pain in the previous year (Magora, 1973, p. 191).

The impact of this health problem on the daily work of general practitioners is considerable. One practice reported an annual rate for the acute back syndrome of 24.3 per thousand patient population for males, and 20.6 per thousand for females (Dillane, Fry and Kalton, 1966). Another gave an annual rate of 14.4 per thousand (Barton *et al.*, 1976), and a third found over a 3-year period that 10.2 per cent of patients complained of low back pain (Frymoyer *et al.*, 1980). These several papers reported different rates because of variability both in the population sampled and diagnostic criteria employed. Acute episodes are not always distinguished from those that are chronic or recurrent. Nevertheless, one can estimate that between 10 and 20 per cent of the adult population experiences back pain annually but that only 1.5–3 per cent of that population will seek medical care for this problem.

There are varying reports of the age and sex distribution of patients with back pain. In one practice the incidence of attacks in females was given at two times that of males, but that ratio was consistent with the female-to-male ratio of the registered patient population (Barton *et al.*,

1976). Data from a survey show 21.1 per cent of females questioned have back pain as opposed to 13.4 per cent of males (Nagi, Riley and Newby, 1973). Two practices, however, report a slight preponderance in male patients (Dillane, Fry and Kalton, 1966; Frymoyer *et al.*, 1980). One can surmise that sex is not an important variable, but that it may be secondary to other factors such as health care utilization and perhaps occupation. Similar problems occur with estimates of age distribution. Although there is an increased frequency of visits to physicians for back pain as age increases from 20–60, with a peak incidence in the 50–59-year-old group (Dillane, Fry and Kalton, 1966), survey data show a virtually equal incidence in all adult age-groups (Dunnell and Cartwright, 1972). These data may indicate that older persons with back pain are more likely to seek medical care than are younger persons with similar ailments.

AETIOLOGY

The aetiology of the acute back syndrome is most often not apparent. Although several causes of back pain have been described including ankylosing spondylitis, senile ankylosing hyperstosis, spondylosis, prolapsed intervertebral disc, spinal stenosis syndromes, spondylolisthesis and others, a specific diagnosis is most often not made in the acute syndrome. Dillane, Fry and Kalton (1966) were unable to find a cause for 79.3 per cent of the 605 attacks of acute back syndrome studies in their general practice. In 47 per cent of approximately 10.7 million patient visits for back pain a diagnosis of sprain or strain was made (National Ambulatory Medical Care Survey, 1980). Barton *et al.*, 1976 made this diagnosis in 32 per cent of their patient group (see also Dillane, Fry and Kalton, 1966). However, 'ligamentous sprains and muscular strains are imprecise diagnoses which do not correspond to the mechanical properties of the tissues. The use of such ill-defined terminology simply perpetuates the confusion surrounding the diagnosis of low back disorders' (Frymoyer and Pope, 1978). Even the most experienced expert has problems in this area, as evidenced by Nachemson (1979) who wrote 'having been engaged in research in this field for nearly 25 years and having been clinically engaged in back problems for nearly the same period of time and as a member and scientific advisor to several international back associations, I can only state that for the majority of our patients the true cause of low back pain is unknown'.

RISK FACTORS

A higher incidence of back pain occurs among heavy industrial workers as compared with those with sedentary occupations; sudden, maximal physical efforts appear to be important aetiological factors (Magora, 1973, p. 186). Truck driving, lifting, carrying, pulling, pushing, bending, twisting and vibration are all associated with an increased incidence of back pain (Frymoyer and Pope, 1980).

The role of psychological factors in back pain is controversial, perhaps because most studies involve patients with established chronic back pain, and the temporal relationship between the pain and the psychological stress is uncertain. There is a higher incidence of low back pain in subjects who are dissatisfied with current employment, feel considerable responsibility for their job, or are tense and tired after work as compared with controls (Magora, 1973, p. 191). Dissatisfaction with the job can prolong work absences in patients with back pain as compared with satisfied workers similarly affected (Berquist-Ullman and Larsen, 1977). Two studies report an increase in behavioural problems or psychological symptoms in low back pain patients as compared with the patient population as a whole (Barton et al., 1976; Frymoyer et al., 1980). High somatic, obsessional, and depression scores on the Middlesex Hospital questionnaire predicted a poor response to therapy for back pain (Berquist-Ullman and Larsen, 1977). On the other hand, in a case-controlled study Becker and Karch (1979) found no significant differences in anxiety, depression or the total number of psychoactive medications received for problems other than low back pain between the two groups they studied.

CLINICAL PRESENTATION AND DIAGNOSIS

For about 40 per cent of patient visits for back pain the problem is new, with a duration of less than 3 weeks (National Ambulatory Medical Care Survey, 1980). Recurrences, however, are frequent with almost half of the patients experiencing another attack within four years (Dillane, Fry and Kalton, 1966). In almost one-half of all cases the onset is sudden, and most are unable to relate the onset to a precipitating cause. The pain is aggravated by movement and the range of movement of the spine is usually limited (Berquist-Ullman and Larsen, 1977). Referred pain is present in about one-quarter of cases (Dillane, Fry and Kalton, 1966).

The contributions of X-ray examinations to the evaluation of patients with back pain appears to be marginal at best. There is no relationship between X-ray evidence of degenerative osteoarthritis and low back pain. Indeed, more patients without back pain had X-ray evidence of osteoarthritis than did those with back pain (Magora and Schwartz, 1976). In a study of 440 patients, of whom 106 received X-ray, the authors concluded that the X-ray examination had negligible diagnostic value and that the use could have been reduced without decreasing the quality of medical care (Rockey et al., 1978).

> In the majority of patients between 30 and 50 years of age X-ray examination reveals little that is not seen or at least suspected on clinical examination and since lumbar spine X-rays are connected with a very high gonadal irradiation risk, we must challenge our patients' many requests for immediate radiographic examination. Radiation is not the treatment for low back pain (Nachemson, 1976).

Nevertheless, 20.5 per cent of the 10.7 million United States patient visits for back pain resulted in X-ray (National Ambulatory Medical Care Survey, 1980). In addition to the radiation risks, the costs at current prices for the X-rays alone is in excess of $125 million.

THERAPY

Among several possible treatments for the acute back syndrome, there is evidence that bedrest has a salutory affect. The duration of the initial acute back syndrome attack is less than 2 weeks for 62 per cent of patients studied, and only 15 per cent of the attacks persist for over a month when patients are given rest, heat, and analgesics (Dillane, Fry and Kalton, 1966). In a prospective study of 200 young adults with a diagnosis of acute back strain which excluded patients with radiating symptoms, bedrest as compared with ambulation decreased time lost from work by 50 per cent. The mean number of days lost from work for those put to bed was 6.6 as compared with 11.8 for the ambulatory group. Although analgesics contributed to reduction of pain, return to work was not hastened by their use (Wiesel et al., 1980).

The effect of therapies other than bedrest is more difficult to assess. In a prospective study which compared spinal manipulation with soft tissue massage, immediate short-term improvement was greater in the manipulated group, but at discharge there were no significant differences. This analysis, however, did not separate patients with acute pain from those with chronic pain (Hoehler, Tobis and Buerger, 1981). In a comparison of treatments given by physicians and chiropractors, the outcomes in terms of functional status and patient satisfaction were generally equal, although patients treated by chiropractors felt that they were more welcome and received better explanations of the problem and its treatment than did patients treated by physicians (Kane *et al.*, 1974). Immediate relief through manipulation is demonstrated in a study by Glover, Morris and Khosla (1974), but subsequent evaluations at 3 and 7 days showed no significant differences in improvement between the two groups. Of interest is their observation that improvement began almost immediately in both untreated and treated groups following entry into the trial. In a multicentre trial of 456 selected patients who were randomly allocated to one of four treatments including manipulation, definitive physiotherapy, corset, or analgesic tablets, no important differences were noted among the four groups of patients. Here, too, patients receiving manipulation tended to respond quickly, although long-term benefit could not be demonstrated. In addition, there appeared to be no method of predicting which patient would respond to manipulation (Doran and Newell, 1975). Frost, Jessen and Siggard-Anderson (1980) compared the effect of three injections of a local anaesthetic with three of saline. Both techniques produced short-term improvement, with saline somewhat superior to the local anaesthetic, but there was no comparison with a non-injected group. The effect of exercise is also difficult to ascertain. In a study of patients assigned to three different types of exercises, isometric flexion exercises appeared superior to general mobilizing exercises and back extension exercises. Few patients in any of the groups became symptom-free, and back extension exercises made several patients worse, but again there was no placebo or comparison group with other types of therapy (Kendall and Jenkins, 1968). Regular participation in exercise programmes had no effect on the duration of subsequent attacks of pain (Berquist-Ullman and Larsen, 1977).

The use of patient education can be an important adjunct. As compared with a placebo group, recovery was hastened by attending a 'back school', in which patients were given four 45-minute lectures during a 2-week period. Lectures included back anatomy and function, instruction in rest in the semi-Fowler position, instruction in isometric abdominal muscle exercises, demonstration on how to lift properly and encouragement to maintain general fitness. Unfortunately, although the initial episode and absence from work were shortened, incidence of recurrence was not affected.

What then is the most rational approach to the patient with an attack of acute back pain? A careful history and physical examination should be performed to rule out pathology originating in the prostate, pelvis, abdomen and other locations. Back X-rays are not likely to be helpful. The formulation of a specific aetiological diagnosis will not be possible in most cases although presence of abnormal neurological findings often are indicative of disc disease.

Bedrest should be encouraged until the pain subsides, and analgesics given as needed. The patient can be reassured that in most cases the pain will be gone in less than 2 weeks, although in those where the onset was insidious the prognosis is somewhat worse (Berquist-Ullman and Larsen, 1977). Patients with a positive straight leg raising test have a longer absence from work than those with a negative test (Berquist-Ullman and Larsen, 1977), but the presence of radiating pain has no significant effect on the time required for resolution of the attack (Dillane, Fry and Kalton, 1966). For patients unwilling or unable to accept bedrest as therapy one might consider rotational manipulation. Although the results are unpredictable, an occasional patient will derive short-term benefit. There is little evidence that injections, corsets, physical therapy, traction or short-wave diathermy are superior to bedrest. Although these therapies can have a placebo effect, medical costs are increased and long-term benefits are lacking. In summary, our current state of knowledge indicates that for the patient with the acute back syndrome a short period of bedrest coupled with analgesics and perhaps most important of all reassurance from an empathetic physician will produce results superior to other interventions.

References

Barton, J. E., Haight, R. O., Marsland, D. W. *et al.* (1976). Low back pain in the primary care setting. *J. Fam. Pract.* **3,** 363–366

Becker, L. A. and Karch, F. E. (1979). Low back pain in family practice: a case control study. *J. Fam. Pract.*, **9,** 579–582

Berquist-Ullman, M. and Larsen, U. (1977). Acute low back pain in industry. A controlled study with special reference to therapy and confounding factors. *Acta Orthop. Scand.*, Suppl No 170

Dillane, J. B., Fry, J. and Kalton, G. (1966). Acute back syndrome – a study from general practice. *Br. Med. J.*, **2,** 82–86

Doran, D. M. L. and Newell, D. J. (1975). Manipulation in treatment of low back pain: A multicentre study. *Br. Med. J.*, **2,** 161–164

Dunnell, K. and Cartwright, A. (1972). *Medicine Takers, Prescribers and Hoarders.* p. 11. (London and Boston: Routledge and Kegan Paul)

Frost, F. A., Jessen, B. and Siggard-Anderson, J. (1980). A control, double-blind comparison of Mepivacaine injection versus saline injection for myofascial pain. *Lancet*, **1,** 499–500

Frymoyer, J. W., and Pope, M. H. (1978). The role of trauma in low back pain: A review. *J. Trauma*, **18,** 628–634

Frymoyer, J. W., Pope, M. H., Constanza, M. C. *et al.* (1980). Epidemiologic studies of low back pain. *Spine*, **5,** 415–423

Glover, J. R., Morris, J. G. and Khosla, T. (1974). Back pain: A randomized clinical trial of rotational manipulation of the trunk. *Br. J. Indust. Med.*, **31,** 59–64

Hoehler, F. K., Tobis, J. S. and Buerger, A. A. (1981). Spinal manipulation for low back pain. *J. Am. Med. Assoc.*, **245,** 1835–1838

Kane, R. L., Leymaster, C., Olsen, D. *et al.* (1974). Manipulating the patient. A comparison of the effectiveness of physician and chiropractor care, *Lancet,* **1,** 1333–1336

Kendall, P. H. and Jenkins, J. M. (1968). Exercises for backache: A double-blind controlled trial. *Physiotherapy,* **54,** 154–157

Magora, A. (1973). Investigation of the relation between low back pain and occupation. IV Physical requirements: bending, rotation, reaching and sudden maximal effort. *Scand. J. Rehab. Med.,* **5,** 186–190

Magora, A, and Schwartz, A. (1976). Relation between the low back pain syndrome and x-ray findings. 1. Degenerative osteoarthritis. *Scand. J. Rehab. Med.,* **8,** 115–125

Nachemson, A. L. (1976). The lumbar spine: An orthopedic challenge. *Spine,* **1,** 59–71

Nachemson, A. L. (1979). A critical look at the treatment for low back pain. *Scand. J. Rehab. Med.,* **11,** 143–147

Nagi, S. Z., Riley, L. E. and Newby, L. G. (1973) A social epidemiology of back pain in a general population. *J. Chron. Dis.,* **26,** 769–779

National Ambulatory Medical Care Survey. (1980). *1977 Summary.* United States, January–December 1977. Data from The National Health Survey, Series 13, Number 44. Hyattsville, Md.: DHEW Publication No. (PHS) 80–1795, April

Rockey, P. H., Tompkins, R. K., Wood, R. W. *et al.* (1978). The usefulness of X-ray examinations in the evaluation of patients with back pain. *J. Fam. Pract.,* **7,** 455–465

Walkind, S. N. (1972). Low back pain: A psychiatric investigation. *Postgrad. Med. J.,* **48,** 76–79

Wiesel, S. M., Cuckler, J. M., Deluca, F. *et al.* (1980). Acute low-back pain. An objective analysis of conservative therapy. *Spine,* **5,** 324–330

Wood, P. H. N. and Bradley, E. M. (1980). Epidemiology of back pain. In: *The Lumbar Spine and Back Pain.* pp. 29–55. Jayson, M. I. V. (ed.) (Folkestone, Kent: Pitman Medical)

Commentary

Backache is the consequence or punishment of human achievement of two-legged propulsion. Probably there are many different causes of the 'acute back'. It is not easy clinically to arrive at aetiological diagnoses and then to apply rational therapies. The clinical trials quoted, used by each side to support their own case, are open to criticisms on selection of cases, on choice of therapies and on assessment of outcomes. Activity enthusiasts quote dramatic improvements but do not publicize their non-successes, and supporters of conservatism emphasize that the natural tendency to recovery should be given a chance.

The two schools of therapy converge with the problem of the persisting backache often with referred nerve pain (sciatica). In these difficult cases too there are no panaceas. The conclusion, therefore, is that each practitioner has to work out his own approach to these common problems.

10 Terminal care – at home or in the hospital or hospice?

The issues

About one-third of deaths in Britain take place at home and two-thirds in hospitals; relatively few spend their final days in hospices, chiefly because there are few hospices.

Not all terminal care is concerned with cancer; prolonged terminal care also is necessary for those dying from cardiac failure, chronic airways obstruction, neurological disorders and crippling rheumatic diseases.

The issues here relate not to whether home, hospice, or hospital care is best, but rather how each complements the other.

The case for home care of the dying
M. Keith Thompson

In the Middle Ages, when the west was populated by young people, 50 per cent being under 20 years of age, so chronically malnourished that the future here on earth meant little or nothing, death itself was feared only should it prove painful, or abnormally frequent. The fact that death came quickly and easily, almost as a daily occurrence, meant that people would know when they were dying, and be able to summon friends and family in order to take leave of them.

In our modern gerontocratic civilization, when the prime causes of death have been narrowed down almost exclusively to heart disease, stroke and cancer, the process of dying is more prolonged and agonizing, due, in no small measure, to medical ethical uncertainty and an unclear prognostic grasp. In some cases patients have been medicated by the practice of skills more appropriate to the resurrectionist than the doctor;

153

and others, who might have exposed unwittingly the limitations of 'scientific medicine', have been subtly punished by being left incommunicado when they most needed interpersonal interaction of a meaningful kind. The explosion of medical technology in this century has focused medical attention in directions that largely exclude the dying, and today's practitioner is under constant pressure to accept an orientation towards the use of science and technology in the 'fight for life' rather than in the understanding of people's needs, and the alleviations of suffering. The inadequacy with which we deal with death reaches its apogee in the strange crematorial ritual, with its highly abbreviated service and canned music, geared to synchronize with the next funeral.

THE HOSPICE MOVEMENT

It was appropriate, therefore, that the tradition of the hospice was introduced in 1905 at St Joseph's Hospice in Hackney at the beginning of the period of enhanced expectation of life which continues today in Britain. There had, of course, been many other earlier hospices in Britain, and abroad, but it was the reception of the first patients at St Christopher's Hospice in 1967 that offered the first serious attempt to balance science-oriented medical practice with equal concern for patient care, research and teaching, in an effort to meet the needs of the whole person.

It is easy to conclude that it is only in the context of such an approach that adequate care for the terminally ill is made possible, particularly in view of the fact that hospice care involves the patient and family as the unit of care. The hospice movement has spread like wildfire, for there are now more than 50 hospices established in the United Kingdom, and over 70 in North America. However, hospices support the contention that many people would choose to die at home if the appropriate supports were available, and it is this aspect that will be examined and promulgated.

It is my contention that, even if resources would allow it, the expansion of hospices to the extent that every terminal illness could be thus cared for, would cause the concept to fail. When the absence of budget constraint allows an activity to be expanded, those things should be done first where the benefit is greatest. Beyond a certain point, if the service is expanded, it will progressively bring in those people who are getting less and less benefit. There should therefore be a strict limit to hospice provision so that it should never become a service provision, for to do so would dilute its impact on the problems it seeks to examine. The hospice movement has arisen as a reform of hospital care, due to the technical and disease-oriented care in which the act of dying has no place. Hospices have become, and must remain, centres of excellence and teaching, and one of the commendable activities at St Christopher's Hospice is the regular series of residential interdisciplinary courses which include, for a period of a few weeks, medical, nursing and theological studies.

As such, hospice care must be closely related to the mainstream of health care activity in order to exist and have maximal impact on care of the dying person, not only to avoid the 'house of death' stigma, but also to make an important statement regarding the direction taken by health care as a whole. What the hospice movement has done has been to advocate the quality of life that should be lived until death, in association with the absence of pain, the maintenance of personal control, and the support of the family. It has demonstrated that larger philosophical framework in which there is renewed recognition that emotional wellbeing is at least as important as physical health. In developing such a system of care, attention has been paid to the importance of the environment, personal privacy, the continuity of care, and family needs.

It is not proposed to argue here that there is a best and second best. Hospice care and home care are complementary alternatives. Yet, the choice between alternatives remains. In making a choice, it must be a real choice, for in modern society there are many people for whom there is no choice between a home and a hospice. Increasingly, it seems there are those who find warmth and fellowship more easily in public houses than in private homes.

THE IMPORTANCE OF ENVIRONMENT

The emphasis in the care of the dying does not lie in clinical competence for diagnostic procedures, or lifesaving techniques; instead the emphasis lies in enabling family and patient to use their remaining time together most comfortably and easily. It must allow those participating in such care to innovate, and participate in care within the resources of the home.

Thus, one of my patients cared for at home with motor neurone disease, remembered having removed servants' bells from the kitchen years before, and stored them on their spring brackets in the garage. No bell could have been better designed for summoning assistance by a man no longer able to raise his arms, and increasingly forced by his illness into a posture of flexion. All those who cared for this dying patient relied on his retained intellectual clarity to devise the best means of management which proved entirely successful. The importance of the home environment is that it allows to the greatest extent supervision and control over the nursing situation by the patient himself.

There is in most people that same sense of territory demonstrated in the behaviour of birds and animals. Even in the conditions of flux and mobility created by modern societies, there is some diapason note in most human beings that draws them ultimately to their origins. Vast sums are paid to return the mortal remains of those who die amidst the alien corn, and for those fortunate enough to build a home it becomes, in later life, a love object and time capsule. However welcoming, architecturally designed and furnished, the hospice for such people must take second place to the individual home as the most desirable environment for the end of life.

THE IMPORTANCE OF THE INDIVIDUAL PATIENT

While the home is the best place for the care of most patients, this is not always so. There is no doubt that the intelligent and involved executive can function very much better during his last days from his own home. Old people, transferred to the care of strangers and a wholly unfamiliar environment, are likely to become confused and dependent. The exception to what is almost a general rule is the mother. It is paradoxical that she who has built her home, and tended it throughout life, should often become at the end of life the one person best transferred away. Yet this is so, from observation, probably because she experiences more mental pain through ceding control of home management to others, while children can often relate to her more effectively in surroundings which allow communication with her to be personal, rather than practical.

THE CONTROL OF PAIN

There is little doubt that pain mirrors the emotional state or spiritual situation of the patient. Much has been learned from modern hospice care concerning the titration of drugs in the relief of pain. But the pain of the dying must be seen in its totality as compounded of physical, mental, interpersonal, financial, and what may be called spiritual pain. It is often observed, when the patient with terminal cancer is returned home, that a reduction can be made in his pain-relieving drugs, and sometimes that simple analgesics can be substituted for opiates.

The great Samuel Johnson, who had always entertained a morbid fear of death, having obtained the truth about his prognosis from Dr Brocklesby then said to him 'I will take no more physic, not even my opiates; for I have prayed that I may render up my soul to God unclouded', and died with so little apparent pain that his death was hardly perceived by those gathered round him. We may interpret this now as a situation in which endorphins are released by conditions of comfort and support, much as the cries of a baby are stilled by the arms of the mother.

THE IMPORTANCE OF RELATIVES

The care of the dying patient cannot be carried out without the mobilization of family resources, and a kind of shift system of operation which ensures that everyone knows roughly what to expect in the way of problems. While it is emotionally taxing for staff to work in a context of exposure to death, the hospice staff has been selected, orientated and trained to provide special care. This involves a training by which doctors and nurses remain calm in situations that would be extremely stressful for the average citizen, and is achieved by altering the psychological level of response in these individuals, and defusing the threatening aspects of events by cognitive reappraisal techniques. Relatives cannot be expected to work along these lines, but can be assisted by professionals to make meaningful contact with the dying with appropriate emotional expression, and catharsis. The best results are achieved by an amalgam of care in which professionals and relatives work together at various levels of input. The skills that need to be used involve an understanding of the biology of illness, methods of stress reduction, communication, counselling, family dynamics, loss and grief, pharmacology, and even transcultural care and comparative religions.

THE THERAPEUTIC COMMUNITY

It is abundantly clear that the centre of interest shifts from the disease to the patient, and from the pathology to the person, in the care of the dying individual. Time and again one is struck by the rich resources within ordinary people in what is a form of crisis intervention, and how well communication takes place when the patient understands his prognosis.

The great advantage of the home situation is the focus it becomes for travellers. This is a cardinal factor. Everyone knows how patients are influenced by visiting, and can become part of the continuing dialogue with beneficial results. On their own territory, and with their own possessions within reach, some patients can be observed, in their own home, to reach levels of social involvement during terminal illness that could hardly be expected to arise within a hospice. Unfortunately, we see in general practice examples of the potentiation of pain in circumstances of loneliness and deprivation, and recognize the need to transfer such patients to the stimulating and friendly community that can be provided by a ward.

CONCLUSION

It can be seen that the complementary provision of home and hospice require flexibility of arrangements, and often a shuttle service between them. There should be careful selection of patients wherever their care takes place, and thorough preparation of resources of personnel and materials. Full advantage should be taken of the outreach services of the hospice, and the advice of those experienced in such care which is always generously given over the telephone.

There are few circumstances in which a well-organized primary care team will not be the best able to deal with the physical and emotional aspects of the dying patient. Pain control, incontinence, pressure sores, vomiting, fistulae, and cough, are symptoms commonly dealt with, while the importance of a relative in states of confusion, and in dyspnoea are well recognized.

It must never be thought that the bricks and mortar qualitatively influence terminal care. Certainly the modern hospice is purpose built, and convenient for that reason, but it is the programme of care and its content that is important. In the support of the individual lifestyle, and the continuum of care, there are obvious advantages in being in one's own home at the end of life.

The dignity of death is a phrase used quite often, but it must surely indicate a situation in which doctors, nurses, and social workers, ministers of religion, physical therapists, and volunteers, are guests in the patient's home. If the claim that the focus should be on life and living, rather than on death and dying, the removal from home must pose questions, if not problems for the dying. Too often the comparison has been made between hospice care, and that in the acute wards of general hospitals, rather than the home. It matters very little what kind of place the home is, so long as it is embraced by the patient and his relatives as such, and is a place in which the family myths can have full reign. The proximity of a hospice is of great assistance, and I have had considerable help from St Christopher's Hospice in South London during the care of patients at home, at various levels.

The care of the dying at home is one of the most difficult, demanding, and worthwhile elements of family practice. In the successful management of terminal illness at home, a subtle factor is that of timing. The family know very roughly what to expect in the way of problems, but they need training and support to do their best. Between a doctor's visits the cohesion of the family can be gauged, and the mixed talents (which are often latent until this majestic event) begin to gel into a group structure, and organization. Invariably it happens differently in each case, so that there is an eventual pride of achievement according to the degree of individual contribution. The educational opportunity is intense, and very often a living memorial is built into the minds of young people around this happening. Grieving is combined with labour, and bereavement counselling becomes superfluous when participation with the deceased has been real.

The dying words of outstanding men indicate that people die as they have lived. We may consider here such different men as Oscar Wilde and William Hunter, whose last words have been recorded. The roles of the hospice and the individual home are complementary, much as the obstetric unit and domiciliary midwifery used to be. It is my view that the hospice gives a great sense of comfort and a feeling of safety to the dying patient. To be able to die with similar standards of care, tended by the doctor with whom one has had a long and deep personal relationship – that is a blessing.

The case for hospital/hospice care (1)
Bridget Matthews

The case for saying that the best place for a patient to die is in a hospital or hospice depends on so many variable factors. 'In the best of all possible worlds' the process of dying should be made as easy and comfortable as is humanly possible wherever it may take place, but in our present far-from-ideal world hospices and hospitals are probably the best places in which to die.

CHANGES FOR THE BETTER

In recent years there has been an increasing tendency in medical teaching towards the concept of whole patient care. There has also been a change in the awareness of the needs of the dying patient. Medical and nursing

Nurses who choose to undertake terminal care are usually dedicated and are those to whom nursing is an art. They find it rewarding, and the standard of care tends to be excellent. In present-day hospices and terminal care wards the ratio of nurses to patients is high. The cost of this is balanced by the savings made on expensive investigations and curative treatments These nurses are encouraged to find time to communicate and talk to patients. They are expected to discover each patient's anxieties and symptoms, so that they may be brought under control. In most hospices no requests from patients are overlooked, and it is such attention to detail that makes life for the dying so much easier. This is often enriched in small ways simply because the nurses do have time and because the more personal wishes of the patient are not frowned upon. For example, grandchildren or family pets are allowed to visit, long-distance phone calls are made to members of the family or friends, who may never be seen again, special recordings of music obtained on tape for individual patients, and other special last requests arranged. Small bonuses like this not only give pleasure to the patient but also to the staff.

DIFFICULTIES OF HOME CARE

With the decline of the nuclear family and the scattering of the extended family, home care can be difficult. In so many families both partners are working and it is not always financially possible for one member of a family to give up work entirely in order to look after another. In many country areas neighbours know and care about one another, but in towns and blocks of flats they may only be acquaintances, not known well enough to be called upon for help.

Busy general practitioners, often in group practices and perhaps using a deputizing service to take out-of-hours calls, cannot always give continuing individual medical care at home, and although a doctor may always be available, it is not necessarily a doctor who is familiar with the problems and with the family. It is not easy for a doctor to hurry a visit to a dying patient; it takes time to cope with the patient's fears and anxieties as well as attempting to sort out and control his symptoms. The patients are often hesitant to take up too much of a busy doctor's time and therefore may keep some problems to themselves.

A dying person is often frightened of being left alone, and at home it may be difficult to provide night and day cover. In a hospital setting one is rarely alone and there is always someone to call upon for help. Junior hospital doctors are permanently on call, as are facilities for coping with unexpected emergencies. 'Home' implies a comfortable, cosy place, surrounded by friends and relations, but so often this is far from the truth. Many people live in bedsitters or in poor housing with inadequate facilities. Very often they are far from the shops or chemist, and many have no friends or relations available to help in a crisis and may have to rely on services which are already overstretched. There may be no access to a telephone and no-one to give the drugs as often as they may be needed. A patient having to be turned frequently may be too heavy for one person to manage alone, and the extra work, washing and broken nights, on top of the strain of having a sick person in the house, are often too much for many families to cope with.

Once things start getting out of hand, families get frightened and worried, the patient distressed and angry, and all too often the situation for all involved becomes a nightmare. Unhappy situations can, and do, occur in hospital, but hopefully, with improved care and better education, these are becoming less frequent. In hospices unhappy situations rarely arise, mainly because all those involved are motivated to prevent them, and consequently the one asset that all hospices share is an atmosphere which radiates a calm cheerfulness and happy cooperation.

HOSPICE CARE

Most cases admitted to hospices are carefully selected. Patients must be known to be in the terminal phase of their illness when active, curative treatment is no longer possible. They usually have distressing symptoms which have not been controlled, or the situation at home has become difficult, or possibly there is no family to look after them. Hospice care includes family care, and relatives are encouraged to visit at any time, or even stay through the night if they so wish. They are encouraged to help with nursing procedures, thus enabling them to understand what to do to help the patient and so lose their fear of not coping properly. The more a family is involved the easier they find facing up to the eventual loss, partly because their sense of guilt about their own inadequacies in caring for the patient has been diminished.

Death being an everyday occurrence in hospitals and hospices, it is dealt with in an efficient and matter-of-fact way. The laying-out of the patient, the issuing of the death certificate and if necessary cremation forms are dealt with as standard procedure. Relatives are instructed what measures to take at a time when they are bewildered and confused if given no guidance. Hospitals can also arrange for social workers or volunteers to give invaluable help to relatives in coping with registration of the death, funeral arrangements, applying for a death grant, solicitors, finances, wills, etc.

Hospice care is obviously only suitable when the course and prognosis of the disease is to a certain extent predictable. With so many illnesses this is not possible, and for this reason most hospice patients tend to be suffering from malignant diseases, the natural histories of which are known. However, people die from many other diseases, or even as a result of trauma. To be in hospital is often essential under these conditions, as all the facilities and equipment for dealing with resuscitation and complications which might arise are available. If death in these cases does occur, then the family knows that all measures that could be taken to help the patient were to hand.

To summarize, the advantage of dying in a hospital or hospice are:

(1) 24-hour medical and nursing cover;
(2) easier symptom control;
(3) availability of special nursing treatments, regular drug and dressing rounds, emergency services if necessary;
(4) the strain is taken away from the family, but the patient is still accessible to the relatives;
(5) help can be given to the family to cope after the death.

'Men must endure their going hence', but this need not be difficult and very rarely need it even be distressing. With increasing education and awareness of the needs of the dying patient, hospitals and hospices can provide a better quality to the end of life.

The case for hospital/hospice care (2)
A. G. O. Crowther

The concept of a place where all or most of the patients are dying seems to be quite wrong and a recipe for disaster, and yet in the last 15 years or so the hospice movement in many places of the world has increased considerably, both in quantity and the quality of care given. While there may be an element of the subject being fashionable in recent years, and this seems to have some truth as far as the interested professions are concerned, there has been large appreciation and acclaim from the lay press and the public. It seems therefore, as in other aspects of life, that the theoretical objections are not as important as are the practical applications and the results from the work.

While perhaps having hospice care available may be desirable, it is expensive on manpower and finances and increasingly dying patients are well cared for on acute wards, as the staff on these wards in recent years have been taught many of the basic skills of terminal care during their training.

SPECIAL TERMINAL CARE UNITS

The siting of hospice care may be in a purpose-built building or a converted building, either of which may be away from the acute hospital, or in the grounds of this hospital, or it may be a ward within the structure of the hospital. There are advantages and disadvantages to all of these, but they all share a similar problem and this is their image, namely that of the death house. This should not be as large a problem as might be expected so long as the staff are aware of this potential problem. They must deliver good and kind care and be known for such attention. It is easy when in good health to dismiss the concept of a terminal care unit, but when one is ill and desperately in need of such care, as a result of the medical and social problems associated with the illness, then, provided the care is known to be good, the patient will usually be only too pleased and relieved to accept the admission suggestion and the benefits therefrom. In many ways, it is comparable to the patient who knows his terminal diagnosis but blanks it off in his mind and gets on with living; similarly if the need is there, the patient and relatives conveniently blank off any preconceived death-house image that they may have had of the terminal unit.

Only exceptionally, in my experience, do patients want to leave their homes when they are terminally ill. It seems far preferable, where possible, to be among relatives and friends as well as in familiar surroundings. An increasing number of patients are able to die at home comfortably and with dignity as a result of home care teams and the increased awareness reflected in the training of the various professions involved (medical, nursing, social worker, clergy, physiotherapy, occupational therapy and others).

Having accepted this, it must be clearly understood that with some patients a home death is just not possible, either for physical or social reasons, or more usually a combination of factors. When considering the patient's needs that demand an alternative to home care, it must be remembered that these are usually multiple in any one family and require the widest spectrum of consideration.

Age is increasingly a factor where hospital or hospice care is needed for the dying patient. A recent survey has shown that with patients dying at home of malignant disease, the main carer was aged 70 or over in 20 per cent of cases. There are many reasons for this, but a shift to this from a figure of 14 per cent only 10 years ago, must mean that an increasing burden is being put on relatives. It is therefore important that hospice or hospital beds are made available for terminal admission where this is considered necessary. It is also very significant in this discussion to realize that, in spite of a large increase in the elderly population in the last hundred years, and a shift in needs due to advances in medicine, the number of beds available for the elderly in the United Kingdom (in hospital and social care homes together) is virtually unchanged since 1880. There is therefore a tremendously increased pressure on relatives to cope at home. It seems that hospice and hospital beds have something important to offer here.

Sometimes other illness in the caring relative, which may be acute or chronic, precludes home management and admission for terminal care is desperately needed. I never cease to wonder at how often chronically ill relatives struggle to manage their dying relative at home; but on occasions this burden is just too much and admission is needed.

Increasing social splitting up of families, not only on a national scale but also internationally, makes for a need for institutional terminal care. Tied in closely within this break-up of family units is tighter career structures making time off difficult or impossible, as well as an increasing number of husbands and wives who both work, leaving little or no leeway for sickness of significance within their family. This is particularly difficult with terminal illness, since this may involve weeks or months of time-consuming care.

As a result of modern methods of treatment of disease, there is an increasing number of patients where the terminal illness is longer and occasionally much more difficult than it used to be. This increased time puts a greater burden on the carers who become even more tired, both physically and emotionally, and require even more support. Also several diseases, notably carcinomas of breast and prostate, often have long natural histories, with many twists and turns in the inexorable move towards death, all of which add tremendously to the burden on both patient and relatives. Short-term, and sometimes long-term, admission is frequently a necessity for these patients.

'HORROR' PROBLEMS

Although only a small proportion of terminally ill patients will have a 'horror' problem, they are an extremely important group and take up a significant part of the bed space and a lot of the professional skills in hospices and hospitals. The form this horror takes varies, but may be as a result of the lesion being grossly fungating; there may be foul smells either from lesions themselves or as a result of the disease process; there may be physical deformity from the disease or as a result of drugs (gross steroid appearances); there may be mental deformities from destruction by disease of the normal personality or mental functions. These add greatly to the burden on relatives as well as on the patient and may be the prime motivation behind a request for the patient's admission.

Many patients are afraid of the path to death and what will happen along it, but seldom are they afraid of death itself. However, many relatives are very reasonably terrified of the dying process, of seeing a dead relative and of what procedures they will be expected to perform at and after death. Understanding here will help a lot, along with careful and simple explanations, but nevertheless in some families it will greatly interfere with the care that they can give to the patient during life, thus leading to a need for admission to hospital or hospice care. The 'what happens if . . .' syndrome, as I call it, frequently operates at home. This is a fear, sometimes conscious, but often unconscious, that the patient has of something happening in the course of his illness with which he will be unable to deal, and neither will his relatives be much help. I believe that it is this fear that makes symptom control difficult, and sometimes impossible, in home management. It is a fear of what happens 'if I choke . . . if I start vomiting . . . if I get severe pain . . . if I cannot get hold of the nurse or doctor . . . or if my relatives cannot cope with my problems'. These fears, often not involving death itself, are most easily and fully dealt with in the relaxed atmosphere of a hospice, although hospital care will go a long way to alleviate them.

SYMPTOM CONTROL

Surely the largest offering that the hospital, and in particular the hospice, can make is in symptom control with the administration of the correct drugs at appropriate intervals, and also occasionally bringing in experts for palliative surgery or radiotherapy, nerve blocks, etc. Care must also involve the relatives since they are often just as desperate as the patient, even though on a different plane. Control of pain, confusion, nausea and vomiting, disorientation, incontinence, dyspnoea, diarrhoea and any other troublesome symptom can be tackled with various degrees of success in hospital or hospice when it has failed or been found to be difficult at home. The management of patients with ununited pathological fractures frequently necessitates admission; also complicated large time-consuming dressings may not be suitable for management at home, with busy community nurses and general practitioners. Acute hospital care may not be ideal for these patients due to staffing levels, but hospice care certainly does allow for this sort of problem.

HOSPITAL CARE

For many patients and relatives the alternative to home care is that of being in an acute hospital ward; this may well be the one in which their initial diagnosis and subsequent treatment has been conducted. These wards vary tremendously in the standards of care that they can give. The staff are very busy and are mainly geared to achieving a diagnosis by investigation, treatment initiation and discharge. This training and the efficient, often impersonal, care required in the acute ward situation is not conducive to being able to give good terminal care. This is no-one's fault, but simply a fact of life. In recent years a few hospitals have introduced oncology liaison teams (usually a doctor, nurse and social worker trained in terminal care) to go to the patient in the ward, at the request of the sister or consultant, and advise on the management of the terminally ill patient and his relatives. These teams have been very successful and result in better care for the patient and his relatives, as well as their expertise being taught to the ward staff for future use. It is an exciting and relatively cheap way of upgrading the care of the terminally ill.

These oncology liaison teams can also operate in the community with similar results, but it is much more difficult to arrange or assess the results as there are so many more variables. Many hospices operate home care teams, or support nurses (often financed by the National Society for Cancer Relief) or day unit care or various combinations of these, thus acknowledging the preference for care at home, but with the addition of the expertise of the hospice-trained staff. A few places operate home care teams of trained staff without a hospice base to work from, but on occasions having to call on hospital beds for intractable problems. These teams are obviously cheaper to finance than hospital or hospice beds, but they do not, in my opinion, make these beds unnecessary; rather do they release them for additional more difficult problems.

Hospital and hospice care for the terminally ill includes care of the relatives who need varying degrees of support, understanding and direction. Bereavement counselling begins before the death and, of course, frequently continues for some weeks, months or years after. To give this sort of care, skilled staff of all disciplines are required, an organization probably impossible to arrange in the home.

FUTURE HOPES

It has recently been suggested in rather sneering terms that hospices are all the fashion in recent years, and certainly it may be that the pendulum from virtually no hospices 15 years ago through the present and on to the future, is at risk of going too far the other way. Nevertheless, nationally less than 5 per cent of malignant deaths occur in a hospice so that this care has only been available to a small proportion of those dying of malignancy. The movement has come a long way since Dame Cicely Saunders started first in St Joseph's Hospice, Lambeth, and then St Christopher's Hospice, Sydenham, but I do not believe it has gone too far. There have been suggestions of a Euthanasia Bill in Parliament, and there is a Euthanasia Society (now called Exit), but there is no doubt in my mind that these are expressions of the dissatisfaction that the public have for the terminal care or absence of care that the medical and nursing professions have offered in the last 40 years or so. Therefore it seems that by improving hospital care and having hospice care available, our society will go a very long way to making any Euthanasia Bill unnecessary and Exit sterile.

Hospices also have a very important role as highlighted in the recent Department of Health and Social Security report on the care of the dying. This is a teaching role for the many disciplines involved; hospices should be centres of excellence not only for the care of the patients and relatives referred to them, but for interested professionals to learn and become themselves knowledgeable so that they may apply this expertise in their own sphere of work.

Thus while acknowledging that hospital and hospice care is only second best to satisfactory home management, this does not mean that this institutional care is not required for the problems which are so large as to make community management impossible. It does mean, however, that the institutional care offered must be of the highest order of skill and understanding, and this I believe to be true of inpatient terminal care today. These units are a necessary and important part of our society as we know it, offering more than just care for the terminally ill patient and his relatives, with expert teaching to involved professions, but also research on methods of symptom control and drug efficacy; in addition they are a resource for day care facilities and to home care teams, who may strive to make the inpatient bed empty and yet are bound, for the reasons given, to fail on occasions.

Commentary

Terminal care is an art and a science with skills that have to be learnt and practised with sense and sensibility. There are advantages to home care, and with the support of a primary care team that now includes professional nursing that can be provided at times of need for 24 hours at a time, many more dying patients can be managed at home – but a time and a state may be reached when admission to a hospice or hospital may be best for the family as well as the patient. Such a move should not be looked upon as a failure on anyone's part.

The hospice movement has had an influence much beyond the sheltered care provided. It has highlighted and demonstrated the problems of the dying and the bereaved and researched into and taught on the best ways of managing them.

The district general hospitals will continue to provide most of the care for the dying. They must accept this as one of their roles and duties in the community. For it to be done well each hospital should create and develop its own services for the dying and the bereaved, which have to go well beyond such care being delegated to the junior residents in side rooms or curtained-off ward areas.

There are few differences of emphasis in the three contributions on this theme – all highlight the problems and suggest how cooperation can achieve optimal care.

11 Compulsory immunization, or not?

The issues

Immunization against infectious diseases has provided protection for millions against unpleasant illnesses, serious complications and death. The dilemmas about compulsion are concerned with those issues that have resulted from the very successes of immunization. But because of the decline of whooping cough are not the complications of immunization greater than those of the infection itself? Similar arguments were being put forward before smallpox vaccination was stopped.

The questions therefore are: What weight should be given to individual freedom of choice and to the needs of the community herd immunity? How much *compulsion* by whom and against whom? How much *persuasion* by whom and at whom? How much *freedom of choice* for whom?

The case for compulsory immunization*
W. O. Williams

Vaccination is not only one of the most efficient tools which medicine can use, it is also the cheapest way to improve the health of the individual.
*Dr Leo A. Kapiro, Regional Director of World Health Organization for Europe –
World Health Day, 7 April 1977*

WHY VACCINATE?

We can kill many types of bacteria with antibiotics but, in some highly infectious diseases such as diphtheria and whooping cough, their use is

* In this chapter the term vaccination is used synonymously with immunization.

171

limited except against secondary infections. The situation is more difficult with virus infections, where no efficient parenteral antiviral agent has been found, although one such agent, amantidine hydrochloride, has been used with some success in influenza, provided it is given early, usually to contacts of known cases within a household.

The best form of protection from infectious disease is by natural immunity following an attack of the disease itself. Although this is a very efficient way of producing antibodies, the patient may suffer a serious illness in the process. However, an adequate production of antibodies can be achieved by vaccination with very little discomfort to the individual. Here an antigen is introduced in an attenuated form and it will protect most people from having the disease. However, a few will have the disease in spite of vaccination, but they will get it in a milder form. Vaccination, therefore, seems to be the most sensible form of protection against infectious diseases. It is usually carried out on a voluntary basis but this approach can be fraught with failure.

FAILURE OF VOLUNTARY VACCINATION

In voluntary vaccination the final decision is left to the individual or a parent or guardian, in the case of children. They may have already been influenced in their decision by a doctor, a nurse, friends or neighbours or even the media. A powerful stimulus to voluntary vaccination is the sudden appearance of a serious or life-threatening infectious illness in the locality. An excellent example of this was the smallpox outbreak in South Wales in 1962. It occurred unexpectedly and long since the country had ceased to be an endemic area for smallpox. There was an irrational demand by the public to be vaccinated. Routine morning and evening surgeries were disrupted while general practitioners dealt with queues of people wanting to be vaccinated. Compulsory well-disciplined epidemiological control with selective vaccination was all that was necessary. Another example of an irrational approach to vaccination is when the public becomes afraid of the vaccine itself and then refuses vaccination.

This happened in the United Kingdom in 1974 when a great deal of adverse publicity was given to the pertussis vaccine both on the television and in the press. There followed a sudden drop in the acceptance rate for the vaccine from nearly 80 per cent in children born in 1970 to 38 per cent in those born in 1974. The lowest figure in the country was in West Glamorgan with a population of 350 000, where it reached 9.5 per cent. Of 2295 cases of whooping cough studied in this area, three children died; 64 children were admitted to hospital and none of them had been vaccinated. Compulsory vaccination of all children at 3 months of age provided they had no contraindications to the vaccine, would have maintained a high herd immunity and may well have saved the lives of those three children who died. The cause of the adverse publicity to the vaccine was that its safety had been in question.

THE RISKS OF COMPULSORY VACCINATION

In the case of the pertussis vaccine it was claimed by the media that brain damage (encephalopathy) due to the vaccine was far too common. A well-conducted study carried out subsequently by Professor David Miller of Middlesex Hospital, London showed that the chance of permanent brain damage was in the region of 1 in 310 000 injections. It was found that there were some doctors who were still vaccinating patients in whom there were clearly defined contraindications.

The risks from compulsory vaccinations would be very small if the rules of contraindications to each vaccine were strictly adhered to. As with any drug, no vaccine is completely without risk neither is it completely effective in every case. The advantages and disadvantages of vaccinating against a particular infectious disease have to be reviewed from time to time, and when the risks from the disease are much greater than from the vaccine, then it is better to vaccinate.

THE RISKS OF TOO LOW A LEVEL OF VACCINATION

We have seen how voluntary immunization cannot always guarantee a satisfactory level of acceptance rate. There is then the risk of the herd immunity dropping so low as to allow an epidemic to occur.

Those who are too young to be vaccinated, and those in whom vaccination is strictly contraindicated, are now at much greater risk of being infected. In whooping cough, for example, these two groups are particularly vulnerable to complications if they contract the disease. The disease will also remain endemic in the country and smoulder on indefinitely with no hope of complete eradication, as in the case of smallpox.

THE ERADICATION OF SMALLPOX

Some infectious diseases can be wiped out permanently. A remarkable recent example was the total elimination of smallpox from the world.

This was made possible by the singleminded effort of the World Health Organization and its members of the smallpox eradication teams. The programme was a complete success. The last case of endemic smallpox occurred in Somalia in 1977, and although two cases occurred in the United Kingdom in 1978 this was due to a laboratory accident.

Smallpox was also eradicated from the United Kingdom by a determined effort which started in the middle of the nineteenth century with the introduction of compulsory vaccination.

COMPULSORY VACCINATION AGAINST SMALLPOX

Smallpox was a dreaded disease, carrying a very high mortality rate amongst the unvaccinated. It had been smouldering on in the United Kingdom for many centuries and it was necessary for someone to take the courageous step and introduce compulsory vaccination.

It was Edward C. Seaton who was mainly responsible for the introduction of the Compulsory Vaccination Act of 1853. This was a serious measure to stamp out a very serious disease. The Act remained until 1948 when it was repealed with the introduction of the National Health Service Act, because by this time the disease had already ceased to be endemic in this country. During this intense vaccination period there were also risks from the vaccine itself but they were far less than the risks from the disease.

SPECIAL SITUATIONS IN WHICH COMPULSORY VACCINATION SHOULD BE SERIOUSLY CONSIDERED

The complete eradication of disease

This is possible by vaccination alone if man is the only vector. It was for this reason that the WHO were able to eradicate smallpox. Although monkey pox is still present in monkeys, and monkey-eating tribes can get the disease, the virus causing it was sufficiently different from the virus of human smallpox to present no problem in the worldwide eradication of smallpox itself.

An attempt is now being made in the United States to eradicate measles. Here again there is no vector other than the human being. Compulsory vaccination with strict adherence to the rules of contra-indications would make such a programme more complete.

The armed forces

Serious outbreaks of infectious diseases in an army can be a more serious problem than enemy bullets or bombs. It should be mandatory when joining the armed services to be vaccinated with the vaccines recommended at the time. It is impossible, for instance in jungle warfare, to control yellow fever by eradicating the vector. The only sensible way to tackle the problem is to have compulsory vaccination.

It should also be important to have compulsory booster vaccinations against the various diseases and especially before entering zones where these diseases are endemic.

The health services

There is nothing more effective than an influenza epidemic to cause a breakdown of every type of service in the country. One of the essential services which is particularly affected is the medical service where the work increases suddenly for those working both in hospital and in the field of general practice. The number of cases of serious chest infections, myocardial infarctions and acute heart failures increase during such an epidemic, and admissions to hospitals are greatly increased. The pressures on the medical services staff are markedly increased. It is therefore important that they themselves should not fall victims of influenza. Young nurses living close together in nurses hospital accommodation would be particularly liable to infection, especially if they have not had a previous experience of that particular strain of influenza. If the hospital staff is depleted through illness, then the pressures are considerable on those left behind to do the work, some of whom may have carried on working through sense of duty, in spite of being ill themselves.

This situation also applies to general practice where the work may increase as much as three-fold. Ill and tired doctors who have carried on working become less efficient and are more likely to make mistakes. There is therefore a case for the compulsory vaccination of health service staff against influenza.

The virus is continually changing during the period of 'drift' so that new vaccines have to be prepared when necessary. However, outbreaks of influenza are not usually as serious during a period of 'drift' as they are when an epidemic due to a major antigenic change takes place. This is due to a complete change in one or both of the surface antigens (neuraminidase and haemagglutinin) – an antigenic 'shift', producing a completely new subtype.

There is usually very little time to vaccinate these people in advance of an epidemic due to a major antigenic change. Sometimes we are lucky, as in the Hong Kong pandemic which started in Hong Kong in 1968, but did not cause an epidemic in the United Kingdom until the winter of 1969–70. In situations like this, compulsory vaccination of health service personnel in advance of the epidemic should be considered.

WORKERS AT SPECIAL RISK

Laboratory workers

Laboratory workers handling infected material for which there is a vaccine should be vaccinated, and it should be mandatory for it to be included in the terms of their employment. Vaccinating such people not only protects them, but it prevents a spread of infection outside the laboratory. It is particularly important with workers who work with dangerous pathogens, but a vaccine is not available against all of these at present. When available, vaccination should be mandatory, and consideration should also be given to vaccinating the members of their household, especially as transmission of the disease may be possible before symptoms have become manifest.

There are a few laboratories in the world where the smallpox virus is still being stored. Although the workers in these laboratories are highly trained, accidents can still occur, as for example a gas explosion, lightning, a fire or flooding. It is therefore important to prepare for such an event.

Special medical teams

For medical teams specially trained to deal with serious outbreaks of infection such as a laboratory accident or the introduction of an exotic disease from another country, it should be made a condition of service to be fully vaccinated before joining such a team. There are no vaccines for some dangerous pathogens, but they should be used as they become available.

One of the duties of such a team is to carry out an epidemiological control in order to contain an outbreak. They would not be able to do this properly without compulsory vaccination of contacts.

Likely rabies contacts

Compulsory vaccination to protect themselves against rabies should be mandatory for those who are likely to handle imported animals or any animal suspected of rabies, for example veterinary surgeons and also airport and seaport personnel handling imported animals.

The new diploid vaccine is superior to and less unpleasant than the previous duck embryo vaccine, and therefore more acceptable.

Post-mortem attendants

All post-mortem workers should not be accepted for employment unless they have had a Mantoux test, if necessary followed by a BCG vaccination.

Workers handling dead animals

For their own safety workers working with carcases, skins and animal bristles should be vaccinated against anthrax as one of their terms of service for employment.

Travellers

People entering the country from an endemic area should not be allowed to enter without producing a valid certificate of vaccination.

This should also apply to travellers re-entering their non-endemic country after a short absence to an endemic area.

CONCLUSION

There should be no 'half measures' in dealing with the prevention of serious, often life-threatening infectious diseases. Apart from good hygiene and creating good socioeconomic conditions, vaccination with the specific vaccine is the most efficient method of prevention. When necessary its compulsory use should be seriously considered.

The case against compulsory immunization
Tommy Bouchier Hayes

Who shall decide when doctors disagree
And sound casuists doubt, like you and me.
Alexander Pope, 1732

The word 'compulsory' has a very solid ring to it, meaning compelling, obligatory or compelled. But compelled by whom? When it is applied to immunization, ought it to be by government, on the assumption that elected representatives know what is best for those under their jurisdiction, or by doctors, who supposedly know what is best for their patients? Indeed ought immunization to be compelled by anyone at all? I would argue that the answer is no.

UNCERTAINTIES AND PRESSURE GROUPS

During the whooping cough epidemic of 1977–79, after doubts had been raised about the safety of pertussis vaccination, an official silence, in effect, was maintained. True, the previous advice of the DHSS – favourable to vaccination – was not changed, but neither was it emphasized. On the contrary, planned publicity was cancelled and doctors were provided with no factual information, let alone explicit support, for vaccination, with which to persuade parents. The implication was that ultimate responsibility for the decision lay with the latter, and this was reiterated recently by the Health Minister who, while in favour of pertussis vaccination except in specific circumstances in which it is contra-indicated, stated that the patient must decide. But making a choice which could in rare instances mean the difference between life and death, or long-term handicap, for one's children is obviously not a burden that all can take lightly and it seems that many patients, having pleaded for years for greater participation in the decisions which affect them so vitally, are now asking us again to be dogmatic.

Vaccination against smallpox was carried out in this country for about a hundred years before its theory was understood, and before the nature and cause of its attendant risks began to be appreciated. During this time strong opposition developed towards vaccination and a campaign of slander and wilful misrepresentation was pursued vigorously by a small and influential group of people. It is still carried on, though less vigorously, by those who are influenced more by emotion than by reason, but in recent years opposition to compulsory immunization has sprung up from a quite different source – that of scientific workers moved not by emotion but by factual evidence.

In any truly democratic country, opposition and the freedom to express opinions contrary to those of the majority are the breath of life and it is thoroughly wholesome for long-continued practices to be submitted to critical scrutiny lest the accumulated weight of precedent is allowed to obscure the need for their revision or discontinuance. My purpose in this debate is not to adopt any partisan attitude but to present such information as we have on the hazards of immunization, to highlight the need for all doctors to be aware of the precautions that must be taken when carrying out immunization procedures and to point out the need for them to consider whether a particular procedure is in fact necessary or desirable.

CONFUSIONS AND DILEMMAS – PERTUSSIS

After years of doubt about the safety of whooping cough vaccination the government has produced its official verdict – that the benefits of vaccination outweigh the risks. Examination of the available evidence leads one to the conclusion that this is indeed the case in general terms, but the problems arise in deciding how one weighs the dangers and the benefits for a particular patient. One patient may obtain from two equally honest and caring doctors two quite differently weighted sets of facts as follows.

From the first, 'An epidemic is expected in the winter of 1981–82 and during the last epidemic about four per thousand of the population were affected and there were 36 deaths in Great Britain. About one in a hundred of those who contracted whooping cough were admitted to hospital, and of those inpatients one in a hundred required intensive care. The illness can last up to 10–12 weeks and is extremely exhausting for both the children and their parents. Vaccination reduces the chances of catching the disease and decreases its severity, though it does not prevent it. Oh, by the way, my children were vaccinated.'

And from the second another true and equally convincing story, 'Whooping cough rarely causes long-term damage and no properly controlled assessment of pertussis vaccine's efficacy and dangers has yet been made. For the years 1959–73, when whooping cough vaccination was in its heyday, the government had to compensate as many as 35 families a year for the harm done to their children, an overall rate of four in 100 000. Oh, by the way, my children were not vaccinated.'

Clearly when the available facts can be used in support of either one of two opposing arguments, the concept of compulsory immunization is difficult to justify.

Whooping cough has an interesting 4-year periodicity which seems to be independent of the prevailing levels of vaccination and this enables the general practitioner to plan his immunization programme intelligently without the need to provide blanket protection. For example, if the next outbreak of whooping cough were to be expected this winter, babies born during the latter part of this year would be particularly vulnerable by virtue of their age. Their vulnerability would be further increased by the presence of siblings of school age as it is they who are the agents by whom infection is introduced into the family unit. These, therefore, are the babies for whom protection by pertussis vaccination would be advisable in the absence of any specific contraindication.

It makes little sense for a procedure to be made compulsory if its efficacy is not guaranteed or consistent. In the case of pertussis vaccination, for example, the vaccine should contain strains of the organism currently circulating in the community if it is to be effective. This principle was demonstrated in 1963 and 1964 when new serotypes emerged against which the vaccines then in use gave little protection. Such events can be neither predicted nor prevented.

Recent litigation relating to immunization procedures has highlighted the need to disclose to the patient any possible complication of a vaccination. To avoid litigation requires one of two steps – either that vaccination be made compulsory and the doctrine of informed consent abolished, or that every patient be given sufficient information to allow him to participate fully in the decision-making. The abolition of informed consent would lead to a return of medical paternalism (or worse) at a time when patients are asking to take more responsibility for their own medical care. Though providing adequate information takes time and requires that all medical staff be fully aware of the available facts, this must seem the better of the two alternatives.

I have used the case of pertussis vaccination to demonstrate the disadvantages of making such a procedure compulsory, but it is my belief that rather than making any vaccination compulsory we should be considering whether some currently available vaccinations are required at all and whether they should be discontinued except in special circumstances.

IMMUNIZATION AGAINST OTHER INFECTIONS

BCG vaccination against tuberculosis

BCG vaccination is carried out routinely in this country, but two recent studies in India and the United States have raised doubts about its true value. A study in the United States showed a protective efficacy of only 14 per cent, and a study conducted in southern India showed no protection at all over a 7-year period. The rate of decline of tuberculosis in Britain since 1950 has been largely unconnected with the vaccination programme and it has been calculated that the 100 000 vaccinations carried out in the years 1971–76 will prevent only 88 notifications in the subsequent 15 years. That is, it will have required 1150 vaccinations to prevent *one* notification. The time has arrived when the number of cases prevented is too small to justify the cost of the schools BCG programme, and interest should now be concentrated on those at greatest risk, such as nurses, doctors and medical students. The marked decline in the incidence and morbidity of tuberculosis in most advanced countries over the last half-century makes it difficult to justify the continuation of mass immunization.

Diphtheria

Diphtheria has almost disappeared from Britain in the last decade, though it remains prevalent elsewhere in the world outside north-west Europe and North America. Though it is currently customary to combine diphtheria toxoid with tetanus toxoid and pertussis vaccine in a triple vaccine given first at the age of 3 months, there is in fact no point in giving it so early in life as the incidence of the disease amongst children below the age of 1 is almost nil. It has been said that infant immunization rates of 80–90 per cent are necessary to protect the unimmunized members of the population in this country, but in 1974, when the acceptance rate for triple vaccine varied between 20 and 40 per cent, there was no outbreak of diphtheria. In addition it is believed to be unnecessary to reimmunize children beyond school-entry age against the disease. Apart from the inconvenience caused to parents and children by adding to the burden of unnecessary immunization, it is important for medical credibility that we cast off the old and redundant so that we are not guilty of being anachronistic. It is of course far easier to introduce a new measure into practice than it is to discontinue one which has been well-established, but the time has come for a review of the position of diphtheria immunization in this country.

Measles

In the United Kingdom measles vaccination is offered routinely in the second year of life. It is doubtful whether the current policy of mass immunization is justifiable in view of the generally low mortality and morbidity of the disease. It can of course be complicated by ear and chest infections, but these are on the whole eminently treatable and short-term, unlike the subacute sclerosing panencephalitis (SSPE) which has been reported following active immunization. Immunization by no means guarantees protection and many are the children who still contract at least an attenuated form of the illness despite it.

Rubella

Rubella, when it occurs as it normally does in adolescence or childhood, is a relatively unimportant disease. About 85 per cent of women are immune by the time they reach childbearing age and are in no danger. The other 15 per cent should be offered the vaccine. It is obvious that rubella causes fetal wastage and much misery. Of the 10 000 congenitally abnormal babies born every year in England and Wales about 100–200 are affected by rubella. Approximately half of these congenitally damaged live births are firstborn, and of the remainder it appears that in most cases the mothers are infected by their own children. It seems therefore that in total about 50–100 rubella-affected abnormal babies could be prevented without mass immunization simply by immunizing those mothers at risk in the postpartum period following their first pregnancy. Some of the remainder could be prevented if those who undergo therapeutic termination of pregnancy were to be tested for the presence of rubella antibodies and offered immunization where appropriate. The answer to the tragedy of rubella-affected babies lies not in compulsory mass immunization of schoolgirls, but in taking the opportunity to test all women who attend family planning clinics and to offer the vaccine to those who are not immune, to vaccinate all vulnerable women in the postpartum period, and to offer vaccination to nurses, nursery staff, general practitioners and the staff of antenatal clinics and obstetric units in order to reduce the chance of transmission of the virus to pregnant women.

Influenza

Influenza vaccine should not be used for routine mass immunization in an attempt to control epidemics, but it may be of limited value in the protection of high-risk groups. The difficulty in producing satisfactory vaccines stems from the biological characteristics of the virus, the antigenic structure of which constantly changes. When a new strain differs only slightly from an earlier strain, the previously prepared vaccine will probably provide protection, but if there is a major change in the antigens the old vaccine will not do. One of the arguments for the use of influenza vaccine has been the assertion that it prevents so much sick leave. The average British workman has 21 days sick leave per year, and I would suggest that even if he were given influenza vaccination he would still take 21 days off though his absence might be attributed to some other illness. Annual vaccination is recommended for the elderly and for those with chronic chest or heart disease. Compulsory immunization would be of benefit only to the manufacturers.

CONCLUSIONS

Rather than considering compulsory immunization – increasing medical paternalism and discouraging the patient from taking some measure of responsibility for his own health maintenance – we should be tending away from the urge to provide indiscriminate blanket protection and towards consideration of the requirements of each patient as an individual. Identifying at-risk groups, acquainting them with the facts and offering them appropriate immunization, is a more satisfying and economically viable method of practising preventive medicine than embarking wholesale upon expensive projects which often fail in their stated aims and are not without risks.

I conclude my side of this debate by quoting Sir Graham Wilson who said 'It is for us and for those who come after us, to see that the sword which vaccines and antisera have put into our hands is never allowed to tarnish through over-confidence, negligence, carelessness or want of foresight on our part.'

Commentary

This dilemma debate demonstrates the needs to consider the question of immunization from more than one point of view. Given the state of information as is known the individual must be allowed his/her views and there have to be opportunities to opt out of a compulsory situation.

The physician who is concerned to promote the health of his community as well as his individual patients will be keen to promote, persuade and even compel individuals towards immunization against infectious diseases.

The lesson from the eradication of smallpox is a strong argument for compulsion. However, the lessons of the possible side-effects of pertussis immunization can be used as an argument against compulsion. In between are the questions of immunization against the many other possible infectious diseases at home and abroad. How far should we go?

12 House calls – more or less?

The issues

Care by family practitioners in the community involves caring for people in their own homes as well as in practice premises, in hospitals and in other units. Home visiting (or house calls) must be an essential part of good family practice.

The issues are: How many home visits are necessary and useful? What conditions are best managed at home? How may home visiting best be carried out, and by whom?

The case for fewer house calls (1)
John Grabinar

One fact stands out in all the published figures about home visits: there is a huge range, reflecting the varied nature of general practitioners and their communities. One study (Fry, 1973) shows a 32-fold range in the number of visits made, per patient, per year, between 14 doctors; another shows a 26-fold range, between 22 doctors (Birmingham Research Group of General Practitioners, 1978). No discussion on the subject can ignore this variation, and it is accordingly difficult to draw general conclusions about the merits or otherwise of house calls. Despite this, commentators have repeatedly drawn attention to a pronounced trend downwards in the number of calls made. Between 1949 and 1971, 60 per cent fewer visits per person, per year, were recorded (Fry, 1973). This trend has continued, and simple extrapolation suggests that no house calls at all will be made within 10 years. American experience shows that this is not fanciful, but I am not prepared to argue that it is desirable or likely to occur in the United Kingdom. We can, however, learn from the

185

practitioners with low visiting rates something about the nature of our work, and the best ways to fulfil our patients' needs.

PRACTICAL DISADVANTAGES

Every practitioner recognizes that many house calls are made for non-medical reasons. Some of these have been given by patients in one practice (Carey-Smith, Dreaper and Jenkins, 1972): lack of transport, difficulty in booking an appointment, lack of a babysitter, private patient, bad weather, requiring a certificate. The medical reasons may be dubious too: fear of catching a 'chill', risk of giving or catching an infection, belief that all ill persons should stay in bed.

None of these irritations would matter, except for one crucial point: home visits are expensive. Admittedly, in the present British system, the doctor receives no fee to encourage visits (except between 11.0 p.m. and 7.0 a.m.); the patient also is offered no incentive to attend the surgery. But home visits take longer than surgery consultations. In our urban practice, a home visit takes about 15 minutes (twice as long, if the doctor is called from home), whereas appointments are booked at 5-minute intervals. About half of this time is spent in wasteful travelling, which is a heavy expense to all doctors. Suppose we examine a practice where the visiting rate is one per patient, per year. This would make a total of 2500 visits per (average) doctor, per year – six or seven a day – requiring an hour or two's travelling time, maybe 300–600 hours a year. If the patients made the same journey, each would travel only once a year – a quarter of an hour. The resultant time saved by the doctor could be used in many ways, perhaps by providing alternative services of benefit to the patients: antenatal, child development or well-woman clinics, for example. And petrol expenditure saved would not be negligible!

PROBLEMS AT HOME VISITS

In a sense, the luxury of a home visit is paid for by other patients, both through their taxes, and through the loss of the services of that doctor for the time taken travelling. There are other advantages in bringing the mountain to Mahomet. Physical examination of patients is often hampered by poor lighting, a low bed, and lack of equipment. Although most consultations can proceed despite these snags, there are occasions when an Anglepoise light illuminates the rectum or vagina, and perhaps the diagnosis; or an ECG can be performed easily, instead of needing a second trip; or an ulcerated leg can be promptly dressed, in clean conditions.

Chaperonage

One problem, which is theoretically important, although in practice usually ignored, is the question of chaperonage. I have frequently visited, and examined, young women in their own homes, with no other member of the family present, and no doubt most of my readers do the same. The risk to the patient is nil, but the risk of a false accusation against the doctor is not. Only the bond of trust between patient and doctor serves as our protection. In a surgery, of course, receptionists or nurses are available to hold a nervous patient's hand, and guard the doctor's reputation. I wonder how my female colleagues appreciate this problem?

EFFECTS OF REDUCTION OF HOME VISITS

Having decided to reduce the visits made, how can we be sure this will not cause distress or inconvenience to our patients, out of proportion to the benefits to ourselves? First, remember that other practices have achieved dramatic changes without loss of patients' goodwill (or, more importantly, patients). Fry (1973) claims a 10-fold drop in his home visiting, between 1949 and 1971, and still manages to care for 4500 patients – no loss of goodwill there! Second, the patients have answered these questions themselves (Carey-Smith, Dreaper and Jenkins, 1972): when offered alternatives to home visits, over 60 per cent said these would be acceptable. The alternatives were: telephone advice from the doctor; a visit by an ancillary worker; and an offer of transport to the surgery.

Factors

Consider these in more details.

Telephone

Many doctors now ask for all visit requests to be transferred to them, even while in consultation with another patient. This allows simple advice to be given, which may be sufficient. It allows an urgent appointment to be offered, which is frequently accepted. And it allows the truly urgent visit to be detected quickly, and acted on at once. At evenings and weekends, when we have no receptionists guarding the telephone, I find only half the requests result in a visit. In our practice, too, the availability of a surgery even on Sunday mornings acts as a safety-valve and prevents several unnecessary visits between Saturday and Sunday morning. Of course, all this presupposes that the patient has a telephone. In our urban area, over 90 per cent of the homes have one. In the whole country, there are enough telephones to make one available to every other person (*Encyclopaedia Britannica*, 1980). Even when the family are not 'on the phone', the local telephone box, or kindly neighbours, fill the gap.

Ancillary staff

Ancillary staff are alleged to save the doctor's time. In real life, we have found they generate even more work than they save. It is however true that many calls, for example, by anxious mothers, can be taken by attached health visitors, who may give advice or call themselves. Routine requests by housebound patients are frequently attended to by the attached district nurse, who can arrange for prescriptions to be collected, and can advise the doctor when a medical visit is really needed. Our attached social workers have proved invaluable in visiting the mentally ill, or chronically disabled, patients and helping them through crises. I think here of one woman, whose schizophrenia was marked by many traumatic admissions to the psychiatric hospital, until our social worker organized a new home, help for the teenage daughter 'in care', and transport and sympathy when the patient's breast cancer needed radiotherapy. How many visits I have been saved by this help I could not exactly say, but it must have been dozens.

The key word here is 'attached'. It is no use the patient ringing the surgery, to be told the district nurses are at another number, or the social workers at a third. The patients lose interest, and simply call the doctor. It is essential for all these attached services to be under the same roof, sharing facilities and experiences. We find the theoretical problems of confidentiality have no meaning, when professional staff are helping to care for a particular patient or client.

Transport

Some practices have set up private minibus schemes, to ferry outlying patients to a central surgery. This is clearly effective in rural areas, and the patients might even consider contributing the equivalent of a bus fare to the running costs. Sadly, public transport is for the fit and able now; the sick, old or frail dare not risk our London buses. In our urban practice, a group of patients have set up a voluntary aid group, one of whose tasks is to provide transport, by private car, to patients in need. Many regular attenders would be unable to come without the generous help given by these people. Some financial backing, to help with petrol and insurance costs, is made available by the local authority. In this regard, it is a good idea to have a local councillor on your list!

BENEFITS OF SURGERY CONSULTATION

There is one subtle advantage in encouraging surgery attendance. It forces mobility on those who are unwilling to move. Elderly patients with mild to moderate arthritis, tend to stick at home and their joints become stuck too. A monthly visit to the surgery, on foot if possible, is a means of providing physiotherapy. The psychological barrier is also overcome, and other journeys may be made, to shops or relatives. This helps the patient maintain a normal, gregarious life. I know several nonagenarians for whom this theory applies. Another group who benefit are the agoraphobics. Once the initial trauma of leaving the home is overcome, the journey to the surgery is therapeutic. A sympathetic nurse, health visitor or social worker may help achieve this end, and the technique is a form of practical behaviour therapy.

NON-REQUIREMENTS

Two points mentioned at the beginning require explanation. In the British National Health Service, a doctor may not refuse to issue a national insurance certificate if the patient requests it. For many years, this required the patient to be seen every time, and for prolonged illnesses monthly visits were required. Now it is possible to issue sickness notes for an indefinite period, or even without seeing the patient, as long as another doctor or hospital has recorded the disability. The 'certificate visit' is no longer required, and only clinical need governs the decision. Secondly, the febrile child is a common reason for requesting a visit. It is surprisingly difficult to persuade parents of the need to cool children in this condition. There is no harm in a febrile child being carried to the surgery, in pram, pushchair or car. Sometimes, when I have given this advice, the parents have taken umbrage and carried the child instead to the local hospital; it is difficult to see the logic of their actions. If the patient appears to have an infectious rash, he or she can be secluded from the other patients in the waiting room, or asked to come at a time when the building is nearly empty.

FINAL COMMENTS

In the 1977 James Mackenzie Lecture, Pereira Gray (1978) made a plea for a return to home visiting, which covered some of the points made by my fellow authors in the opposing essays. But even Dr Pereira Gray concedes that his visits have decreased, from one per patient, every 2 years, to one every 3 years. There is no patient who is completely unable to travel. Urgent cases may require a stretcher and ambulance to take them to hospital. Even the dead can have a hearse! Each request for a visit should be considered individually, and the doctor must assess the advantages and disadvantages. Provided a reasonable alternative is offered, a home visit is not obligatory under the terms of the national health service. In a previously unknown case, where the diagnosis is uncertain, a visit may be judicious. But we know most of our patients, and can often suggest surgery attendance, provided their fears of fresh air can be overcome. If we can reduce our visiting rates to the level of, say, one per patient, every 10 years, we would have an average of 250 per year, per doctor, or less than one a day. This is more than adequate to cover the genuine emergency, while freeing the doctor's time for more fruitful work.

References

Birmingham Research Group of General Practitioners (1978). Practice activity analysis. 6: Visiting profiles. *J. R. Coll. Gen. Practit.*, **190,** 316–317

Carey-Smith, K. A., Dreaper, R. E. and Jenkins, C. W. (1972). Home visits – the patient's viewpoint. *J. R. Coll. Gen. Practit.*, **125,** 857–865

Encyclopaedia Britannica (1980). *United Kingdom Year book for 1980*, pp. 682–685

Fry, J. (1973). *Present State and Future Needs of General Practice. 3rd edn.* (London: Royal College of General Practitioners)

Pereira Gray, D. J. (1978). Feeling at home. *J. R. Coll. Gen. Practit.*, **28 (186)**, 6–17

The case for fewer house calls (2)
George Davie

The value of home visits must be judged on two planes:

o The purely scientific: whether important information, relevant to the patient and his disease can be gleaned more readily at his home than in your office?
o The public relations exercise, demonstrating the general practitioner's willingness to serve.

Many other reasons trotted out defending the practice of home calls are not valid. Are the surroundings of the patient's abode more indicative of his hopes and aspirations than the personality he presents to you in your consulting rooms? Has the way you see his home more relevance than the way he describes it when he tells you about it? Should the environment of the patient influence you at all, or is it the appraisal and analysis of the person sitting opposite you that will determine an appropriate therapeutic response?

If observing the patient in his own setting has proved so valuable, why do psychiatrists and clinical psychologists not insist on making more use of this tool?

Patients often communicate ineffectively at home, when surrounded by other people. The face put on for others is usually different from that presented in private consultation. Surely it is communication with the patient and not his shell that is important? I recently heard a doctor who was extolling the importance of home visits mention that he made a point of following the lady of the house into the kitchen when she made tea. There, away from the others, she was free to be herself and could speak.

Perhaps it is a physician who is uncomfortable in his own environment who finds it easier to converse with people in their homes. A patient visiting the doctor in a territory where he enjoys complete control must share the best of the doctor's abilities if he has also taken the trouble of creating an atmosphere in which the patient can feel secure and comfortable. If the overall character of the practice is so hurried that no-one could penetrate the doctor's haste, a home visit now and again may be the only way that one could justify the claim to being a family physician with all that it implies.

As far as the adequate examination of the patient is concerned, no home evaluation can compare with that undertaken in a reasonably equipped consulting room. Here a urine sample can be spun and microscopically examined, stool specimens can be analysed, throat swabs plated immediately and an electrocardiograph reliably produced. I would rather be the dogged scientist who diagnosed little Jane's urinary tract infection in my rooms than the kind fellow who treated a fever at home and left the diagnosis to the paediatrician in his rooms the next day.

The patients' reasons for requesting a home call are often illogical. Not wanting to expose a feverish Jane to the outdoor cold reflects an ignorance of what she would experience in hospital in a cold oxygen tent.

The effort contributed by the patient and his family in bringing the sick one to the rooms, even after hours, is often therapeutic to the doctor. I have no qualms in getting out of bed at midnight to see an ailing child in my consulting rooms, because I know that the parents have supported their conviction that it was neccesary by putting in an equal amount of effort. I do not relish going out at night to find the whole house asleep after an irate father had felt that he should not have to suffer his child's whimpers alone and chose to share them with the doctor.

The case for more house calls (1)
William Stewart

A great deal has been written about house calls, both pro and con (Carey-Smith, Dreaper and Jenkins, 1972; Colling, 1974; Elford *et al.*, 1972; Fleming, 1980; Fry, 1978; Goldsmith, 1979; Khan, 1980; Marsh, McNay and Whewell, 1972; Morton, 1979). After being in rural practice 15 years, I have acquired a very strong belief that there should be more rather than fewer house calls, particularly in the United States. Rather than citing the literature, in which one can find articles to support any point of view, it might be more instructive to cite some personal examples of house calls that made a critical difference in individual problems of patient management, producing results that would have been most difficult to obtain in any other manner.

DYING IN PEACE

The first case is that of a 78-year-old widow who was still living on her farm with her grown children. Years before, she had had her uterus and one ovary removed. I first saw her for an abdominal mass which turned out to be a malignancy in her remaining ovary. Shortly after surgical removal, she developed bilateral pleural effusions from metastases. Finally, after she had received the maximum amount of irradiation and chemotherapy for a person of her age and condition, she was sent home for terminal care. The specialist who had taken care of her in the hospital sent a note stating that her pleural fluid was reaccumulating at a rapid rate and she would probably need thoracenteses on at least a weekly basis. Because she was much too weak to come to the surgery, I visited her at home only to find a cachectic elderly woman who begged me to let her die in peace. However, with some reluctance I tapped both sides of her chest and gave her a medication for pain to be taken regularly. Before leaving I also informed the family members that I would return the next week and wanted all of them there for a conference.

On my arrival the next week I first went to see the patient, who reiterated her plea to be allowed to die in peace. This time I did not tap her. After spending some time with her, I talked to the assembled members of the family. I explained to them that it was only a matter of days before their mother would die. We talked about her expressed wish to die and her opposition to repeated thoracenteses. It was obvious that I was only prolonging a life in pain. When I asked the family if they wanted me to continue with the thoracenteses, they all gave me a look of gratitude and asked me not to pursue that course.

I suppose it could be argued that I could just as easily have met with the family members in my surgery. However, I would obviously have had to continue seeing the patient in her home. Furthermore, I would have inconvenienced all her children, who were farmers or farmers' wives who would have had to take time off at a busy time of the year to come to my surgery.

ORGANIZING CURE

Another patient for whom house calls proved very rewarding was an elderly farmer who had suffered a stroke and was left with a residual paralysis on his left side. He had just returned home from the hospital where he had received what was determined to be maximum benefit. Since it was a weekend, all of his concerned relatives were able to be present for a family conference.

It was soon determined that the patient's wife would be unable to turn him and care for him at home by herself. The family also immediately rejected the idea of putting the patient in a nursing home. The relatives finally decided to come to the home on a rotating basis to assist his wife. It was also decided that he would spend some period of time at their various homes.

Again, it would have been possible for the family to have met at my surgery; however, I do not know where I would have put them all! It also raises the question of the advisability of leaving the patient out of the decision-making process. It was important in this case for the family to know that the physician's support was going to be there on a regular basis, as well as when necessitated by a change in condition. I seriously doubt if the relatives would have been willing to take care of the patient at home without the guarantee of the availability of this support. Interestingly, although the patient had received daily physical therapy while hospitalized, no one in the hospital had thought of the necessity of showing members of the family how they could perform passive exercises with the patient in order to prevent his getting contractures. Home visits made it easy for me to assess the patient's physical condition and demonstrate to the family the appropriate passive exercises and proper turning of the patient.

RESIDENTS' EXPERIENCES

House calls are relevant in urban as well as rural situations. Two such instances occurred in one of the residency training programmes that I directed. I was supervising in our family practice centre one afternoon when some relatives came struggling through the front door with an elderly female patient in a wheelchair. I have never seen anyone with more severe permanent joint deformity from burned-out rheumatoid arthritis. After the resident had taken her history and examined her, he presented his findings to me. We discussed her case at some length and finally agreed on a course of action. I then asked the resident when he thought he should see the patient again. He responded that he wanted her to come back in a month. He was somewhat taken aback when I suggested that he make a house call rather than putting this very ill lady through the torture of coming to the surgery. He pointed out that he could not possibly do any blood studies on a patient at home; I replied that this was one reason why we had needles, syringes, and bottles with anticoagulant in them. Reluctantly he agreed to make a house call in a month's time. Some time later he admitted that actually it was a rather enjoyable experience to make house calls; it got him out of the clinic once in a while, and he learned a great deal from the experience. Parenthetically, that first and only office visit had been occasioned by the receptionist telling the family that we did not make house calls, a misperception that was soon corrected. I do not believe that the patient's care would have been improved by forcing her to come to the surgery, but I *am* sure that it would have caused her a great deal of mental and physical discomfort.

TERMINAL CARE

Another urban case was that of the 52-year-old wife of a university professor. This patient was first seen for pneumonia by an alert resident who discovered that she also had a neurological deficit. She had had a two-package-per-day habit of cigarette smoking for many years. During hospitalization we soon found that she had a carcinoma of the lung with three cerebral metastases as determined by computer axial tomography (CAT) scan. The situation was explained in detail to both the patient and her husband. Both of them were quite insistent that they wanted her to die at home. Therefore, after the initiation of radiation therapy and appropriate chemotherapy, the patient was discharged from the hospital, her case to be followed by the resident. She was able to come to the surgery for visits over a period of time. Finally, she became too weak to do this and the resident began to make house calls at increasingly frequent intervals. The patient died quietly and peacefully at home. After the funeral, her husband came to the clinic to personally thank the resident for taking such good care of his wife and for allowing her to die at home. This patient would not have been able to have her final wish fulfilled if it had not been for the availability of a medical support system.

CONCLUSIONS

From the standpoint of economics and efficient use of time, house calls are impractical. However, as we have seen, there are valid reasons to make them – reasons that seem more important than practical considerations.

There is absolutely no other way in which the clinician can gain so much information about a patient's surroundings, economic circumstances, and mode of living. It is sometimes a revelation to find that someone who dresses up for a surgery visit is really in rather dire economic straits. (I have also seen the reverse situation.)

One also gains a perception of the limitations that a patient's household facilities impose. I was greatly embarrassed on one occasion to have recommended sitz baths for a patient with haemorrhoids on earlier surgery visits, only to find on a home visit that he did not have indoor plumbing in his house.

The home visit also provides the physician with great insight about other relatives in the household and their relationships with the patient. Strengths and weaknesses of the family support structures can only be adequately assessed by a home visit. I received a surprise when I made a house call on the mother of a patient whose hypertension I was completely unable to control. During my conversation with her, I found that she did not believe that there was such a thing as hypertension and had persuaded her son that taking the medication I had prescribed was a complete waste of money. I spent a great deal of time enlightening this lady about hypertension and the necessity for her son to take his medication regularly. She became completely cooperative, and the hypertension immediately came under control.

My final reason for making house calls is the increased bonding that takes place between the patient and the physician as a result. Bonding is an extremely important and unique experience that takes place between the family physician or general practitioner and his or her patients (one that does not usually occur between specialists or subspecialists and their patients). After a period of repeated contact between the family physician and his or her patient a reciprocal caring develops. The physician no longer looks on the patient as just a patient but as a person and a friend. The patient also begins to look at the physician as a trusted friend and counsellor.

I know of no better way of enhancing this bonding relationship with a patient than by making a house call.

References

Carey-Smith, K. A., Dreaper, R. E. and Jenkins, C. W. (1972). Home visits – the patient's viewpoint. *J. R. Coll. Gen. Practit.*, **22**, 857–65

Colling, A. (1974). What could the G.P. treat at home – with proper support? *Br. Med. J.*, **2**, 390

Elford, R. W., Brown, J. W., Robertson, L. S., Alpert, J. J. and Kosa, J. (1972). A study of house calls in the practices of general practitioners. *Med. Care*, **10 (2)**, 173–78

Fleming, H. A. (1980). Domiciliary visits by consultants (letter). *Br. Med. J.*, **1**, 406–7

Fry, John (1978). Home visiting: more or less? *J. Fam. Pract.*, **7 (2)**, 385–86

Goldsmith, Seth B. (1979). House calls: anachronism or advent? *Publ. Health Rep.*, **94 (4)**, 299–304

Khan, M. A. (1980). Domiciliary visits by consultants (letter). *Br. Med. J.*, **1**, 649

Marsh, G. N., McNay, R. A. and Whewell, J. (1972). Survey of home visiting by general practitioners in northeast England. *Br. Med. J.*, **1**, 487–92

Morton, D. J. (1979). Night calls in a group practice. *J. R. Coll. Gen. Practit.*, May, 305–8

Wood, R. A. (1980). Domiciliary visits by consultants (letter). *Br. Med. J.*, **1**, 51

The case for more house calls (2)
Andrew Fraser

House calls, home visits – call them what you will – used once to be an integral part of primary care and we, as family doctors, were almost the sole providers of this form of medical practice.

But times have changed; less and less often does the patient invite us to his home to look to his illness – even in a life-threatening emergency – preferring it seems to visit us on our ground or, lamentably, that of his nearest hospital. Maybe it is the economics of present-day medicine which has influenced him. In immediate postwar practice 'half-a-guinea' was the common fee for care either in one's surgery or at the patient's home, and we seemed well rewarded and the patient well satisfied. It was a gentlemanly sort of exchange – more an honorarium than a fee created, as it now is, by statisticians and computers.

As one who mourns the decline of home visiting and has made strenuous, but by now sporadic, efforts to retain it and to whom machine-medicine becomes more and more an anathema the points following are put forward in support of a return to visiting in the home.

ORGANIZATIONAL ADVANTAGES

Aside from emergencies to which we *are* called and which we recognize need immediate attention, such as suspected myocardial infarction, or bleeding from trauma, or other reasons, home calls may be planned to fit the day depending on the pathology you suspect your patient may have.

The child, or adult, with recent onset of abdominal pain can be visited early – before surgeons are hard to find or hospital theatres closing up for the day. The man whose 'diarrhoea' you suspect may be melaena, or the old lady who fell out of bed that morning, too, can much more easily be properly assessed or X-rayed early rather than late. Left to your receptionist or, worse, arriving without an appointment at the end of a busy day, as patients still occasionally do in most practices, increases 10-fold the mechanics of dealing with the problem.

Most of us – or perhaps it is only those nearing the geriatric years themselves – have a list of patients who expect, and usually need, to be visited at regular intervals. A few, such as the patient dying slowly of malignancy, need to be visited weekly; a few with cardiac failure need monthly supervision; and just a few with restricted mobility and handicaps deserve continued interest and support through home visits. These visits can be planned geographically, and it is surprising when you know your patient and his illness well and where to find him, how many such home calls can be done within the hour.

The matter of time is always raised by opponents of house calls. They forget that in this sort of setting you are the protagonist – the actor who holds the stage and who can depart from it as he wills. Contrast this with the dilatory or anxious patient who 'knows you are busy, doctor' but continues to hold the fort. House calls are *not* time-consuming – 10 minutes will often cover a full history and examination.

CLINICAL ADVANTAGES

We, as family doctors, subscribe to, and laud the concept of, 'whole-person medicine'. How one can really know someone, without actually seeing the background and environment in which he spends almost two-thirds of his day, is hard to conceive.

A neglected house and garden, an obvious unconcern for reasonable hygiene, actually seeing the kind of foods on which the household subsists, can often tell one more than the most detailed history sought in consulting rooms. I remember severe ketosis in sudden-onset diabetes first suspected because five 2-litre bottles of lemonade consumed that afternoon were still on the table alongside the patient's bed; or the lady with 'recurrent hepatitis', being managed by an infectious disease hospital, with a stack of gin bottles at the bottom of her garden attributed, by her husband, to diligent collecting for the Red Cross. Or the woman seen during an epidemic of viral pneumonia whose diagnosis was immediately changed, and subsequently proven, when several sick parrots were discovered surrounding the visiting doctor as he washed his hands in the kitchen.

Quite apart from signs, the history can often be amplified by a relative in the home who recounts that your patient really buys cigarettes by the carton and that his stated consumption of 10–15 daily is more than usually underestimated. A mother corrects the story of a teenager with tonsillar exudate which makes the diagnosis of infectious mononucleosis almost certain; or a husband, met for the first time, presents to you as an entirely different personality from the one painted for you for years by his wife. One of the changes in patient habits is the prevalent tendency of members of a family not to rely on the same doctor for their individual care – a change which makes for difficulties in developing a complete picture of a family and its relationships.

The patient, unless he is an individual who greets you at the door with the sort of excuse that he has called, rather than visited, you because the weather is too cold (or too hot), is already completely undressed and in bed. This saves time, too, now that the patients appear to remove such garments as brassières with reluctance and shoes and socks scarcely at all unless specifically invited to. How one is expected to examine movement, let alone auscultate the chest, or examine peripheral pulses, or elicit plantar reflexes, makes one wonder occasionally whether this area of clinical examination has perhaps gone out of fashion.

Finally specimens may be immediately available for examination: purulent sputum, perhaps with blood, between the fold of the ubiquitous 'Kleenex' in a heap on the bedside table; an abnormal stool which the patient has thoughtfully preserved by not flushing the toilet; or a specimen of urine retained in the pot under the bed. This is an element of home visiting fast disappearing – it was handy immediately to detect bilinuria or to take away, without the delay and uncertainty of obtaining it, a specimen for microscopy. It has its disadvantages, of course, for the unwary who, if the china model were kicked as he leant to examine his patient, unwittingly announced to all concerned that the consultation had begun.

OTHER ADVANTAGES

Compliance is one of these terms which makes the older practitioner wince. Until it was introduced, simple souls that we were, we used to think our patients followed advice implicitly and took every tablet and drained every bottle that we prescribed. Not so, the researchers tell us but perhaps they failed to appreciate that home visiting provides an ideal situation for monitoring whether proper and complete drug dosage is being adhered to. Two experiences, one where an elderly patient was taking both digoxin and digitoxin in maximum dosage because both her own doctor and the hospital outpatient department thought she required digitalization – which incidentally she did not; and another where a lady with a large liver, being investigated for suspected melaena, proved to be taking Ferro-Gradumet (dried ferrous sulphate) when frusemide had been prescribed, makes one wonder how else could such an important therapeutic error have been uncovered.

Seeing one's patient in an environment differing from his usual surgery visit is often rewarding. The pill-rolling tremor of one hand as the patient with pneumonia lies fairly still in bed might be noticed for the first time, or the sacral oedema of the old lady now in bed for 3 or 4 days makes you realize that you should have suspected her early cardiac failure many weeks before.

At least a passing glance at other members of the family present is an essential part of a house call. A boy of 10 standing in the corner of the room while his mother was being examined had such an obviously productive cough that the diagnosis of his bronchiectasis was no further delayed beyond the several years that it had been already. The wife of a man who had fallen and sustained a Pott's fracture while erecting new curtains looked paler than the incident warranted; the recognition of her lymphatic leukaemia a day or two later probably prolonged her life in more comfort than it might have been otherwise.

Home visiting of course, involves driving about the district in which you practice. A man apparently crippled with backache to the extent that he was about to be retired from his job as a railway shunter moved so smartly across the road in front of my car one day as to make his further claims for certificates useless; and a woman whose symptomatology and general affect always seemed suspect of having an hysterical basis was seen progressing down the main street with as flaunting a walk as one who found it an essential part of her profession.

The changing face of practice – have we changed it or has the patient? If we want high quality and complete primary medical care let us teach and encourage young graduates to return to home visiting – and the patient to ask for it.

Commentary

Whatever physicians think and feel, their patients want house calls; public expectations must be heeded.

Family medicine exists in a state of social and medical changes. More families have telephones, and access to private motor transport. Advice can be given by phone and sick persons can be brought more easily and in more comfort to practice units. Advances in medicine have made it possible for more care for ambulatory persons than for bed-bound patients. It is more possible to treat children with measles, for example, by a diagnostic visit at the practice centre followed by advice and guidance on the likely cause of the illness and with a follow-up check in a week or so – with the proviso that possible complications might be reported and dealt with either by a home visit or further attendance at the practice centre.

There are special and particular conditions and situations that are best managed by home visiting: care of the dying; care of the severely disabled housebound; visits to possible at-risk individuals (elderly isolates) to promote preventive measures; care of the acute-sick who are too unwell to attend the practice centre.

Home visiting may be carried out by others than physicians – nurses, health visitors (public health nurses), midwives, social workers and various other voluntary and professional workers are all involved in home visiting. Collaboration and cooperation between all these home visitors is very necessary.

13 Teamwork – delegated or shared?

The issues

The acceptance of the *primary care health team* idea raises the issues of the various members of the team working together. *Delegation* implies hierarchical levels, leaders, directives and responsibilities. It raises sensitive interprofessional issues and decisions on who is 'boss'. *Sharing* implies greater equality and democratic associations between colleagues who respect one another. It raises the same pertinent issues as to who should act as leader and whether his/her role will be accepted by the others.

The case for delegation (1)
John D. Williamson

The Director-General of the World Health Organization, Hafdan Mahler, debating the spiralling costs of medical care throughout the world, asked if all current medical activity should remain the domain of the medical profession. 'If these activities can be described in such a way that the knowledge and skills required for them can be objectified, is it not possible that some of them will be found to be entirely within the competence of lesser qualified people' (Mahler, 1975)?

Of the disease-related workload of general practice, only 15 per cent is related to serious or life-threatening conditions. Is it so ridiculous to suggest that at least some of the remainder might be delegated to others?

SELECTION OF CARE

If the therapy required by a patient is available freely then the only real reason for requiring a doctor's involvement is that the disease seriously incommodes the patient (Williamson and Danaher, 1980). And since the most obvious consequence of illness is anxiety it should not surprise us that the commonest reason prompting consultation is the desire for reassurance (Danaher, 1977). When this is not present there is often little or no reason to visit a doctor, and since not every illness is worrying it is no surprise to note that only 21 per cent of complaints are ever presented (Fry, 1978). The remainder are either self-treated (63 per cent) or ignored (16 per cent).

Even when problems are referred self-treatment may be continued. No fewer than 60 per cent of presented complaints will be treated by both the doctor and the patient. It is debatable, however, that the former recognizes either the scope or the potential of self-treatment. Too often is the patient's own effort to heal himself seen as injudicious meddling. And yet, with a little encouragement, and not a little education, much of the symptomatology brought to the average general practitioner could be easily and safely managed by the self-caring layman.

SELF-CARE

The obvious barrier to self-care is that the patient will often need something obtainable only through the doctor. Some medicines are available only on prescription even though the patient is as well qualified to assess his need for them as the doctor. Other medicines are considerably cheaper on prescription than they are over the counter, especially if the patient is one of those lucky people who receive medicines free of charge. Finally some patients need a doctor's signature to prove that they have been ill. None of this encourages self-care. Yet from my own experience I know just how much one can cut one's workload by encouraging self-treatment and by not mocking the failed self-carer who has had to resort to the doctor's potions.

FIRST-CONTACT CARE

Assuming that a self-treatment remedy is readily available patients' dilemmas revolve round the need for reassurance. Do they need to see a doctor or will a nurse do? Or a neighbour? It is only the lamentable lack of knowledge about illness and health care in the population at large which prompts many people to bring trivial problems to the consulting room. If they knew that help was available from other, less-elevated, sources than the doctor surely many people would tap those first. And perhaps there would be fewer doctors complaining that 65 per cent of their workload was for minor illness (Royal College of General Practitioners, 1973), with up to half of that 'trivial' (Cartwright, 1967).

THE NEW PRACTICE NURSE

Doctors are, of course, used to working with nurses, but it was not until the early 1960s, when attachment schemes became popular, that tasks other than basic nursing duties came to be delegated. About half the work of the home nurse now relates to technical procedures like electrocardiography, audiometry, venepuncture or taking cervical smears (Hockey, 1972). And given that some 77 per cent of home nurses were attached to general practice as early as 1973 (Department of Health and Social Services, 1974), it is clear that many doctors have grasped the opportunity of saving their clinical time by asking the nurse to undertake additional duties which are quite within her capacity.

In my practice it has been possible to stop sending patients to the nearby hospital for laboratory investigations altogether. No referrals are now necessary for electrocardiography or for skin testing; and my own clinical activities have been expanded by virtue of a nurse's presence. I can now undertake minor surgery, sigmoidoscopy, and injections into arthritis joints in the sure knowledge that the time-consuming part of that work – the preparation, tidying-up and dressing – are all going to be done by a nurse. The doctor is busier, but happier, and the patient's time is saved. The benefits are very clear.

In the field of preventive medicine, the nurse is invaluable. In my practice all attending adults over 30 years of age have a blood pressure check and all over-60s a urine check, if there is no record of this in the previous 12 months. My record on cervical cytology has improved considerably since patients realized that there was a nurse available to take the smear. New patients are asked to complete a questionnaire, and basic health data analogous to that needed for insurance medicals (for example, height, weight, peak-flow, audiometry, visual acuity, urinalysis) is collected so that baseline data are available on each new patient *before* he or she falls ill.

A more recent development has been the research nurse. She has taken on all manner of extra duties but without any shadow of doubt the most important of these has been in clinical decision-making. My own research nurse, who is working on the treatment of mild hypertension, is the sole person to see most patients in the trial. After a medical examination the patient's progress is monitored, and his drugs dispensed, by the nurse herself. Naturally the limits of her autonomy are strictly laid down but she does have a degree of autonomy virtually unknown to the old-style district nurse.

Professional autonomy in nursing is not entirely new, though. The midwife and the health visitor have jealously guarded their right to act independently of the doctor without any apparent hazard to the patient. But there is no real overlap between these roles and those of the average general practitioner. Since their work is complementary there is less need for superordinacy in the doctor. The extension of the home practice nurse into clinical medicine, on the other hand, is a significant invasion of the medical domain.

PROTOCOL TECHNIQUE AND THE NURSE

Perhaps because of its financial implications, most of the work on these physician extenders, or nurse practitioners, has been done in other countries. And the approach has been found useful. Useful, that is, for those disorders whose management is clear-cut, whose control can be adequately and objectively monitored, and whose requirement for a medical professional opinion can be easily and speedily identified (Cross, 1974; Komoroff et al., 1974). The most obvious application of this 'protocol technique' is in chronic disorders whose natural history and response to therapy is well established, but it is equally valid in acute diseases where similar objective management plans can be devised. Indeed, it has been shown that lay-assistants with minimum training can be right more often using such a protocol than doctors who are not using it (Essex, 1976).

NURSE-CONSULTATIONS

Success in these pastures has encouraged some doctors to experiment with nurse-consultation as an alternative to doctor-consultation in the primary care field. This has been found acceptable to patients and a useful adjunct to the practice (Cunningham, Bevan and Floyd, 1972; Lees and Anderson, 1971; Marsh, 1969; Smith and O'Donovan, 1970). However, when I tried this out I found that patients only sought the nurse's advice for things they would not have taken to a doctor anyway had the nurse not been available. It is questionable whether the nurse's intervention in this setting actually reduces workload. Nonetheless the Royal College of General Practitioners (1968) has confidently asserted that 27 per cent of the doctor's time could be saved by the nurse undertaking additional duties.

BURLINGTON TRIAL

The Burlington Trial of the nurse-practitioner is the most significant experiment in this field. In this, patients could choose whether to see a nurse or a doctor on their first visit, and a good proportion did in fact choose the nurse. Only 40 per cent of the nurse's work then had to involve a doctor at all (Spitzer *et al.*, 1974). But even here it is not clear that the conditions referred to the nurse *would* have been presented to the doctor. People learn of new procedures and services very quickly; they soon become attuned to higher levels of expectation.

THE NURSE AND HOME VISITS

The same argument can apply to home visits, though here the nurse has a most obvious role to play. Nurses are very competent at assessing sick people from the point of view of deciding whether medical aid is needed. So, it might be expected that nurses are very good at screening first home visits. Experience supports the expectation, and it has been estimated that only a tenth of nurse-visits need be followed up by a doctor (Smith and Mottram, 1967). This is a consistent finding (Carey-Smith, Dreaper and Robinson, 1972; Moore *et al.*, 1973; Nisbet, 1977; Wallace, 1973) which should not surprise us if we recognize that the commonest reason for requesting a home visit is not the illness itself but the anxiety that this engenders (Williamson, 1980).

PSYCHOSOCIAL MATTERS

Nurses can be very good in dealing with anxiety, but so too can others. The staggering increase in the use of initially professional but latterly lay-counsellors is one of the major innovations of modern general practice. The recognition that many anxiety states are related to social, and occasionally psychological, states within the understanding and succour of lay-people is undeniably one of the greatest breakthroughs in medical practice. It is no longer considered that only a doctor can help a patient who presents with a physical symptom regardless of aetiology, and that is both a considerable boon in workload terms and a restraint on the more enthusiastic doctors who insist on a hot-pursuit approach to their work. Medical practice is increasingly viewed as *medical*, non-medical considerations being regarded as the purview of others even if the doctor can, or wants to, be involved.

The fundamental of counselling is that the patient is being helped to be more self-sufficient – to be more able to cope with life. Today we recognize that fellow-travellers have just as much to offer as professionals or volunteer helpers. A major phenomenon of the past decade has been the rise of the self-help group (Robinson, 1979; Williamson and Danaher, 1980). Where self-help groups exist the doctor has a supremely effective tool for helping some of the more intransigent cases on his books. But what self-help exists determines what benefits accrue.

Most communities boast an Alcoholics Anonymous, an AlAnon, a Gingerbread Group and an Age Concern. Beyond that there is great variation. When I arrived in my present practice I found that that was it! So I set about establishing self-help groups for asthmatics, coronary patients, depressives, diabetics, epileptics, nephritics, mastectomates, psoriatics and mothers of handicapped children, to name but a few. It was fairly easy, though I had to be beware of the danger of becoming involved and therefore prime-mover and leader (Williamson, 1979). The groups have thrived and enable me to refer an increasing number of patients to them – not out of a desire to 'ditch' the more difficult patient, but in the sure knowledge that self-help groups educate him better than I could and influence me in a way that little else could.

REALITIES AND THE FUTURE

As the Director-General of WHO said (Mahler, 1975) it makes good social, economic and professional sense to take the choice of options as far down the professional tree as possible. It encourages a greater community involvement in health care. It encourages more realistic expectations of the doctor who ceases to be seen as the automatic arbiter of every ill. It is relatively cheap to use non-doctors to do the non-medical work. And it increases the doctor's job satisfaction to be reserved for tasks requiring his unique blend of knowledge, experience and skill.

The basic objection is that delegation is a threat to the doctor (Bowling, 1981). Many doctors fear that too much worksharing with lesser-trained personnel, or with untrained laymen, will seriously undermine their own prestige. There is a not altogether unjustified fear that if you remove the non-medical tasks from the doctor's workload it will be clear that there is considerable overmanning in general practice.

The counter-objections are more encouraging than this. First, it is by no means certain that the public's attitude to the medical profession as a whole is conducive either to good health or satisfactory medical care. There are many who argue quite the opposite (Abse, 1967; Bradshaw, 1978; Carlson, 1975; Illich, 1974; Mechanic, 1979; Williamson and Danaher, 1980). It is more than likely that more realistic perceptions and expectations of the doctor will bring tremendous benefits in terms of appropriate consultation, greater compliance, and more self-sufficiency in health and in illness.

It is equally questionable that ridding the doctor of inessential work will result in overmanning of the health service. All the available evidence suggests that only a minority of perceived symptoms are taken to a doctor (Last, 1963), while the commonest expressed reason for not consulting is that the doctor is too busy (Fitton and Acheson, 1979; Townsend and Wedderburn, 1965; Williamson and Danaher, 1980). By removing non-medical work the doctor can be fully utilized in practising medicine. The main result may be that there is simply less hidden illness in the community.

Finally, the suggestion that delegation will undermine the prestige of the medical profession fails when you look at fundamentals. Above all else, medical practice is based on judgement. While this is dependent on the doctor's knowledge it is heavily influenced by that intangible we call 'experience'. Only those tasks where the doctor's management is clear-cut can legitimately be delegated to lesser qualified workers. Thus, delegation is no threat to medical professionalism. On the contrary, the gains are too great to be lost by faintheartedness.

References

Abse, D. (1967). *Medicine on Trial*. (London: Aldus Books)

Bowling, A. (1981). Delegation to nurses in general practice. *J. R. Coll. Gen. Practit.*, **31,** 485–490

Bradshaw, J. (1978). *Doctors on Trial*. (London: Wildwood House)

Carey-Smith, K. A., Dreaper, R. E. and Robinson, N. A. (1972). Home visits – the patient's viewpoint. *J. R. Coll. Gen. Practit.*, **22,** 857–865

Carlson, R. (1975). *The End of Medicine*. (New York: John Wiley and Sons)

Cartwright, A. (1967). *Doctors and their Patients*. (London: Routledge and Kegan Paul)

Cross, H. D. (1974). The case for problem-orientated medical records. *Br. J. Hosp. Med.*, **11,** 65–68

Cunningham, D. J., Bevan, J. M. and Floyd, C. B. (1972). The role of the practice nurse from the patient's point of view. *Community Med.*, **128,** 534–538

Danaher, K. (1977). Research memorandum from the Guy's Self-Treatment Project.

Department of Health and Social Services (1974). *Health and Personal Social Services Statistics for England* (London: HMSO)

Essex, B. (1976). *Diagnostic Pathways in Clinical Medicine.* (Edinburgh: Churchill Livingstone)

Fitton, F. and Acheson, H. W. K. (1979). *Doctor-Patient Relationship: A Study in General Practice.* (London: HMSO)

Fry, J. (1978). The place of primary care. In Fry, J. (ed.) *Trends in General Practice 1977.* (London: Royal College of General Practitioners)

Hockey, L. (1972). *Use or Abuse – A Study of the State Enrolled Nurse in the Local Authority Nursing Services.* (London: Queen's Institute of District Nursing)

Illich, I. (1974). *Medical Nemesis.* (London: Calder and Boyars)

Komoroff, A. L., Black, W. L., Flatley, M., Knopp, R. H., Reiffen, B. and Sherman H. (1974). Protocols for physician assistants. *N. Engl. J. Med.*, **290,** 307–311

Last, J. M. (1963). The iceberg. *Lancet*, **2,** 28–30

Lees, R. E. M. and Anderson, R. M. A. (1971). Patient attitudes to the expanded role of the nurse in family practice. *Can. Med. Assoc. J.*, **105,** 1164–1168

Mahler, H. (1975). Health: a demystification of medical technology. *Lancet*, **2,** 829–832

Marsh, G. N. (1969). Visiting nurse – analysis of one year's work. *Br. Med. J.*, **4,** 42–44

Mechanic, D. (1979). *Future Issues in Health Care.* (New York: Free Press)

Moore, M. F., Barber, J. H., Robinson, E. T. and Taylor, T. R. (1973). First contact decisions in general practice – a comparison between a nurse and three general practitioners. *Lancet*, **1,** 817

Nisbet, E. (1977). Assessing the urgency of home visits. *Nursing Times*, September 22, 1427–1474

Robinson, D. (1979). *Self Help in Health.* (London: Martin Robertson)

Royal College of General Practitioners (1968). *The Practice Nurse.* Report from GP 16 (London: Royal College of General Practitioners)

Royal College of General Practitioners (1973). *Present State and Future Needs of General Practice. 3rd edn.* (London: Royal College of General Practitioners)

Smith, J. W. and Mottram, E. M. (1967). Extended use of nursing services in general practice. *Br. Med. J.*, **4,** 672–674

Smith, J. W. and O'Donovan, J. B. (1970). The practice nurse – a new look. *Br. Med. J.*, **4,** 673–677

Spitzer, W., Sackett, D. L., Sibley, J. C., Roberts, R. S., Kergin, D. J., Hackett, B. C. and Oylnich, A. (1974). The Burlington Trial of the nurse practitioner. *N. Engl. J. Med.*, **290,** 251–256

Townsend, P. and Wedderburn, D. (1965). *The Aged in the Welfare State.* (London: Bell and Sons)

Wallace, C. M. (1973). Assessment of the elderly by a district nursing sister attached to a group practice. *Health Bull.*, **31,** 258–267

Williamson, J. D. (1979). Self help and the doctor. In Hatch, S. (ed.) *Mutual Aid in Health and Social Services.* ARVAC Pamphlet no 1. (London: NCVO)

Williamson, J. D. (1980). *Patient-initiated home visits in general practice.* Unpublished thesis. London Faculty of Community Medicine

Williamson, J. D. and Danaher, K. (1980). *Self Care in Health.* (London: Croom Helm)

The case for delegation (2)
John Smith

INTRODUCTION

'Health for all by the year 2000' is the goal that has been set by Dr Hafdan Mahler, Director-General of the World Health Organization. Though this goal may sound utopian, it is a goal worth pursuing as ill-health is a costly burden to the patient, to the family, to the community and to the state. He has stated that half of the health care expenditure of the western world is still directed towards people who will be dead within the space of the next 12 months.

Governments realize that the major threat to world economic and therefore social stability is inflation. They are becoming increasingly aware of the anti-inflationary benefits of good primary health care on the one hand and the price paid for bad health care on the other. For economic reasons, if for no other, health care concepts have probably changed more in the last 30 years than in the previous 3000 years.

With rapidly rising costs without visible and meaningful improvements in services, there has been an inability of health services to meet patient wants and needs. This state of affairs has been attributed to financial restrictions. This is a comforting thought for it implies that the difficulties will largely disappear if funds can be provided.

Sir Harold Himsworth (1980), former secretary and deputy chairman of the British Medical Research Council, queried whether this was not a too simple solution to the problem. Shortage of funds may create problems for a service, but it does not create problems in it, merely aggravates those that are actually or potentially already there.

Today forward-looking planners are inverting the health care pyramid. No longer can the super-modern hospital occupy its traditional safe place at the top of the pyramid where it monopolizes most of the attention and most of the expenditure. The majority of health intervention should be undertaken at the most peripheral level of the service by health professionals most suitably trained for performing these tasks. That is to say that if a service is to be cost effective no one should perform a task which someone less qualified can carry out as competently and implicit in that statement is the assumption that there must be patient acceptance, professional acceptance and legal acceptance.

Health wants are infinite, resources finite. We must face economic realities and become good managers. Good management implies delegation of duties and optimal utilization of resources. Unless increasing workloads are delegated, standards must drop.

DELEGATION

Not only is the gap between ideal doctor-to-population ratio widening in developing countries, but in all countries we must face the realities of the maldistribution of doctors between rural and urban areas which cannot be resolved by simply training more doctors. The government of the United States has increased expenditure on health manpower programmes 10-fold in 10 years and in spite of this has not succeeded in persuading enough doctors to live in rural areas. Consequently, more emphasis must be given to roles of activity rather than staff categories. For health care to be effective it must reach a very high percentage of the population.

The obvious person to delegate work to is a nurse. The essence of a nurse's professional role is to care for people; the extension of this role occurs by delegation and it is important that the delegation is clearly defined as to what can be treated and by whom and what must be referred to a senior health professional.

Effective delegation depends on training before undertaking the job, training on the job and refresher courses. As David Morley (1973) has stressed in *Paediatric Priorities in the Developing World*, effective delegation is only possible with good communication and answering what are often the unspoken thoughts of the person undertaking the delegated work.

(1) Let us agree clearly what I am to do.
(2) Give me a real chance to do it.
(3) Give me knowledge of my progress.
(4) Give me help when I need it.
(5) Give me recognition when I have done it.

Good management (Cherrington, 1971) also involves planning, organizing, motivating or training for providing the service and finally evaluating that service.

PLANNING, ORGANIZING AND TRAINING

The catalyst which has sparked off successful organizations and services is that their strength has been built on simple principles which everyone can understand and world trends in successful health service systems have evolved along similar lines. The cornerstones of health are housing, nutrition, education and employment, with containment of population growth. On this foundation has been added the four levels of care.

The term 'primary care' was first used to describe the general practitioner level of care, but today this level includes any contact between patient and any primary health professional.

While it has become necessary to delegate work to other health professionals in order to provide maximum coverage of the population, so it has also become necessary to train lay people as 'health auxiliaries' on a paid or voluntary basis to work at the most peripheral level, that is the level of self-care. Such interested people, preferably chosen by the neighbourhood or community, should be trained in basic health matters, accident prevention, first aid and home nursing and this knowledge they should be able to pass on to their neighbourhood or community. They should be available to advise families where to seek help for their problems, and to be able to mobilize community resources to fill the gap between what the state can provide and what the community needs to improve the quality of life for its elderly, handicapped, chronically ill and less fortunate members. In this way the service through the extended role of these workers can have viable grass roots.

Traditionally health services have expanded from hospitals outwards with the result that hospital solutions have often been applied to community problems; also communities often do not understand nor contribute to resolving such problems. We must work *with* people and not only *for* people. At least half the health problems seen are either preventable or could be better managed if individuals were better informed. Patients must become active partners in the health team in regard to their own and their families' health. Health education plays a significant role in primary care.

SERVICE

The Cape Peninsula (South Africa) covers an area of approximately 40 km by 20 km and has a population of $1\frac{1}{2}$ million people. While there is not a unified health service, there is a comprehensive one. For the more affluent members of society and those covered by medical insurance primary care is provided by general practitioners on a fee-for-service basis. There is also a network of local authority preventive clinics available to all the people free of charge.

In 1969 the Day Hospitals Organization (Smith, 1981) was started in the Cape Peninsula to provide a primary health care service for the people in the lower income group not covered by medical insurance, who were attending the overcrowded outpatient departments of the general and teaching hospitals. These units equate more with community health centres than with specialized day hospitals. Today there are 18 such centres strategically placed in the communities. Our staff carry out over a million and a half consultations a year including 100 000 home visits, over 3000 same-day surgical operations and 5000 confinements. Our referral rate to specialist services is 2 per cent.

The primary health care teams which staff these centres consist of general practitioners, nursing personnel including district sisters, midwives, social workers, physiotherapists, radiographers and pharmacists, as well as a community paediatrician and obstetrician. There are full pathological facilities, with specimens being sent to a central laboratory.

In 1973 the first Midwifery Obstetric Unit (MOU) (Van C. de Groot, 1978) was opened. Previously low-risk deliveries were done on a domiciliary basis. At the antenatal clinics patients are placed into high-risk and low-risk categories. Those in the high-risk category are followed up and delivered in the specialist units at the teaching hospitals, while those in the low-risk category are followed up and delivered in the MOUs by midwives. Should abnormalities arise during or after labour the patient is either transferred to the specialist unit by ambulance or the obstetric flying squad is called. Normally mother and child stay at the MOU for a few hours after delivery and are then followed up at home.

In the obstetric field, booking and referral criteria (Van C. de Groot, Dommisse and Howland, 1981) can be grouped into the following categories:

(1) Booking criteria for hospital care and/or delivery
(2) Booking criteria for MOUs
(3) Referral criteria from MOU to hospital – antenatally
(4) Referral criteria from MOU to hospital – in labour
(5) Referral criteria from MOU to hospital – third stage and puerperium
(6) Referral criteria from MOU to hospital – for the neonate

Since 1973 Dr J. D. Ireland (Ireland and Power, 1979) of the Red Cross War Memorial Children's Hospital (RCWMCH) has been training Advanced Paediatric Clinical Nurses (APCN). The course consists of 6 months of lectures, clinical and tutorial training. The candidates are selected from applicants with adequate paediatric training, or with the paediatric nursing diploma. The standard expected at the examinations is that of a final-year medical student in the areas of paediatrics and child health. After having passed the examination they undergo a further 6 months 'internship'.

At our health centres the APC nurse takes full histories, examines and treats the patients. The prescriptions are written up by the doctor. The optimal number of patients that can be seen by the clinical nurse is 30 per day. It has been found that she consults the doctor on less than 20 per cent of cases. Not only is she involved with the presenting problem, but also in other aspects of comprehensive care often overlooked by the busy practitioner. This includes developmental screening, early detection of other handicaps, growth problems, checking vital senses, nutrition and immunization status, family planning and relevant social problems. Consequently the APC nurse relieves the doctor of much routine work, so that he can have more time for the major problems.

Since the APC nurse is a highly trained person and insufficient numbers can be trained a more basic and shorter course has been started and already our staff have been impressed with their competency in lightening the doctor's workload.

In the field of adult medicine our staff have trained nursing staff along similar lines. Subjects covered have been the common acute and chronic conditions seen at the health centres. These clinical nurses have been very effective in running the hypertensive, diabetic, asthmatic and obesity clinics amongst other duties. While health education should be a part of every consultation, these clinical nurses are ideally suited to inform patients about diets, medication and how changing lifestyles can improve their health.

Finally, delegation down to the community and family: unless we harness the energy and resources of voluntary organizations and communities we shall be unable to meet the WHO goal. Through community health liaison committees interested and active members of the community, representatives of voluntary organizations such as the Red Cross Society, the Child Life Society, Meals on Wheels and others meet the community health professionals. In addition the Red Cross Society has expanded its training programme to include basic health education and accident prevention and these health auxiliaries will be playing a significant role in the health scene in the 1980s.

EVALUATION

It has been stated that 10 per cent of any organization's time and money should be spent on evaluation. Evaluation of performance may lead to modification and improvement of the service provided. Only by evaluating a service can it become dynamic.

Today, the Cape Town Municipality has one of the lowest birthrates in South Africa, 21 per 1000 in 1979. Perinatal mortality at our MOUs has dropped from 30 per 1000 in 1975 to 13 per 1000 in 1979, a figure which excludes high-risk cases at initial booking. While at the Retreat

MOU, our first purpose-built unit, there was only one perinatal death of all cases delivered where fetal heart sounds were present on admission, a perinatal mortality rate of 0.75 per 1000. This confirmed once again the efficacy of our protocols.

Deaths from gastroenteritis are one of the most sensitive indices of health status. The drip-room statistics at the RCWMC hospital have dropped from 17 156 cases with 158 deaths in 1971 to 9367 cases with only six deaths in 1980; the infant mortality (white and coloured) in the Cape Town Municipality has dropped from 45 per 1000 in 1969 to 18 per 1000 in 1979.

SUMMARY

If we wish to have cost-effective 'health for all by 2000' the family practitioner must not only be a leader and coordinator of a health team, but also a good manager. We must place more emphasis on working with people and not only for people so that our patients become active partners with us in their own health.

The use of health teams and community involvement may well rival the more sensational technological advances in the next two decades by mobilizing communities at the grass roots and activating them in decision-making and self-care. If we take our patients' health more seriously, maybe we can persuade them to take their health more seriously too. Not only will we be providing more economical health care, we will also be providing more effective health care.

References

Cherrington, P. (1971). *Management and the Health Services.* p. 27. (Oxford: Pergamon Press)

Himsworth, H. (1980). On the integration of expert knowledge into the machinery of government. *Br. Med. J.*, **281,** 1197

Ireland, J. A. and Power, D. J. (1979). The paediatric primary care clinical nurse in South Africa. *Curationis*, **2,** 33

Morley, D. (1973). *Paediatric Priorities in the Developing World.* (Sevenoaks: Butterworths)

Smith, J. (1981). The day hospitals organization. *S. Afr. Med. J.*, **59,** 609

Van C. de Groot, H. A., Davey, D. A., Smith, J. A. *et al.* (1978). The midwife obstetric unit. *S. Afr. Med. J.*, **53,** 706

Van C. de Groot, H. A., Dommisse, J., Howland, R. C. (1981). Trends in obstetric practice at the University of Cape Town, 1967–1977. *S. Afr. Med. J.*, **59,** 824

The case for sharing
David Brooks

> To the leader of the team:
>   When in charge – PONDER
>   When in doubt – MUMBLE
>   When in trouble – DELEGATE!
>   *A. Bloch (1979)*

INTRODUCTION

A primary health care team is an interdependent group of general medical practitioners and secretaries and/or receptionists, health visitors, district nurses and midwives who share a common purpose and responsibility, each member clearly understanding his or her own function and those of the other members so that they all pool skills and knowledge to provide an effective primary care service.

Joint Working Group (1981)

The above definition of a 'core team' excludes the 'extended team' which could include social workers, clinical psychologists, occupational therapists, dieticians, community psychiatric and colostomy nurses, dentists and community medical officers. This list is rarely static and varies geographically and in time according to the needs of different communities.

Team work has much in common with groupwork (*Update*, 1979) and teams can function either coactively or interactively. An example of coactive team behaviour might be a hospital outpatient department with medical and surgical clinics taking place during the same afternoon. Members function quite independently, there is little need to coordinate their special tasks and they have independent learning needs. An example of interactive team behaviour might be a football team or an operating theatre team. Although each member has a different role each is dependent on the others. Part of their shared task is to coordinate their activities and they have common learning needs.

The verb '*to delegate*' is defined by *Chambers 20th Century Dictionary* as to entrust or commit a representative. Delegates require authority or a delegacy, and it might be argued that the doctor's authority to delegate could be founded in his longer training and in the fact that the team's patients register primarily with him.

'*Sharing*' is defined by the same dictionary as participating in or having in common. A primary health care team by definition shares a common purpose and responsibility; this chapter will explore and develop the nature of teamwork by outlining its historical development, discussing the primary health care needs of the community, examining the concepts of delegation, sharing and leadership, and finally by discussing the education of the team.

HISTORICAL DEVELOPMENT

Reedy (1977) describes the development of the team concept. In his view it was inevitable that with the rapid development in technical medicine in the 1950s and 1960s general practitioners would seek to shed 'lower status activities' and widen their spheres of influence and competence. During the same period and often as a direct consequence an increasing number of patients were cared for entirely or largely in the community, a process which continues to this very day.

Before the late 1950s the general practitioner services and the professional nursing services had pursued a policy of separate development. The general practitioners as independent contractors were responsible for employing their own staff whereas the nurses were employed by the local authority. It was comparatively rare for nurses and doctors working in the community to even see each other. Indeed the author entered practice in 1965 and recalls that it was several months before he was even aware of the existence of district nurses and even longer before he actually met one. If an appropriate task was identified by a doctor it could be delegated to a nurse by leaving a message at a local authority centre.

If the team concept was to become a reality it was clear that doctors and nurses would need to work together, and in the late 1950s the first experimental schemes were started in Hampshire and Oxford as a result of the initiative of the respective Medical Officers of Health. This involved the '*attachment*' of health visitors to general practice but by the early 1960s district nurses and midwives had also been included.

In 1963 the report of a subcommittee of the Standing Medical Advisory Committee of the Central Health Services Council (1963) recommended that 'Field workers such as the nurse, midwife and health visitor should be attached to individual practices'. In 1965, as a result of reorganization of services and remuneration general practitioners gained financial incentives to improve their premises, form group practices and employ adequate staff. This development catalysed both the attachment of local authority nursing staff and the direct employment of nursing staff (Figure 13.1). By 1966 an amendment in the terms of service of general practitioners allowed them to delegate appropriate work to nursing and lay

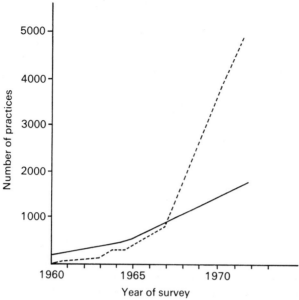

Figure 13.1 Association between nurses and doctors in general practice 1960-73. Practices starting attachment (– – – –) or employment (————) of nurses. Source: Reedy, Philips and Newell (1976)

staff in their own employment. The Standing Medical Advisory Committee (1971) issued a report on the organization of group practice which recommended that much of the medical work required by the community should be undertaken by a doctor supported by nurses and secretarial staff caring for a defined population. In 1972 the general practitioner's terms of service were extended further to allow him to delegate to nursing staff employed by the local authority. Indeed it can safely be claimed that attachment has now become the norm for local authority staff and many studies have been published describing the difficulties and problems that they have in working with doctors in primary health care teams (Beales, 1978; Gilmore, Bruce and Hunt, 1974).

THE PRIMARY CARE NEEDS OF THE COMMUNITY

Since the only possible reason for the existence of primary health care teams is to service the primary care needs of the community it might be helpful to consider those needs in more detail, as this process might shed some light on the proper functioning of teams and whether function might be aided by delegation or sharing.

Metcalfe (1979) has emphasized that primary medical care must embrace the changing needs of society. We are serving a rapidly changing society. There are population changes resulting in a shift towards an ageing society which will be particularly acute by the end of the century. Morbidity changes have characterized the last 50 years. Deaths from acute infectious disease have declined rapidly to be replaced in significance by the chronic degenerative diseases which have been so neglected at primary care level and which will demand so much more of our attention in the future. Society is changing its structure; not only has the nuclear family replaced the extended family with consequent neglect of the elderly but we have a changing mixture of ethnic groups. Politicoeconomic change has resulted in an era of high unemployment and dwindling financial resources. These problems have been particularly acute in the inner cities. The recent riots at Toxteth and Brixton in the United Kingdom provide startling and alarming evidence of this process and reopen the debate about the role of the primary care services in the inner cities. Perhaps most significant of all are the educational and attitudinal changes of recent decades. People know a great deal more about medical care and the movement for patient participation and self-care reflects the consumer-orientated age in which we live and the desire of many general practitioners to share care and provide a need-orientated service.

Metcalfe (1979) goes on to point out that hospital-based care is capital-intensive, labour-intensive and hierarchical. People working in this system have prescriptive skills, which means that they train to acquire certain skills and then provide a service to those whose needs happen to fit those skills. There is as a result fairly clear demarcation between the roles of different hospital-based specialists whether doctors or nurses. All this makes hospital care expensive, slow to change and relatively inflexible but none of this detracts from its role which is to find, define and correct pathophysiology in a referred population. Primary care, however, should have low capital costs, be lean on manpower and non-hierarchical, characteristics which make it more flexible and ready to adapt to change so that skills can be adapted to the changing needs of the population rather than to the interests of the examiners.

DELEGATED CARE OR SHARED CARE?

If the above model of a changing society is anywhere near correct and if the changing emphasis in health care from a demand-orientated system towards a need-orientated system and prevention is to become a reality, primary health care teams have got to work. No one discipline could embrace all that is involved in the delivery of primary care in terms of health maintenance, illness prevention, diagnosis and treatment.

At the present time primary health care teams have problems. The increasing numbers of directly employed practice nurses over a period when area health authority nurses were being attached to practices (Figure 13.1) reflects these problems as does the trend towards geographical rather than practice attachment of health visitors. Beales (1978) after a 5-year study of health centres and primary care pointed out that the failure of teams to develop effectively has to do not only with environmental and administrative difficulties but with the inadequacies of team members. In the first place some did not believe that full teamwork was necessary for patient care. Others saw it as a threat to their own status or professional standing. Others saw it as a means of increasing the number of people under their control. Where they function at all too many teams function in a coactive way, content to work with a few delegated tasks and minimal interdisciplinary contact.

The concept of delegation to nurses has a long and respectable history. Traditionally, nursing has always been a reactive rather than an initiating profession. Florence Nightingale in her book *Notes on Nursing* warned 'Let no woman suppose that obedience to the doctor is not absolutely essential'. Even today, at least away from centres where students are taught, many nurses have happily seen themselves as existing largely to carry out delegated tasks and functions that do not require the expertise of a doctor. This situation, which encourages coactive team behaviour, has been largely responsible for the failure of today's teams.

Bowling (1981) has shown that a significant minority of the doctors and nurses whom she studied were reluctant to have minor clinical tasks delegated and a majority did not think that nurses should carry out delegated diagnostic procedures. If teams are to meet the health care needs of a changing society (and today's young team members will be working to provide care well into the next century) it will mean new ideas of what it means to be a general practitioner, a district nurse or a health visitor. A shift from coactive to interactive team behaviour will aid this process. District nurses, health visitors, general practitioners and other team members must see themselves as providing health care to a registered practice population within the full limits of their skills as team members and in full consideration of the nation's economic resources. Before this ideal can be achieved there must be a change of emphasis away from delegation and towards sharing.

THE NATURE OF SHARED CARE

For many general practitioners the term 'shared care' is synonymous with the extended role of the primary care nurse. An increase in the capacity for independent decision-making is indeed one of many benefits which would flow from shared care but the term implies a great deal more than this. The concept of care involves independent decision-making not only in problem-solving but also in problem identification and interactive teamwork requires participation in the latter as well as the former process. Interactive teamwork requires that the health care needs of a practice population be analysed and broken down into health care objectives at practice level by nurses and doctors together as recommended by the Panel of Assessors for District Nurse Training (1978). This will ensure that changing needs within society are identified at practice level and that there is then motivation for changing ideas about what it means to be a general practitioner, a district nurse or a health visitor.

Those who would argue that such activities are beyond the skills of the nurse ignore the profound changes now taking place in nursing methods which could lead to a redefinition of the boundary between medicine and nursing (*British Medical Journal*, 1981). We have seen the introduction of the 'nursing process' into many teams and its development and usage is likely to have the same effect on nurses as the conceptual thinking involved in producing a job definition had on general practice. The nursing process involves four stages – assessment, planning, implementation and evaluation. Assessment is regarded as the key to good nursing care. It must include not only a medical history provided by the general practitioner (which may be good, bad, accurate or inaccurate) but must also include the nursing history which concentrates on the effects of the illness rather than on the disease itself. Many approaches to assessment have been developed but a comprehensive physical, mental and functional approach is the essence of any of them. It will include personal information, information on the present illness, experience of previous illnesses, personal lifestyle, social and interpersonal information, medical nursing and social care received before the current episode and the planned medical care for the present illness. Whatever system is used will involve self-recording by the patient and both structured and semi-structured interviewing techniques. Discrimination between what is important and relevant and what is not will allow actual and potential problems to emerge according to a hierarchy of needs. Assessment and diagnosis have much in common, and with the development of a job definition for a nurse which encourages an independent contribution to patient care, the nurse's role in the eyes of the patient could extend and merge to some extent with that of the doctor.

Interactive behaviour and the sharing of care will encourage the sharing of other things. The sharing of premises and the development of treatment rooms are already well advanced but sharing implies more than this. We have yet to see experiments extending this theme, such as nurse partnerships, although some practices do include the names of some team members on their letterheading.

The sharing of responsibility is an area which is confused at the present time, there being few legal precedents; new developments are likely. The report of the Joint Working Group (1981) points out that the general practitioner has a contractual responsibility to provide medical services to patients on his list, and that he is professionally responsible for the advice and treatment that he provides. His legal liability in the view of the committee is limited to those actions he performs himself or vicariously to those performed by the staff over whom he has some measure of control. He will have no direct liability in respect of actions performed by a nurse if these relate solely to nursing duties for which she has been properly trained and will have vicarious liability only in so far as the nurse is employed by him, or can otherwise be said to be under his control. Delegation therefore implies a greater legal obligation on the general practitioner than sharing.

Shared care and shared responsibility imply shared rewards. A sharing of status will automatically follow a shift from delegation to sharing and increased status will allow developments such as first contact appointment with nurses when patients themselves request this, and prescriptions issued by nurses for items used in their work. Increased responsibility and status deserve financial recognition and nurses involved in nurse partnerships, whether full time or salaried, would have a full professional role in a practice. Through their work they would make a significant contribution to the practice income and their share of the practice profits should reflect this.

SHARED CARE AND LEADERSHIP

The concept of shared care does not require leaderless teams. However, leadership of a primary health care team does not mean telling other professionals what to do or how to do it. Nor does team leadership necessarily equate with clinical responsibility for the patient. Leadership does imply a particular personal responsibility for the achievement of optimum team function.

Team leadership has much in common with small-group leadership and requires certain interpersonal skills. Team motivation, moral and coordination are important aspects of leadership, as is the ability to audit the work of the team and monitor patient care. It follows, therefore, as recommended in the report of the Joint Working Group (1981), that no attempt should be made to relate leadership automatically to any particular profession; rather each team should look at the abilities and skills of its members.

It should be noted that leadership of the team on the view of its members does not necessarily equate with leadership of the team on the view of the patient. On this view, purely because of his longer training and his professional relationship with the doctor, leadership is likely to be offered to the doctor. One marker of the progress of the team towards interactive behaviour is likely to be greater patient education about the roles of team members and the offering by the patient of leadership to other team members when problems identified seem to suggest this.

EDUCATION FOR SHARED CARE

If interactive teams are to become a reality sharing must commence with education for teamwork. It has been demonstrated (Brooks, Hendy and Parsonage, 1981) that when trainee general practitioners, student health visitors and student district nurses are brought together for a joint study day, attitudes inimical to the success of the primary health care team have already been acquired. Even before they have joined teams of their own student district nurses do not trust general practitioners and general practitioner trainees doubt the value of health visitors; many are unenthusiastic about the team concept.

Beales (1981) has concluded that producing an education programme that has much chance of success is going to be very difficult. He points out that many of the problems start at medical school because anything that cannot be translated into strictly medical terms is given very little teaching time. More emphasis needs to be placed at undergraduate level on the delivery of medical care.

In the author's view the evidence of the last couple of decades points overwhelmingly to the fact that delegation has failed. Indeed it had to fail. How could one discipline possibly assess needs lying within the expertise of several others? Even if such a paragon existed how could he or she persuade his nursing colleagues to accept a delegated role. Bowling (1981) interviewed a random sample of inservice primary care nurses and found significant opposition to delegation. One nurse said: 'Delegation may save the doctor's time but by implication the nurse's time is seen as less valuable. I think all this business of delegation is really pure pig headedness on the part of the doctor with only his time being saved.

There is no way we are going to be treated as equal health professionals with that attitude.'

The author and his nursing colleagues have brought together over 300 young doctors, nurses and health visitors over the past 4 years during training programmes for primary care, and we have learned that young nurses are too proud of their professional competence to be task-dependent on general practitioners.

The emphasis must now be on education for shared care. The teaching practice geared to provide care to a practice population should become the training base for at least core team members so that trainees of all disciplines have the opportunity to acquire positive attitudes together rather than negative attitudes in isolation. Release to appropriate on-going courses should be seen as a necessary part of each training programme. Only in this way can trainees and students identify common learning needs.

Perhaps the final argument should be left to Beales (1981):

A good teacher should surely teach his students humility, to recognize their own limitations and the necessity of working with other people with complementary skills and training. All too often those who teach are preoccupied with their own professional standing and the identity of their own professional group and passing that concern to their students. They cannot teach humility if they have none themselves. In fact individuals often acquire during their training programmes negative stereotypes of the people they should be learning to work with and see them as outsiders or even enemies. This is no less insidious when conveyed in traditional lecturer's jokes. Somehow somebody has to reach an approach that looks at all the patient's needs and then say what can't I do for this patient? What can other people do?

References

Beales G. (1978). *Sick Health Centres – and How to Make Them Better*. (Tunbridge Wells: Pitman)

Beales, G. (1981). *Education for Co-operation in Health and Social Work*. RCGP Occasional Paper No. 14, p. 5. (London: Royal College of General Practitioners)

Bloch, A. (1979). *Murphy's Law and Other Reasons Why Things go Wrong*. (London: Magnum Books)

Bowling, A. (1981). Delegation to nurses in general practice. *J. R. Coll. Gen. Practit.*, **31,** 485

British Medical Journal (1981). Leading article. Doctors and nurses. *Br. Med. J.*, **283,** 683

Brooks, D., Hendy, A. and Parsonage, A. (1981). Towards the reality of the primary care team: an educational approach. *J. R. Coll. Gen. Practit.*, **31,** 491

Gilmore, M., Bruce, N. and Hunt M. (1974). *The Work of the Nursing Team in General Practice*. (London: Council for the Education and Training of Health Visitors)

Joint Working Group (1981). *The Primary Health Care Team. Report of the Standing Medical Advisory Committee and the Standing Nursing and Midwifery Advisory Committee*. (London: HMSO)

Metcalfe, D. (1979). *Education for Co-operation in Health and Social Work*. RCGP Occasional Paper No. 14, p. 11. (London: Royal College of General Practitioners)

Panel of Assessors for District Nurse Training (1978). *Curriculum in District Nurse Training for State Registered Nurses and Registered Nurses*. (London: PADNT)

Reedy, B. L. E. C. (1977). The health team. In Fry, J. (ed.) *Trends in General Practice*. p. 111. (London: Royal College of General Practitioners and *British Medical Journal*)

Reedy, B. L. E. C., Philips, P. R. and Newell, D. J. (1976). Nurses and nursing in primary medical care in England. *Br. Med. J.*, **2**, 1304

Standing Medical Advisory Committee (1963). *The Fieldwork of the Family Doctor. Report of the Subcommittee, Central Health Services Council* (London: HMSO)

Standing Medical Advisory Committee (1971). *The Organisation of Group Practice. Report of Subcommittee DHSS/Welsh Office*. (London: HMSO)

Update (1979). Leading article. The primary health care team. *Update*, **19**, 505

Commentary

Achievement of 'health for all by the year 2000' depends more on good generalist primary health care than on specialist care at district general hospitals. Good primary health care depends on teamwork and on defining and accepting roles and duties. But interprofessional sensitivities cause difficulties and must be resolved to make best use of resources.

'Sharing' and 'delegation' complicate and hinder our endeavours to better primary health care teamwork. Their problems have to be spelt out and resolved if we are to improve. *Delegation* implies the family practitioner as the team leader who also has to function as the co-ordinator, manipulator, manager and delegator. It also implies vertical up-and-down relationships amongst non-equals. *Sharing* implies lateral–horizontal relationships amongst equals.

Who does what?

Sharing and delegation both have to accept the many others involved in the primary health care team: individuals and families with responsibilities for self-care; non-professional lay-workers who can be stimulated and trained for local tasks in health promotion and disease prevention. Such workers have roles in developed as well as in developing societies. Disease-centred groups of victims and their families offer great scope for collaborative care within the community.

There is need for new breeds of primary nurses, health visitors and social workers who, based in primary care health centres, can undertake more extensive and intensive work. There is also need for a new breed of family physician who is ready and willing to work more closely in sharing care and in accepting delegation as well as giving it.

In order to achieve such better care be it through delegation, sharing or both there has to be training for all involved in how best to do it.

14 Patient participation – more or less?

The issues

The relationships between patients and doctors have changed and are changing. There are more demands from patients to be better informed about their own problems, about the nature, risks and outcomes of medical/surgical procedures, and more involved in their own care, particularly in long-term disorders, and in the organization and delivery of health care services.

The medical profession feels uneasy and threatened if it loses its distinct mystical, magisterial and dictatorial roles. It is anxious over the increasing volume and expense of medical complaints, litigation and costs of insurance against such actions.

The issues here are:

For *each practitioner*: How much information and explanation to give at each consultation? How much patient-participation to allow and encourage?

For *each practice*: How much patient involvement should there be in the practice organization? How to obtain and act on patients' wants? Whether the patients' groups or committees should be encouraged?

For *all*: What are the real *benefits* of more patient participation? What are the *hazards* of more patient participation?

The case for less patient participation (1)
Alfred O. Berg

INTRODUCTION

Increasing the quality and quantity of patient participation in medical practice is rapidly becoming one of those primary care icons in which the negative view, if voiced at all, is indignantly shouted down as yet another proof of medical paternalism. In this respect the situation is not unlike that surrounding other issues in primary care medicine, such as continuity and comprehensiveness, in which the energy expended in advocacy seems inversely related to the quality of evidence available.

I shall state the case *against* increasing patient participation in medical practice, pointing out the inevitability of limits on the participation of patients in medical decisions, and the hazards to both doctor and patient if the limits are breached. After a brief overview and discussion of current trends, I shall examine in some detail the lines of evidence which have led me to conclude that patients and physicians should retain their unique roles in medical decisions.

SEEING THE ISSUE IN PERSPECTIVE

Participation of patients in medical decisions is best viewed against the rich tapestry of the patient–physician relationship more generally. I shall weave my backdrop by examining two topics: the social role of physicians, and the patient–physician relationship.

The very fact that our dictionaries divide us into two classes of people, patients and physicians, evidences the important social role of each. Our modern view of these roles, however, is heavily filtered by current practice of high technology scientific medicine. We have increasingly viewed the physician as a technician who somewhat impersonally plugs the patient into the appropriate health-dispensing technology. A little thoughtful reflection, of course, warrants that patients visit physicians for many reasons, only one of which is hope for cure of disease. Indeed, some patients seek physicians who will certify them as ill so that the patient may legitimately assume the sick role, relieved of responsibilities reserved for the healthy. Thus the social role of the physician is that of the healer and certifier of ill-health, historical roles for which current scientific medicine has changed only the technique. Modern physicians would do well to ponder whether, if all of scientific medicine were swept away, we could still successfully play the role as did our professional ancestors.

What of the patient–physician relationship? Cure has not been its only goal, and technical skills have not been its only currency:

> Some patients, though conscious that their condition is perilous, recover their health simply through their contentment with the goodness of the physician.   *Hippocrates*

It is our duty to remember at all times that medicine is not only a

science, but also the art of letting your own individuality interact with
the individuality of the patient.   *Albert Schweitzer*
One of the essential qualities of the clinician is interest in humanity,
for the secret of the cure of the patient is in caring for the patient.

Francis Peabody

He had surrendered all reality, all dread and fear, to the doctor beside
him, as people do.   *William Faulkner*

I conclude that the social role of physicians and the patient–physician
relationship both involve a timeless dimension. Societies sanction roles,
patients approach physicians with complex expectations, and the
patient–physician encounter has a complex relationship to the eventual
outcome.

Current trends toward increasing patient participation in medical
decisions imply a changing perception, both of the physician's role and
of the patient–physician interaction. Increasingly, the physician is seen
as a technician dispensing expert but impersonal prescriptions, while the
patient–physician interaction is seen as a business transaction with predictable outcome given a precise presentation of symptoms, signs, and
laboratory results. Viewed against these trends, more patient participation seems sensible, much as does the consumer movement in advocating
more participation in product quality, safety, and service. As I will
discuss more fully below, these views ignore traditional social roles and
minimize the obvious complexity of the patient–physician relationship.

PROBLEMS IN INCREASING PATIENT PARTICIPATION

My concerns about increasing patient participation in medical practice
are philosophical (see above), and, if practical, theoretical, since no one
seems to have done a randomized controlled clinical trial to settle the
issue. I will divide my comments into four sections, the 'it' in each case
referring to increasing patient participation in medical decisions: (1)
Does anybody want it? (2) Can it be done? (3) Are there hazards in doing
it? and (4) Would it work?

Does anybody want it?

Not wishing to appear unenlightened, I frequently ask my patients which
of several diagnostic or therapeutic options they might prefer. The (so
far) unvarying response has been something to the effect of 'You're the
doctor, whatever you think best'. Undaunted, I then launch into further

erudite explanations of reasons for and against each option, watching as I do so my patient's smile fade and eyes slowly glaze. This has now happened with sufficient predictability that I am given to wonder who it is that really wants to have patients participate more in medical decisions. I do not believe it is the majority of patients. Even in the most dire and extreme circumstances, patients seem willing, if not eager, to have the physician decide using his best judgement. Further, the rare patient who wants to actively participate makes the tacit assumption that options are determined by the physician, and that if the decision actually made a difference, the physician would limit options to those medically acceptable.

I am also not impressed that physicians would like more patient participation. If anything, most physicians I know are indifferent, willing to humour the patient if indicated by stating the options, but in most cases comfortable in making the decision with patient concurrence.

If not most patients and physicians, who then wants patients to participate more? I, at least, suspect a small but vocal group of social critics. The secretive, arrogant, and patronizing physician has been caricatured by authors, playwrights, and others throughout history, and the tradition remains a rich source of social critique today. That physician stereotype, although undoubtedly present in some irreducible quantity, has never been the norm except in the wishful thinking of those polemicists eager to pull down the whole house of medicine. Of course, like all good satire, such critique has elements of truth which we should heed (try Molière's *The Apothecary*). It does not, however, obligate wholesale changes in the structure of the medical profession and the patient-physician interaction.

Can it be done?

Quite apart from any philosophical problems with the concept, increasing patient participation in medical practice raises formidable questions about its practicability. Here I believe there are at least two major issues. The first is whether most patients are capable of learning the complexity and subtlety of medical information to participate effectively. The second is whether the cost of full patient participation is a reasonable one for a society to bear.

Patient participation in medical practice raises issues similar to those in informed consent for treatment and research. Can any patient fully comprehend the significance of one diagnostic or therapeutic option over another? For complex decisions (such as coronary artery bypass surgery), full comprehension would require a lengthy didactic curriculum. Aside from the obvious objections about adult learning capacity in stressful situations (the patient education literature is not encouraging), the sheer volume of material to be assimilated surrounding a given decision would quickly change our health care institutions into educational ones.

The costs of implementing a patient participation policy have not been addressed. Current health professionals certainly do not have the time to spend in preparing patients for each participatory decision. What society can afford to train and employ the personnel necessary? A serious effort to bring all patients to the necessary level of sophistication could expend enormous resources, resources which in today's economic climate would need to be extracted from other important programmes. Costs of longer physician visits and hospitalizations would be further reflected in lost productivity of patients, another economic burden which a society would absorb. The point here is simply that the costs would be high and the benefits unknown. Even if small improvements in patient satisfaction and medical outcome could be demonstrated, would they be worth the expense?

Are there hazards in doing it?

Increasing patient participation in medical practice may have negative consequences beyond the economic ones mentioned above. Raising the overall level of medical sophistication of a society may, paradoxically, have untoward effects on overall health. Current medical professionals, presumably on the higher rung of medical sophistication, do not have the highest levels of health. In fact, they are rather worse than average for such common problems as alcohol and drug use and suicide, and no better than average for heart disease and cancers. Further, the consequences of applying limited knowledge gained by a patient in a given interaction to general problems encountered at a later time are unknown. Experience suggests caution here.

Would it work?

Increasing patient participation in medical structure would fundamentally alter medical practice. Throughout history, the role of the healer has included the possession of expert, at times mystical, information and skill in dealing with health problems. In visiting a physician, patients have approached the encounter with the view of the healer as in possession of special powers. The interaction between physician and patient exploits these expectations to achieve a positive outcome. Call it the placebo effect, the doctor as therapy, or what you will, the effect on outcome is real. Changing the balance so as to maximize patient participation and minimize such placebo effects stands the substantial risk of destroying the relationship altogether. Given the historical record, one might well expect that patients would seek out some other individual to fill the role of healer. The answer, then to 'Will it work?' is likely to be 'No'. Full patient participation in medical practice flies in the face of observed patterns in health-seeking behaviour.

SUMMARY

Increasing the level of patient participation in medical practice is a modern-day primary care icon in need of closer examination. The concept is ill-defined, and the need for it undemonstrated. Its implementation is a new technology inadequately studied, with the potential for a variety of untoward effects. Its likely cost far outweighs reasonably predicted benefit. Finally, its implementation would blunt one of the physician's most powerful interventions – himself.

The case for less patient participation (2)
Patrick Kerrigan

The advocates of involving the patient more and more in his own medical care have become increasingly vociferous in the past decade. It is not enough for doctors to encourage their patients to take a more active role in managing their own illnesses, which is a laudable concept; there is now a move to encourage patients to take a greater part in the management of other peoples' illnesses.

As medicine has advanced in the past 20 years there has been an increasing awareness by general practitioners that there were certain areas of primary care in which they could effect a 'cure', certain areas in which they could still do very little, and large portions in which with their recently acquired knowledge they could modify and affect their patients' lives. Unfortunately these simple statements are not appreciated by the general public who have been hoodwinked by the media into believing that every complaint except death has a cure, and even death should be postponed.

Against this background there is an increasing need for health education and involvement of the patient in the management of his own illness, whether it be self-limiting or modifying the effects of a chronic long-term pathological process. At every consultation the general practitioner needs to actively seek out the cooperation of his patient if his advice is to be effective. Some doctors carry this cooperation a stage further and feel the need to set up a formal patient participation group.

In the past 10 years about 30 patient participation groups have been set up and continue to function within Great Britain. For them to succeed it has been shown that a general practitioner needs to be the instigator of such a group, and they are not successful if the doctors in the practice are unsympathetic towards their aims. The only common factor linking these groups is that they all hold meetings but the majority take as their role that of a 'troubleshooter' in dealing with the difficulties of practice organization which concern patients; several involve themselves in voluntary work to help patients who have difficulty in getting to the surgery, and a great proportion see themselves as performing some form of community health education.

PRACTICE GROUPS

I will now describe five such groups which are probably representative of others throughout the country, bearing in mind that they all appear to have slightly different aims and objectives.

One practice in Wales has a practice list size of 10 000 patients and declares that its sole aim is 'to build up a close relationship between doctor and patient. Medically there is already a close relationship but we are trying to increase this.' They have a committee of 26 members with an average attendance of 22 at meetings and an annual general meeting with about 75 patients attending. They appear to be covertly political – but not on party lines – and see themselves as a pressure group to produce changes in the working conditions in collieries and factories and so modify the effect of industrial disease on the health of the community.

In a practice in the West Country a list of 8000 patients, with three male doctors and a part-time female doctor (appointed at the request of the association) have a committee of twelve patients and an average attendance of 20–30 at evening meetings. Few of the staff who work in the building ever attend one of these meetings, the reason postulated being that it 'encroaches on an already full schedule'.

In a three-man practice in the Midlands with 7000 patients a group was started consisting of nine founder members who are now down to seven. They stress their health education role but 'seek eventually to monitor the operation of the health centre and ... move into the area of review and audit'. Perceptively they make the point that the practice 'does not really need patient participation because the doctors are already keen to develop and improve their services and provide monitoring and screening systems'.

Nearer London a practice has an association which meets three times a year, concerns itself with health education and the implications of 'training' in the practice. They have posed two questions: (1) How representative can such a group be? (2) Although there might be greater sympathy between the 'representing' patients and the doctors, how far does this communion spread?

Finally, a smaller practice of 5000 patients who live mainly in high-rise flats and middle-class housing has a committee of eight, mainly young professional people and attracts an audience of between 12–50 at their monthly health education meetings.

THE PRACTITIONER'S RESPONSES

What is the typical response of the British general practitioner to the suggestion of such a group? 'No way – you only get neurotics and the practice pains in the anatomy.' 'Patients' committees are full of non-representative local worthies who are even more reactionary than the doctors.' 'Ambivalent – they might want me to do Saturday evening surgeries or they might rise up and destroy the creator of the practice!'

These responses are seen by many general practitioners to touch on the real issues which lie at the heart of professional practice, in other words accountability, responsibility, freedom of practice, and control over one's professional life. The desire to maintain independence from outside interference has always been fiercely defended in the National Health Service and is at the heart of many a bout of political infighting.

The advocates of such associations see themselves in a different light. They feel they should be accountable to their patients, and because they are not feel a sense of guilt; they do not think these groups pose a threat to their clinical independence. Because society is changing, the community is now made up of a competent core with an incompetent periphery; in this periphery lie our major social problems with housing and unemployment of overriding importance and this modifies the presentation of illness to the practitioner. Patient associations may well be aimed at helping the incompetent periphery but by definition they will be run by those belonging to the competent core.

WHY LESS PATIENT PARTICIPATION?

Why then do I advocate less patient participation? My main objection is the waste of time and effort and the misdirected energy that is freely given by the doctor to an unrepresentative group of middle-class, articulate patients who are well able to resolve their own problems and who by their excess of missionary zeal alienate those very patients in greater need.

Study of the various practices shows that somewhat less than 1 per cent of patients are involved in any of the decision-making or are influenced by the health education programme. The laudable aims of delivering prescriptions to those who cannot reach the surgery, by one group, may have an inverse effect. Those who normally cannot reach the doctor's premises might have to make the effort to persuade a relative or friend to take them – a therapeutic excursion in itself. Some groups ferry patients to and from the surgery – surveys in the past see this as being of little value to the health of the community.

These patient associations may well develop into political pressure groups identifying with some local cause. The doctor may feel that parish pump politics can be discussed in the pub and the waiting room but should not intrude into the consulting suite.

As one patient participation group pointed out, those practices which least need a patient association are the very ones to follow this concept. When one studies those doctors who are advocates of patient involvement one will surely find that they *are* the ones who are already studying the dynamics of their surgery organization, the facilities that they offer and the standard of care produced. To devote time in the evenings or at the weekend to reach a small minority of people to assuage part of the guilt that general practitioners feel (am I doing *enough* for my patients?) seems to smack of an adolescent identity crisis. There must surely be a more time and cost-effective method?

I liken patient participation groups to parent–teacher associations. In theory they are a fine concept but in practice they either tend to be a social fund-raising machine, which helps to keep our rates down when they provide a swimming pool, or they demean professional standards by coming into classrooms as unqualified peripatetic pupil teachers (and, dare one say, on occasions they are semiliterate themselves). Their danger is that they become the tail-waggers of the dog instead of the head. Parent-teacher associations are also organized and run by a select band of enthusiasts. I wonder whether these people are 'failed' teachers, and likewise those in patient associations are harbouring repressed childhood desires to play at doctors and nurses?

One practice left a suggestion box in a prominent position in the waiting room. Over the course of 6 years there were two simple suggestions which were easily implemented. That box was impersonal but it did accurately reflect the practice population's interest in the running of the surgery.

The area where greater patient involvement is required is in health education. Monthly meetings of thirty 'regulars' does not seem to show a good return on the doctors' time. The Health Education Council have the resources to mount effective national campaigns with possibly the community health councils providing local facilities. National associations concerned with chronic illnesses such as diabetes and epilepsy have local organizations which could work more closely with general practitioners and provide a far more efficient base for the dissemination of knowledge.

The topics raised by patient participation groups concerning the surgery fall mainly into five categories: structural problems, staffing, organization, services provided, practice policy. They see themselves as a planning tool, a safety valve for the minor irritations of day-to-day life, a means of giving additional social support in the community, in short the eyes and ears of the practice. A group of concerned and interested general practitioners with all the facilities now available to the primary care team do not need yet another group to liaise with and be presented with yet another committee to sit on.

How can doctors and patients be convinced of their usefulness? How can they be made to work? Are they effective? Nobody has as yet been able to answer these three questions and until they do I would suggest less patient participation in family medicine.

The case for more patient participation (1)
Peter Pritchard

I did not get involved in patient participation from lofty ideals nor academic theorizing. I and my partner had lately moved to a new health centre, and we were worried that the pace of change might be too rapid for some of our patients.

General practice is altering all the time, as is the population served by each practice. Doctors and staff have to provide their service against the background of a rapidly changing society. When, in addition, we make deliberate innovations in the way we work – such as delegation to nursing staff, and preventive care – then we may be in trouble.

WHY DID WE START A PATIENT GROUP?

It was in this anxious state that we found ourselves in 1972. Our response to it was to ask a group of our patients such questions as: Are we producing the service you want? Do you understand our emphasis on prevention, and agree with it? Can you help *us*?

We had been encouraged to question our function in society by such publications as Ann Cartwright's (1967) *Patients and Their Doctors*. The climate of opinion at the time favoured the consumer viewpoint in health care, though community health councils had not yet been set up. It was not surprising that two other practices had the same idea quite independently of each other at about the same time (Aberdare, South Wales; and Whiteladies, Bristol).

HOW DID WE GO ABOUT IT?

We had no model to work on. Two alternative strategies suggested themselves: (1) to build up a representative consumer group specifically for the health centre; and (2) to use existing groups and networks in the community. Because of the difficulties inherent in the first, we chose the second strategy. We wrote to every group, club or organization which we could identify in the seven rural parishes served by the practice. These included: parish councils; women's institutes; clubs of all kinds (youth, older people, country wives, young farmers, etc.); voluntary surgery–car groups; single-parent groups, etc.

It was hoped in this way that a much larger section of the community could be reached by using existing organizations many of which had an electoral base (such as parish councils) or a large and active membership (such as women's institutes). Both these organizations have shown an interest in the way health care is provided. We were fortunate in getting a brisk response. Meetings held three or four times a year have been well attended and lively.

Before the first meeting I asked a friendly psychiatrist who was an expert in group dynamics what pitfalls lay ahead. He suggested three:

(1) That if I took the chair at the first meeting I would be stuck with it.
(2) That the group would want to raise money instantly.
(3) That it could easily become a cosy therapeutic group.

He was wrong over chairmanship. A lay chairman was elected to take over the second meeting, and this arrangement has continued.

He was right about raising money! We resisted the temptation, as we thought it would distort the way the group functioned, and divert a lot of energy.

I hope he will be proved wrong in his third prophecy. Patients tend to be too kind to their doctors, and need to be encouraged to suggest improvements – let alone criticize or complain, which they do rarely. My belief is that the group would not have kept its vitality over 9 years if it was only a mutual admiration society.

WHAT PURPOSE HAS IT SERVED?

Our early objective (apart from relieving our anxiety) was to obtain feedback from patients about the service being given, in order to check on how we were doing, and to aid future planning. This was amply achieved. Many suggestions for improvement have been made and implemented. For example, a postnatal support group, and window-cards for isolated people needing help were provided, on their suggestion and with their help. Sometimes they could succeed where we had failed – for example in getting an adequate chiropody service provided by the health authority.

There were many practical ways in which the group helped the doctors – in providing a voluntary car-service from the outlying villages to the health centre, in delivering prescribed medicines, in wording of questionnaires inviting women patients to come for cervical screening.

In many ways they helped the doctors and staff to decide what was appropriate and acceptable – to help them to keep a balance between too much anxiety and too much confidence. One dilemma was the teaching of general practitioner trainees and medical students. Discussion was lively, and patients had very clear views about the extent to which teaching could be allowed to affect the privacy of consultations.

The group raised no objections to trainee general practitioners sitting in with the principal, or consulting on his own. He was accepted as one of the 'family' for his or her year's attachment (incidentally they preferred a female trainee in an all-male practice). They did not like the idea of ordinary consultations being videotaped for teaching, even with prior notice. They thought this would affect the quality of the doctor–patient relationship, which they regarded as a higher priority than teaching – important though it was. They agreed to come as 'simulated' patients.

At an early meeting of the group, the doctors and staff were asked to produce a booklet which patients could read while waiting to see the doctor, containing advice on how to keep well. This was provided as a joint staff effort, and has proved very popular.

It has been shown that health education is less effective if it does not take account of people's 'health beliefs' (King, 1982). A group of this kind helps doctors and staff to explore health beliefs and to decide what is appropriate. It also helps doctors to know how far they can push people to give up smoking. They had no objection to the doctor putting the case strongly if their reason for attendance was linked to smoking (such as a cough). They objected to a lecture on smoking if it came 'out of the blue'.

Information needs to flow between doctors (and their staff) and the community in both directions. It includes more than 'health education'. Doctors and staff learn more about the needs and aspirations of the people served. In rural areas the community can be identified more easily than in cities where many practices overlap. A patient groups helps the doctor to identify his community, and this can be a source of satisfaction to him. Though it is probably easier to start a group in the country, many patient groups are functioning successfully in inner cities.

Doctors who do not have a patient group often imagine they will be overwhelmed with complaints. This is not the case. It is even possible for the doctor to get a few grumbles off his chest, so that patients come to understand the very real difficulties involved in providing a sensitive and responsive service. From this sort of dialogue there arises a better level of understanding, and mutual esteem, and confidence.

ARE PATIENT PARTICIPATION GROUPS REPRESENTATIVE?

It is important that all the members of a practice should know about the group and have access to it. Some groups such as adolescents and the elderly-housebound are difficult to represent. Even elected bodies like parish councils cannot represent the views of all their electorate: however, every voter knows about them and can express his views if he feels strongly. It has always been a worry that patients might not know about our group, in spite of its mention in the handout to all new patients, and the display of the minutes in the waiting room. A recent drive was made by the group to inform every household of the existence and aims of the group, and the names of their local representatives. Suggestions, comments and complaints were invited: very few appeared, which suggests that people are either content or apathetic – or perhaps both. This apathy does not spread to members of the group whose enthusiasm is unabated.

EVERY GROUP IS DIFFERENT

So far I have mostly been giving my personal experiences of the Berins-field community participation group. But all groups have certain features in common, and there is a broad congruence of aims, often not formulated, but implied from the way they work and the topics they discuss. However, each group is unique in the way it does its work, and this is a reflection of the different populations served, the great variety of general practice, and the individual personalities of doctors and staff.

Once a group starts, it tends to adapt to local needs and circumstances. It is a listening post in the community, an action group, a vehicle for health education, an aid to planning, a safety valve, and many other things besides. Many new groups are starting up, now that word has got around about them. Very few have failed.

Critics are to be found mostly among those who have not experienced it, and are afraid of anything so new and threatening! Yet we started a group to meet the threat of change, and found that it was helpful to us.

PHILOSOPHICAL TRENDS IN HEALTH CARE

That consumers have a right to be consulted about their health has always been a cardinal principle of general practice. Illich (1976) has underlined the necessity to return the responsibility for health to the individual whose health it is. Patient participation meets both these desiderata.

The style of general practitioners' consultations has tended to become less authoritative and more in the nature of 'counselling'. It implies that the doctor listens to the patient, encourages him to suggest solutions, and helps him to implement them. Patient participation works on similar lines outside the consultation.

General practitioners are encouraged to audit their clinical work as well as their finances. Some prefer to call it 'performance review'. Should not doctors and staff review the performance of their organization in discovering and meeting health needs, as well as in health maintenance and the prevention of illness? How much better is it for doctors, staff and the community they serve to approach these issues together?

CONCLUSION

Has it been worthwhile in my practice in the last 9 years? Would I start a group now, if I had not done so earlier? My personal answer to both is an emphatic *yes*.

Should every practice have one? That is for each to think about and decide. But in my view every practice should benefit from such a group as it should benefit from any attempt to share knowledge and experience, to listen and to plan together.

References and further reading

Cartwright, A. (1967). Patients and their doctors. *A Study of General Practice.* (London: Routledge and Kegan Paul)

Illich, I. (1976). *Limits to Medicine. The Expropriation of Health.* (London: Marion Boyars)

King, J. (1982). Health beliefs in the consultation. In Pendleton, D. and Hasler, J. (eds.) *Essays on Doctor–Patient Communication.* (London: Academic Press.)

Pritchard, P. M. M. (ed.). (1981). *Patient Participation in General Practice. Occasional paper No. 17.* (London: Royal College of General Practitioners)
   (A collection of papers and references which is, to date, the only source booklet on this topic.)

Pritchard, P. M. M. (1975). Community participation in primary health care. *Br. Med. J.*, **3,** 583–4

The case for more patient participation (2)
G. J. Pistorius

Venturing into definitions is always dangerous, but the definition of 'patient participation' can be simplified by describing it as participation by the patient in the decision-making process regarding his own (or his fellow men's) problems and in the actual management of these problems.

The mere fact that the question of 'more' or 'less' patient participation arises is proof of the fact that such participation already exists. After all, the decision by a patient to consult a doctor is the first step in his participation in the process – without patient participation the whole medical care system as we know it would not have been possible. The only question is: taking it for granted that patient participation exists, must it be 'more' or 'less' for optimal results?

Two main reasons can be stated for more patient participation – economics and more effective medical care.

ECONOMIC ASPECTS

The 'insoluble equation' in health care (Fry, 1979) with

$$Wants > Needs > Resources$$

is universal and speaks for itself. Although insoluble, the problem can and should be alleviated by more patient participation. A well-informed and motivated patient will know which ailments to manage himself, and will not exert pressure for series of costly and sophisticated special investigations. *Self-care* is the first level of the medical care system, and the common diseases at this level are relatively minor and self-limiting or chronic and persistent (Fry, 1979). The more conditions that are managed at the self-care level, the fewer will proceed to the primary care level, which is the first level of professional care. Of those that do proceed to the primary care level, many could be managed on a more economical basis by means of more patient participation.

Taylor (1978) states:

> We are all anxious to achieve the best and most advanced medical care available. However, we are fast arriving at a point of no return, where the cost of medical technology and resources reach a level incompatible with other desirable necessities. Health care costs, which reach a third the amount of an unbalanced national budget, give cause for reflection. Yet, doctors or the general public have no answer or solution.... To reverse this trend is no easy matter. One very definite improvement which has been suggested is to bring the patient into the situation in making decisions as to just how much laboratory work or even hospitalizations are warranted. This is not meant to imply that the patient should become the doctor but that he should be made to realize that increasing the interval between such tests may incur only a minimal risk.

It is obvious that the patient will have to be correctly and fully informed in order to make his own decision. It is also obvious that the doctor will still have the final word where such an investigation is of life-or-death importance.

Often special investigations are being requested due to a lack of communication between the doctor and the patient. An illustrative case presented itself a few days ago:

A qualified nurse lost her first baby shortly after birth due to congenital polycystic kidneys. Her next baby was born perfectly normal, and was progressing very well – all parameters being well within normal limits. The baby was just $4\frac{1}{2}$ months old when the mother received a note from the paediatrician that an intravenous pyelogram examination (i.v.p.) had been arranged for the baby the next day.

The mother was shocked – was there anything wrong? Why this sudden examination? She did not think the i.v.p. was necessary at this stage, as the baby was clinically perfectly normal. The only reason she could think of was that the paediatrician had some valid clinical reason for requesting the i.v.p. It transpired that the paediatrician did not consider it necessary to have the i.v.p. done either – he had thought that the mother, being a registered nurse, was expecting him to do something at this stage.

Communication between the two parties solved the matter eventually. Had the mother been allowed to participate in the decision-making from the start, the whole problem would not have arisen. Had they not communicated in time, yet another unnecessary, expensive special investigation would have been performed, and the 'insoluble equation' would have become more 'insoluble'.

MORE EFFECTIVE MEDICAL CARE

The field of the family practitioner/primary care physician can be divided into four main areas:

(1) Clinical family practice
(2) Family medicine
(3) Community medicine
(4) Practice management.

The levels of care inherent to each of the first three areas are:

(1) Preventive care
(2) Promotive care
(3) Curative care
(4) Rehabilitative care.

Preventive care tries to maintain the present level of health by preventing the onset of a disease process. Promotive care attempts to raise the present level of health through the adoption of a better lifestyle. Should the level of health be lowered as the result of a disease process, then curative care tries to elevate it again to its previous level. In the event of certain functions being permanently damaged or lost, then rehabilitative care is necessary to boost the remaining facilities to their optimal level.

Patient participation is important in each of these areas and levels.

PREVENTIVE AND PROMOTIVE CARE

Fry (1979) divides the social factors that underlie social pathology into the following factors: *'macro'* (adequate food, clean water, efficient sewerage, good hearing, good communication services and appropriate clothing); and *'micro'* (safe environment, happy and sound family base, and healthy personal habits and hygiene). These factors cover to a large extent the areas of clinical family practice and, in particular, family medicine and community medicine.

He states that:

cigarette smoking, overeating, excessive alcohol consumption, lack of exercise, overweight, inadequate sleep and multiplicity of mini and maxi-stresses are all accepted factors leading to general ill-health and major diseases.... The dilemma is who should be responsible for avoiding these factors. Should it be the individual, the family, the medical profession or society in general? ... The answer surely must be that all these must be involved but that the ultimate responsibility must be with the individual, who must know and understand the risks of the factors, and must be helped, encouraged and included by the rest to comply with the rules of good and better health. In other words society has the major responsibilities of dealing with macro social factors, the individual and the family with the micro factors and the medical profession with both sets of factors.

It is thus quite clear that individuals, as well as the community, have to participate in total medical care. In the field of preventive and promotive care this participation centres mainly around the most important aspect of health education. Only one aspect – cancer – will be discussed.

More and better health education about cancer must lead to better patient participation, especially in the promotion of early detection, and of prevention by healthier living. The more informed the patient is, the better he will be able to cooperate in this important matter.

Misconceptions by the patient can hamper the efficiency of his participation. In a study by Spelman and Ley (1966) of laymen's knowledge of lung cancer it was found that although 91 per cent knew of the connection with smoking, 56 per cent the symptoms and 73 per cent the treatment, nearly a third thought that the condition was easily curable. This type of misconception can easily lead to more dependence on the doctors' involvement in the curative process and less self-participation in the preventive process.

During a workshop on doctor involvement in *Health Education about Cancer* (Turin, September 1979), Isele (1979) made the plea that the family doctor should instruct his patients about early signs of cancer and occupational or lifestyle hazards. In particular, he should tell people about the need to have a medical opinion if changes from normal bodily functioning appear. He must also stress that early cancer is curable, manage his own fear of cancer and understand psychological processes relevant to this problem.

Knowledge is power. If the patient has the knowledge, he has the power to use this knowledge. This principle is valid through the whole field of preventive and promotive medicine.

Doctor–patient or doctor–community communication is an absolute requisite for effective health education. Hill, Hefferman and Rice (1979) conclude that there is a need to improve communications between doctors and patients in the field of health education. Better communication will produce more knowledge, which will lead to more efficient patient participation. The plea is thus for the latter.

An informed patient can play an important and essential role in preventive care. 'It is no accident that the growing emphasis on self-care comes hand in hand with an increased interest in preventive medicine. An informed and responsible lay person can do a great deal to prevent disease and achieve positive health. Health workers are developing new strategies by which they can encourage good health practices' (Ferguson, 1980). This self-care goes even further – from the preventive to the promotive field. 'One such strategy is the teaching of wellness self-care. In the traditional medical model, health is defined in a negative way – as the absence of disease. The idea of good health as a positive quality – wellness – goes beyond preventing illness to living in a way that is experienced as more fulfilling and rewarding' (Ferguson, 1980).

In short, the main battleground in preventive and promotive care lies in the presymptomatic field – that is, in the patient's own environment before he even consults the doctor. It is therefore logical that this battle will only be won by more active patient participation.

CURATIVE CARE

The curative aspect will be discussed in relation to the consultation model: history, examination, assessment and management.

Patient participation must not only be looked at in a global sense, but also as a personal experience of the individual patient. Nowhere is it more relevant than in the subjective part of the consultation – the history-taking. At that stage, the first step in patient participation – the decision to consult the doctor – has already been taken.

These first few minutes of the consultation are the crucial moments where patient participation must be optimal. At this stage the patient speaks (participates) and the doctor listens. If the doctor interferes too soon, his whole process of hypothesis-formation will most probably be wrongly founded with catastrophical consequences to his whole plan of management – and therefore to himself and to the patient.

Case history

This is best illustrated by an actual case history described by Heffernan (1981):

> The doctor was really good at history-taking. When a patient complained about any symptom, such as pain, he immediately knew which further questions were necessary to clarify that specific symptom – duration, location, type, distribution, associated factors, etc. However, although he noted pages and pages of carefully elicited histories, he always had the feeling that he was missing out on something – that he did not really penetrate to the core of the problem.
>
> Then a friend suggested some active listening during the first five minutes of the consultation, with no interference in the patient's participation. He agreed to that because five minutes is not such a long time after all – it would be easy just to listen for that short period.
>
> The next patient arrived – a woman in her thirties.
>
> 'Doctor, I am suffering from headaches.'
>
> The five minutes have not passed yet – clarification of that headache will have to wait for a while.
>
> 'Yes. . . .'
>
> 'Doctor, it is not really a headache – it is more like a pain in the back of my neck.'
>
> One minute has passed.
>
> 'Yes. . . .'
>
> 'Doctor, it is not exactly a pain – it is more like a feeling of tenseness.'
>
> He glanced at his watch – five minutes seemed such a long time.
>
> 'Yes. . . .'
>
> 'I get this feeling especially at night. . . .'
>
> 'Yes. . . .'
>
> 'When it is bed-time.'

The doctor kept his promise. Three minutes have passed.
'Yes. . . .'
An undertone of empathy has crept in.
The patient burst out in tears.
'Doctor, please help me. I am as cold as a rock, and I hate myself for
   it. . . .!'

The message is clear. The patient was allowed to participate freely, and the very deep and personal problem came to the surface in 4 minutes. Had the doctor not granted her that opportunity for self-participation, and decided to go for the headache, she would have left his consulting room with an analgesic, a tranquilliser and a bigger problem than before.

Examinations

It is impossible for a doctor to be physically present every time a patient needs an examination. The frequency of such examinations is also a relative factor. A bridge must be built to overcome this problem – this bridge is patient participation by self-examination. Patients can be taught to palpate their breasts, measure blood pressure, test their urine or blood, to name a few self-examinations.

Once a woman has mastered the technique of breast self-examination (BSE), this method holds some advantages over sporadic physician examination of the breast. Greenwald *et al.* (1978) indicated that tumours found during routine self-examination averaged 6.1 mm smaller in diameter than those discovered accidentally, and they estimated that breast cancer mortality might be reduced by 18.8 per cent through regular self-examination.

Blood pressure monitoring

Compliance in long-term blood pressure control is a major problem. A Working Group of the National High Blood Pressure Education Programme in Bethesda, Maryland (1979) defined behaviours critical to hypertensive patients achieving therapeutic control and assuming active responsibility for their own care. They remark:

The difficulty of maintaining faithful adherence to drug regimens is the major current problem in prolonged control of BP. Successful ways to achieve adherence over a long period of time are not yet certain. If the task were to supply the patient with more information it would be relatively simple. Achieving and maintaining BP control, however, involve additions to and changes in behaviour for which knowledge alone is not sufficient. Patients must be motivated to adopt and maintain a long-term and possibly bothersome therapy.

They conclude that 'patients must also have the skills necessary to assume active responsibility for their therapy'. These skills do not only include tasks like renewing prescriptions before supply is exhausted and home measurement of blood pressure, but also of monitoring progress and rescheduling appointments when necessary.

Blood glucose monitoring

Technology has made home measuring of blood glucose levels possible. If it is impossible to stabilize and monitor diabetic patients in hospital without measuring blood glucose levels, it seems logical that patients would also manage themselves better if they were able to measure blood glucose during their ordinary life. Tattersall (1979) lists the advantages of this important aspect of patient participation as follows:

(1) That it gives information about the pattern of blood glucose fluctuations while patients are going about their ordinary life.
(2) It enables the physician to advise on changes of treatment, over the telephone if necessary, on the basis of solid information. It eliminates the need to admit the patient to hospital for stabilization.
(3) Patients are motivated and become more active partners in their management.

Asthma

As regards assessment, the patient's opinion should never be disregarded. Special note should be taken when an asthmatic patient makes any subjective statement regarding his own condition. It is of the greatest importance to the patient with chronic airways obstruction how breathless he feels and how fast he can walk. Williams and McGavin (1980) found that both these observations correlated with changes in vital capacity after steroids. It would seem reasonable to use a combination of these assessments to judge the response of patients with chronic airways obstruction to steroids. In their study, the forced expiratory volume (FEV_1), an objective and reproducible measure of the performance of larger airways on forced expiration, seemed to have less clinical relevance.

Clinical assessment by the physician of the severity of asthma is also less accurate than the patient's own subjective assessment. Shim and Williams (1980) confirmed the fact that experienced physicians are very inaccurate in the assessment of the severity of airways obstruction in patients with asthma. Experienced patients were far more accurate in assessing their own peak expiratory flow rate than were the physicians, and they were quite accurate in judging whether the obstruction was better, worse or the same from day to day. They feel that this ability of patients to assess the severity of asthma has not been fully exploited by clinicians, and may be quite useful in evaluating the clinical state and adjusting therapy, particularly in outpatients – clearly a plea for more patient participation.

Paediatrics and obstetrics

Another warning: Never disregard a mother's assessment of her child's condition. Although the child may appear clinically normal at the time of the examination, be on your guard when the mother insists that 'there is something wrong with the child'. In my own practice, the mother always proved to be right in the end.

Patients can also participate much more in the management of their problems. The introduction of an antenatal progress graph in my own practice led to a great improvement in the efficacy of management. Each patient was handed the chart at the first consultation, and brought it at every visit for all the relevant parameters to be plotted on the graph. She could thus actually see her mass gain, uterine enlargement and blood pressure reading – with considerable motivation to do something about it. At the time of delivery she brought the chart to the hospital, and I immediately had all relevant and important data concerning the whole antenatal period available. Both doctor and patient gained a lot through this example of more patient participation.

Obstetrics in itself is another field where more patient participation should be allowed. I do not plea for patient interference in a doctor's sound clinical judgement, but is that judgement, in fact, always 'clinical' and 'sound'? How many inductions have been done because it suits the doctor, but does it always suit the patient – or the baby, for that matter? Obstetrical analgesia is often forced on a patient against her will. More than once patients have complained to me that they did not really experience the birth of their child in its fullest sense because of a spinal or other analgesic which they did not request. The doctor had never bothered to ask them their opinion.

Sexual problems

Management of interpersonal, family and sexual problems is impossible without intensive patient participation. In these cases the real problem is never the aloofness, or the frigidity, or the impotence, but the relationship. A relationship, by definition must consist of more than one element – in this case, human beings, patients. A third party – the doctor – can only advise; the solution is only attained through 'homework' – that is maximal patient participation.

The converse also holds true. If, for example, an apparent sexual dysfunction comes to light during a routine consultation, what right has the doctor to try and force his values on the patient? If the couple is happy with sex once a month, why make them unhappy by pointing out that their frequency is much below the average, and instituting a course of sex therapy? I feel that this couple has the right to decide for themselves how their relationship functions best.

Debilitating illnesses and nursing home placements

Lack of participation in debilitating illnesses, like cancer, can cause a depressive reaction in patients (Editorial, 1979). They do not feel effective or even have control over their own bodies. 'Their very cells seem to be rebelling and going crazy. It is essential, therefore, for them at least to exercise some form of control over their treatment and their hospital environment. If they are not given appropriate ways for participation, they may see no alternative except resistance to therapy as a means of exercising control.' It is suggested that therapists should be encouraging exuberance, independence and individual responsibility, rather than keeping patients compliant and sedated.

Most elderly patients dread the nursing home or hospital (Anderson, 1979). Great emotional trauma can be caused when one is faced with actually having to live in the home. 'The final decision for nursing home placement is often made by the patient's family, who in turn, rely on the judgement of the doctor, nurses and hospital social services.' Often this decision is 'overprotective' and 'unjustified'.

Although he may be taking medical risks by returning home, his life may not be worth living, to him, in a nursing home. Too often, the aged are treated like children who have no voice in their future. Yet, they are adults who are responsible for making their own decisions. Our job is to make an elderly patient aware of available alternatives and the probable consequences of his decision when we believe transfer to a nursing home is indicated. If he can comprehend this, whether senile or not, he has the right to decide where he wants to live (Editorial, 1979).

Informed consent is just another term for patient participation. The patient has the inalienable right to take part in the decision 'what should be done?' after it has been determined 'what can be done?' Zawacki (1979) also feels that this is not a scientific decision and does involve the patient: 'It weighs the patient's versus the caregiver's values, and at its best it involves doctor and patient sharing in the process, listening as well as talking rather than the doctor just doing what he judges should be done.' He concludes that 'nothing in our training confers upon us the right or expertise to weigh the patient's personal values for him. We cannot produce patient consent; we can only be given it.'

Even the dying patient must still be allowed to participate. Zawacki (1979) states that such a patient 'must be treated maximally, unless, being competent and after being fully informed, they voluntarily refuse. If they do so, I believe we do not have the right to give them such treatment against their will.'

REHABILITATIVE CARE

Rehabilitation must not only be looked upon as the fitting of an artificial limb or the attaining of cardiovascular fitness after a myocardial infarction. More important are the losses in the psychic sphere – the loss of a spouse after a divorce, the loss of a beloved who has passed away, the loss of his self-esteem by an alcoholic.

The doctor is only able to initiate the rehabilitation process, especially in the latter cases, but the family, relatives and friends will have to carry it through. Patient participation in these cases is therefore much more important, relevant and effective than anything the doctor can offer on his own.

PRACTICE MANAGEMENT

Patient participation is not only desirable in the clinical field but also in the administrative area. Fry (1977) stresses the need for more patient involvement in the provision of primary care: '... we will need more data and information on the ways in which our practices are organized, and to take careful note of our patients' views.'

'Taking note of patients' views' can range from listening to the odd patient remark to the institution of a full Patient Advisory Council (PAC), as being utilized by Seifert (1981). The PAC participates in managing most of the non-clinical aspects of the practice, from fiscal management to patient satisfaction. Rather than relinquishing control over his practice, says Seifert, he is sharing the load of responsibility with PAC members.

The most practical way to obtain patient participation in your practice management is to supply a 'suggestion box' in your waiting room. This form of continuous self-evaluation can only do the practice good. Some form of two-way communication, based on the 'suggestions', can then be instituted. Such communication will prove to be very fruitful – there is no other way for the doctor to look at his practice administration from the patients' viewpoint.

A questionnaire is another method to involve patients. In my own experience, such a questionnaire proved its worth in gold. It gave me a very clear concept of my patients' expectations, fulfilments and frustrations, and aided me in meeting them in many ways – with tremendous mutual benefit. Without this participation – initiated from my side and accepted from their side – it would not have been possible.

DOCTORS' AND PATIENTS' OPINION

Is the idea of more patient participation acceptable to the actual consumers – the doctors and the patients?

Seventeen family practitioners attending a postgraduate course of the Department of Family Practice, University of the Orange Free State, Bloemfontein, South Africa were requested to complete the following questionnaire:

(1) Do you feel that patient participation in the management of their own (or their family's or their neighbour's) problems should be *more* or *less*?
(2) Motivate your reply.
(3) Give some practical examples to confirm your motivation.

They were also asked to hand out the same questionnaire to 20 of their patients at a random base.

Of the doctors, thirteen (76.5 per cent) voted for more patient participation, three (17.6 per cent) decided that in some cases it should be more and in others less, while one (5.9 per cent) replied that it should stay as it is. Some of their motivations and practical examples are as follows:

Alcoholism, depression and psychosomatic problems will be much more comprehended by the physician when there is more participation by the family. The converse also holds true: the effective management of these cases is dependent on intense participation by the family. A rehabilitated alcoholic, whose problem originated from domestic problems, fell back into his old habits when he returned home to his nagging wife.

More patient participation in the management of chronic diseases is absolutely essential. Indifference towards and perseverance with the smoking habit in patients with chronic bronchitis or ischaemic heart disease will almost nullify all the doctors' efforts.

Doctors and patients are partners in the management of diseases. It is both the doctors' and the patients' duty to supply each other with all relevant information. In spite of lack of medical education, patients do have common sense.

One doctor struggled for months to motivate a certain patient to reduce her mass in order to obtain better control of her hypertension. During a routine examination he discovered that she had developed diabetes mellitus. After receiving the glucose tolerance test, he paid her a special visit and discussed her condition in detail with her and her husband. He handed her the necessary diet charts and a booklet on diabetes, and discussed all the possible consequences and complications of her disease. She immediately gave her full participation, now sticks to her diet, and is already reducing her mass and has no glucosuria at the moment.

Another of his patients had the same problem, but he only saw her at his consulting rooms, and did not spend the same time with her. Her mass and blood pressure only increased, and she developed a retinal thrombosis. She lost an eye, and he lost a patient.

In the first example the 'partnership' functioned effectively, in the latter there was no partnership at all.

The doctors who voted for 'more and less' participation felt that there is need for more patient participation, but that some patients overdo their participation.

Of the patients' questionnaires, 140 were received back. More participation was requested by 117 (83.6 per cent), less by four (2.9 per cent) and 'more and less' by two (1.4 per cent). Maintaining of the status quo was requested by seventeen (12.1 per cent). All of the latter stressed the importance of patient participation, but remarked that they were satisfied with the degree of participation that they enjoyed in their own patient–doctor relationship.

Some of their remarks were as follows:

The doctor is unacquainted with the emotional problems and undercurrents of the family. Other members of the family must be involved to obtain a clear view of the whole situation. The doctor is not always present to watch the patient's behaviour at home.

Many patients feel that more patient participation will lead to a greater trust and confidence in their doctor, and to greater compliance. One patient was very depressed, and kept on finding fault with others, and blaming them for his condition. His doctor advised him to do some heart-searching and that gave him perspective. In that way he was considerably motivated to self-participation, and his depression cleared up.

They ask for more participation in decision-making, especially where operations or procedures are concerned. A mechanic writes: 'My index finger, right hand, was amputated without my being given a chance to discuss the matter. Probably due to shock I consented to the operation. Only after amputation the next day I thought that my finger could have been saved.'

The importance of communication is also stressed. Because the doctor was behind schedule, he did not pay full attention to what the patient had to say. The patient immediately sensed the doctor's attitude, and consequently did not feel free enough to reveal all her symptoms. She left the consulting room with a few tablets and the knowledge that her problem had not even been identified by the doctor. Lack of communication can lead to repeated unnecessary consultations.

The more the patient becomes involved, the less he feels like a puppet. The realization that he has to make his own contribution to the management of his disease allows the patient to digest his problem much better on the emotional level, and augments his lowered level of self-dignity. Patients should know more about early symptomatology in order to know when to and when not to consult the doctor. The two 'more and less' patients both made the point that some patients can assimilate information regarding the severity or outcome of their diseases, while others will not be able to.

Arguments offered in favour of less patient participation by four patients boiled down to the fact that they have enough trust in their doctor, and that the patient is a layman in medical affairs.

CONCLUSION

Patient participation already exists, and is initiated by the first decision of the patient either to manage his own problem or to consult a doctor. It figures in every aspect of the modern medical care system, but especially so in the field of primary medical care.

I am convinced that patient participation should be more, without being too much. The doctor must still remain the managing director and coordinator of the 'partnership', but he must be able to delegate intelligently and consult with receptivity. In order to do this, he will have to divulge information with discretion, and allow a mutual trust to be established. This should not be too difficult, providing one big truth is always borne in mind. In his first epistle to the Thessalonians (1 Thess. 5:23) Paul writes: '... and I pray God your whole spirit and soul and body be preserved blameless ...' Your partner – the patient – therefore consists of a spirit, a soul and a body, in that order of importance. Ignore any one of these three elements in your mutual contact, and the communication will break down. Regard them as a unity, and the partnership will flourish. More participation by each member of any partnership according to his own capabilities and responsibilities, and on his own level, must lead to the ultimate goal of successful achievement.

In conclusion, this quotation (Llewellyn-Jones, 1979):

> In the past decade, increasing numbers of people expect to be able to discuss their medical problems with their doctor. The older concepts of a compliant patient who was instructed by an uncommunicative doctor is slowly being replaced by a partnership between the sufferer and the healer.... The trend to participation in health care will increase, and should benefit rather than damage the health of the nation.... We feel uncomfortable if we have to step out of our accustomed authoritarian, dogmatic role, have to admit our ignorance, and have to communicate clearly with our clients, avoiding the use of medical jargon.... Yet, health care in the last years of this century will depend increasingly on the involvement of the sufferer in the alleviation or cure of his own illness, and we must be responsive to this change.... If we fail to meet this challenge we have no right to claim the courtesy title of 'doctor'.

References

Anderson, C. A. (1979). Home or nursing home? Let the elderly patient decide. *Am. J. Nurs.*, **79(8)**, 1448

Editorial (1979). Patient participation – a treatment for depression. *N. Engl. J. Med.*, **300(6),** 286

Ferguson, T. (1980). The self-care revolution. *Am. Pharm.*, **NS 20(6),** 13

Fry, J. (1977). Commonsense and uncommon sensibility. *J. R. Coll. Gen. Practit.*, **27,** 16

Fry, J. (1979). *Common Diseases: Their Nature, Incidence and Care.* (Lancaster: MTP Press)

Greenwald, P., Nasca, P. C., Lawrence, C. E. *et al.* (1978). Estimated effect of breast self-examination practices on breast cancer mortality. *N. Engl. J. Med.*, **299,** 271

Heffernan, M. W. (1981). Communication Skills in Communication. 53rd South African Medical Congress Pretoria 6–11 July 1981

Hill, D. J., Heffernan, M. W. and Rice, D. I. (1979). *Involving Doctors in Health Education About Cancer, International Union Against Cancer: Geneva.* (UICC Technical Report No. 44)

Isele, H. (1979). *Dipec Newsletter, International Union Against Cancer No. 1*, p. 11

Llewellyn-Jones, D. (1979). Participation in health care (editorial). *Aust. Fam. Physic.*, **8(5),** 450

Seifert, M. H. (1981). Sharing practice management with patients. *Patient Care*, **15(9),** 142

Shim, C. S. and Williams, M. H. (1980). Evaluation of the severity of asthma: patients versus physicians. *Am. J. Med.*, **68,** 11–13

Spelman, M. S. and Ley, P. (1966). Knowledge of lung cancer and smoking habits. *Br. J. Soc. Clin. Psychol.* **5,** 207–210

Tattersall, R. B. (1979). Home blood glucose monitoring. *Diabetologia*, **16,** 71–74

Taylor, F. W. (1978). Patient responsibility (editorial) *Surg. Gynecol. Obstet.*, **147,** 588

Williams, I. P. and McGavin, C. R. (1980). Corticosteroids in chronic airways obstruction: can the patient's assessment be ignored? *Br. J. Dis. Chest*, **74,** 142

Working Group (1979). Patient behaviour for blood pressure control. *J. Am. Med. Assoc.*, **241(23),** 2534–7

Zawacki, B. E. (1979). The doctor-patient covenant. *J. Trauma*, **19(11),** 871–3

The case for more patient participation (3): self-care benefits for primary care practitioners

Keith W. Sehnert

INTRODUCTION

Ten years ago the first report appeared concerning medical self-care in the United States (Sehnert, 1971). It described how primary care physicians and the allied health professionals who worked with them in a family practice group in Virginia started an educational programme to create 'activated' patients. That article defined an activated patient as 'a person whose clinical skills and an understanding of health is upgraded in order that laypersons could become active participants in their own health care rather than assuming the passive one traditionally assigned to them by health care professionals.'

Throughout the years since, in classes held in over 40 states in the United States, in Canada, Colombia, Great Britain, Denmark, Mexico and elsewhere, the four educational goals have been to help participants:

(1) Accept more individual responsibility for their own care and that of their families;
(2) Learn skills of observation, description, and handling of common illnesses, injuries, and emergencies;
(3) Increase their basic knowledge about health problems and health promotion skills to improve their own health status and that of their family;
(4) Learn how to use health care resources, personnel, services, insurance and medications more economically and appropriately (Sehnert, 1980).

The planners and teachers who created the Course for Activated Patients (CAP) made these three basic assumptions:

(1) Ordinary people with clear, simple information can safely handle in their homes many common health problems earlier, cheaper and sometimes better than health care professionals.
(2) Lay people with little formal medical education can be trusted just as much as persons with much formal education in wisely handling such common problems.
(3) Medical and nursing knowledge should not be the guarded secret of professionals but shared with the laity.

During the decade since CAP was started, there have been significant shifts in the United States regarding roles of the physician and the patient; the numbers of working women who were breadwinners for their family; senior citizens living in specially constructed housing facilities; the number and quality of family doctors and allied primary care practitioners and so on. All these societal shifts made impacts on the programmes that were taught and the types of audiences interested in learning self-care skills, the types of teaching required, the special needs for new types of information about nutrition, fitness, stress management and 'wellness skills'. Health care professionals who taught such classes and the participants who attended learned about 'consumers', 'providers', 'encounters', 'authoritarian doctors', 'wiser buyers/users of health services', 'HSA',

'PSRO', 'HMO', 'medical marketplace' and all the new economic jargon that swept America in the 1970s.

This chapter identifies some of the positive viewpoints about self-care programmes and presents everyday applications.

HISTORICAL TRENDS

The do-it-yourself trend that has swept America in home building and repair, car maintenance, development of independent energy resources, farm animal care, 'quality-circle' management methods, gardening and so on was bound to affect the medical world. When the do-it-yourself trend for self-treatment and diagnosis received additional pushes from disease prevention and health promotion efforts plus the fitness movement, the inevitable result was the concept of medical self-care.

One observer of the scene, Tom Ferguson (1981), editor of the quarterly magazine, *Medical Self-Care*, noted recently that there are now five distinct self-care components seen in the United States:

(1) High-level wellness (with emphasis on running, fitness, nutrition and stress management).
(2) Health promotion/preventive medicine (with emphasis on prospective medicine, health risk analysis, corporate health programmes).
(3) Home health care (with emphasis on parenting, child care, decision-making by women, home remedies).
(4) Medical consumerism (with emphasis on doctor directories; wiser use of medications, health resources, hospitals; health insurance, HMOs and health planning).
(5) Illness intervention (with emphasis on monitoring, self-diagnosis and management of common acute and chronic ills).

Despite the increased scope of self-care, the definition originally developed at a conference sponsored by the National Center for Health Services Research in August 1977 is still appropriate: 'Self-care and self-help are parts of a matrix in the health care process whereby lay persons can actively function for themselves and/or others to (1) prevent, detect or treat disease, and (2) promote health so as to supplement or substitute for other resources.'

At the same conference there was much discussion related to the many medical, social and economic factors behind the consumer self-care movement in the United States. Lawrence W. Green of Johns Hopkins Hospital, Baltimore noted (Green *et al.*, 1977):

... The increased popularity of patient education programs and the growing awareness on the part of consumers that they are indeed capable of rational, sophisticated self-help. Such factors as the movement toward consumer participation in government programs and community development, the self-directed behaviour modification movement, the evolution of nursing theory and practice from 'helping the helpless' toward facilitation self-care and the evolution of group dynamics and self-help groups have all contributed to the trend.

There are many other theories and suggestions about the reasons for self-care and the rapid development of an interest in health promotion activities. These include the women's lib movement, the Counterculture revolution of the 1960s and the change in the nuclear family. One of the explanations, offered by DeFriese, Sparks and Barker (1982), might be associated with what they called 'a reaction against the over-medicalization of society; from this perspective, the health promotion is an "alternative" to conventional forms of health and medical services'.

Whatever the factors and reasons may be, self-care is perceived by its adherents, both from the professional and lay ranks, as being part of the health improvement process. An interesting conceptual diagram was recently developed by Steven R. Mosow (1981) of the Health Futures Institute, Minneapolis (personal communication, 1981):

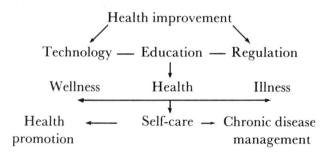

As noted in that diagram some improvement in health status has come from technological advances. Improved technology since the Second World War has made dramatic changes in the way medical care is delivered, in general, and is now making specific changes in the tools available not only to the professional workers but also to the man (or woman) in the street.

A recent report by Sobel (1980) stated:

Until recently, the public has had few diagnostic tools at its disposal other than the thermometer. Lately, however, increasing numbers of home diagnostic tests, from pregnancy kits to blood pressure cuffs have been marketed. The transfer of technology from professionals to the public is both promising and problematic. These tests hold great potential for empowering people in their own health care regarding earlier, more accurate diagnosis; for improving home monitoring of chronic diseases and for substituting cost effective self-care for more expensive professional care.

The growth of such technology with miniaturization, telephone transmission options, home computers and increased sophistication of lay people about medical and nursing knowledge will continue to grow with exponential speed. A recent market survey,* *The Overall Home Medical Testing Market* (1981) shows a current market in the United States of $151 million and a projected market of $183 million by 1982.

Another report from *US News and World Report* (9 February 1981) said that sales of do-it-yourself diagnostic tools surpassed $100 million in 1980. It also reported that Marshall Field and Company of Chicago, Macy's and Broadway department stores in California, People's Drug Stores in the eastern United States and many surgical supply stores across the nation are developing self-care and medical supply services for the consumer public. Marshall Electronics, a major medical device company in Skokie, Illinois, reported that blood pressure units for home use now net $50 million each year.

THE BENEFITS

In the decade since the CAP programs started, many questions have been raised:

(1) Of what benefit is medical self-care to the average person?
(2) What is its current or potential value to a physician or nurse?
(3) Are there economic benefits or mainly psychological ones?
(4) Is there a medical or financial reason to incorporate self-care in a medical or hospital setting?
(5) Is there a payoff beyond improved public relations?

There are four well-documented studies that have focused primarily on the economics and cost-effectiveness of self-care programmes.

---

* Packaged Facts, 274 Madison Avenue, New York, NY 10016

The Ohio studies

Martin A. Evers of Dayton's Health Skills Association (personal communication, 1979) developed a five-session, family-based programme and began a 3-year study in 1976. It involved several hundred Blue Cross/Blue Shield participants. The costs of services to experimental and control groups were compared. The members in the experimental group who took self-care training in 1977 and 1978 experienced medical care costs that went *down* $38 per family. The costs for the control group went *up* $21. An independent analyst with the Miami Valley Health Systems Agency reported, 'I believe that it can be said that to date your program has been cost effective'.

The Idaho study

Donald Kemper (1979) conducted a study with the Gem Valley HMO of Boise, Idaho. The study involved 217 enrollees who all received their primary care from that health maintenance organization. The experimental group took the self-care training provided by Healthwise, Inc. of Boise. Table 14.1 shows the results at the end of 1 year:

Table 14.1

	Experimental	*Control*
Cost of primary care services per family	$80.62	$85.98
Cost of referral care to specialists	$37.19	$49.23
Total	$117.21	$135.21

The Washington DC study

This study done at Georgetown University was directed by Keith Sehnert (1977). Participants and control members were persons who received Medicaid assistance and lived in Metropolitan Washington, DC. The major focus in this research effort was educational design and methodology, but there were some studies related to health care costs – those for drugs, laboratory tests and the number of primary care visits. Table 14.2 shows the results obtained in the 1-year study.

Table 14.2

Average for 1 year	Experimental	Control
Drugs		
Pre-test	$2.23	$1.45
Post-test	$1.97	$2.16
Laboratory		
Pre-test	$4.21	$2.77
Post-test	$2.77	$4.66
Primary care visits		
Pre-test number	5.8	4.5
Post-test number	5.3	6.0

The Maryland study

A study of asthmatic patients who were served at the Johns Hopkins Hospital Emergency Room and lived in nearby Baltimore were divided into experimental and control groups. The experimental group attended five meetings that lasted 75–90 minutes. Patients learned to alleviate symptoms and increase their understanding of asthma. At the end of 4 months, the experimental group had reduced emergency room utilization. Assuming a cost of $20 per visit, the experimental group had a total of $1100 lower costs than the control group.

In addition to the economic factors, there are other benefits reported in other studies around the world. A few of these mostly in USA included:

(1) Dr Haigh P. Fox and Gerald M. Rosen of Providence Family Medical Center in Seattle used do-it-yourself treatment books to cut down on the uncompensated time they used on patient education. They established a registry of such books and materials.

(2) Dr James Strain, a paediatrician with the University of Colorado, developed a successful programme for parents and children and taught them to take throat cultures at home. Dr Harvey Katz of Columbia Medical Plan in Columbia, Maryland instituted a similar plan in 1969.

(3) Dr John Fry of Beckenham, England has developed programmes that improved patient compliance, optimized benefits and minimized dangers of taking medications.

(4) Ross L. Egger, MD, of Daleville, Indiana used a combination of telephone contact, checklists and educational programmes in his office to help him handle his patient load more effectively. In 1971 he averaged 29 daily visits for 4800 patients. In 1978 he averaged 22 per day with 4000 patients under his care.

(5) Tim Rumsey, MD, and his staff at Helping Hand Health Center

in St Paul provided a full spectrum of self-care classes, books and materials as part of standard clinical procedure for the 10 000 low income patients who get their care there each year.

(6) The self-care book report by Moore, LoGerfo and Inui (1980) at the University of Washington has been well publicized. Moore reported that the self-care book, *Take Care of Yourself: A Consumer's Guide to Medical Care*, had no significant effect on the number of physicians visits during a 6- and 12-month study. He summarized his findings in this way, 'Large scale distribution of this self-care book therefore did not result in significantly less dependence on physicians for treatment of acute medical problems'.

EVERYDAY APPLICATIONS

The purpose of this portion of the chapter is not that of attracting clinical practitioners to a wholly different mode of practice, but to raise some questions:

(1) Are there parts of the educational philosophy of self-care that can be used to improve doctor–patient relationships and professional satisfaction in the field of primary care?

(2) Can 'teachable moments' in clinical practice be used not only for primary intervention but even 'pre-teachable moments' as an integral part of primary care?

(3) Can physicians learn something from dentists who have made prophylactic care a major component of primary dental practice?

(4) Are there some aspects of the way the Problem-oriented Medical Record was integrated into everyday clinical practice that can be applied to the self-care educational process?

Improving public relations and professional satisfaction

The educational philosophy behind self-care can help improve the doctor–patient relationship. The 'health partnership' needed in these days of more complex treatment, chronic diseases and multiple social changes in all our families can be enhanced by increasing lay responsibilities and setting realistic professional goals. Such a partnership, using education as a regular clinical tool, will tell patients what the doctor is doing and what is expected and allow frank questions – with honest, direct answers – which could lessen the chances of malpractice suits.

Another byproduct of self-care education is increased professional satisfaction through better communication and improved quality of care. 'Garden variety' illnesses and injuries, over the years, offer little challenge to most primary care practitioners. 'No challenge remains in my practice' is the common complaint of many family doctors. But if an injury or ailment can be linked with lifestyle faults, family stress and personal conflict, the incidents can become 'teachable moments' – even 'pre-teachable moments'. Then, the challenges of health behaviour modification, motivational change and improved communication will challenge most professionals. Then, and only then, primary prevention will start becoming an integral part of primary care.

Putting prophylaxis up front

The Framingham, Massachusetts, studies over the past two decades have identified and documented the major coronary heart disease risk factors. These are all related to lifestyle practices which are subject to change. Risk reduction methods that include nutritional counselling, exercise and diet, stress management and medical treatment and smoking cessation programmes can be instituted. The clinical laboratory support needed to do the various tests and analyse them are available directly or indirectly in all parts of the United States. The educational resources to change behaviour are becoming increasingly available through private vendors, hospitals and other health agencies and are available in most major cities. The new field of prospective medicine, that came out of the work of Robbins and his co-workers at Methodist Hospital in Indianapolis, assists physicians, nurses and allied health professionals in developing analytical methods of the data.

When these clinical approaches are coupled with the educational methodology that has developed in the new field of self-care, with classes, self-care guides and other materials, a broad range of new resources can make prophylaxis as important to primary medical care as it has been to dental practice over the past two decades.

Making medical records focus on prevention

One of the dilemmas that faced most primary care practitioners in the 1950s and 1960s was that of maintaining good records in the paper flood associated with consultation, laboratory and X-ray reports. It took the pioneering work of Larry Weed at the University of Vermont in the early

1970s to bring some order out of chaos. He developed the problem-oriented medical record based on algorithms and other concepts used in developing computer programs. Out of this came the famous SOAP* process now used in all medical schools as part of the logical preparation of good medical records.

Weed (1975) pointed out in one of his recent books that physicians should not only educate patients about their health problems but encourage them to keep and read their own records and states: '... He must be involved with organizing and recording the variables so that the course of his own data on the disease and treatment will slowly reveal to him what the best care for him should be. Crippling dependency states in patients will be fewer. Needless repetition of expensive and dangerous medical activities will be controlled.'

With this in mind, Weed and his co-workers at Burlington and the PROMIS Clinic in Hampden Highlands, Maine have developed a wide variety of flowsheets, questionnaires and other clinical materials. All of these can be adapted to individual practice needs – and all emphasize education as a primary clinical tool, *not an afterthought*.

I have used such concepts in developing what I call the SOAP self-care system. In it participants learn skills in *describing* common health problems with 'what – when – where?' questions, needed in developing their medical history (Subjective); *measuring* vital signs and clinical events with thermometer, stethoscope, sphygmomanometer, otoscope and other equipment (Objective); *comparing* such observations with self-care guide-books (Assessment); and *planning* home treatment and *developing* call-'the-doctor-signals to determine when, and if, professional help is needed (Plan).

CONCLUSION

Programmes developed to enhance the capacity of laypersons to perform self-care skills have been viewed by some sceptics as efforts to 'take away' traditional functions from professionals. It is more accurate to conclude that such educational efforts seek to enhance the capabilities of laypersons to do for themselves – with training – what people have always done – without training. Viewed in this way, self-care may be considered part of the 'health care system'. It is neither opposed to nor the same as profes-

---

* S = subjective information gathered from the history and patient's symptoms;
  O = objective information from laboratory and physical findings;
  A = assessment or analysis of information; and
  P = plan of therapy and medical care.

sional care. Self-care is one part of a continuum. Professional care is another. Both are alternatives for meeting personal health care needs.

My experience over the last 10 years has convinced me that medical self-care is a clinical resource that provides several economic and professional benefits. Its incorporation into the office routine primary care practitioners should be considered.

References

DeFriese, Gordon H., Sparks, Robert D. and Barker, Ben D. (1982). Integrating a Concern for Health Promotion/Disease Prevention with the Clinical Practice of Medicine and Dentistry (In press)

Ferguson, Tom (1981). *Second Midwest Self-Care Workshop*, Spring Hill Conference Center, Wayzata, Minn., 4 May

Green, Lawrence W., Werlin, Stanley H., Schauffler, Helen H. and Avery, Charles H. (1977). *Consumer Self-care in Health*, DHEW Publication No. (HRA) 77-3181, p. 20

Kemper, D. W. (1979). Medical Self-care Education: Impact on HMO Costs. *Abstract in 107th meeting of the American Public Health Association*, November 5

Moore, Stephen H., LoGerfo, James and Inui, Thoma S. (1980). Effect of a self-care book on physician visits. *J. Am. Med. Assoc.* **243,** 2317–2320

NCHSR Research Proceedings Series (1977). *Consumer Self-care in Health*. DHEW Publication No. (HRA) 77-3181, p. 4

Sehnert, Keith W. (1971). Activated patients: a unique course in patient education. *Medical Group News*, August, 16–17

Sehnert, K. W. (1977). A course for activated patients. *Social Policy*, **November,** December, 40–46

Sehnert, Keith W. (1980). The new physician and the theory of well-activity. *Case Western Reserve University Medical Alumni Bulletin*, Spring/Summer

Sobel, David S. (1980). *Self-diagnostic tools, Medical Self-Care*, Summer, 14, 15

Weed, Lawrence L. (1975). *Your Health Care and How To Manage It*. Burlington, Ver. PROMIS Laboratory, p. xiii

Commentary

'More patient participation' is a current modern medical bandwagon that has to be noted and taken note of. It represents a public unease with the medical profession and with the less-than-optimal services provided and the less-than-perfect outcomes of modern medical technology and of modern personal care.

The 'doctor–patient relationship' has been sacrosanct and full of mystery and mystiques. The medical profession has been accused of being a great secret society with secrets that will not be divulged even to the patients under care.

The relationship involves social as well as medical roles. The difficulties of diagnosis, decisions on appropriate treatment and on the management of individual patients by personal physicians is not easy. It is complex and requires for its success certain professional independence and uninvolvement with personal relations. Self-care may lead to difficulties in these matters.

There are benefits from patient participation in promotion of health, disease prevention, self-care of minor ailments and collaboration in chronic and long-term disorders. There are benefits in discovering problems in practice organization, in highlighting deficiencies that may be corrected through voluntary actions within the community, through organizing self-help groups and by better understanding of what is possible and what is not possible in medical care.

Those who have had experience of patient participation tend to be enthusiastic and satisfied with what it achieves. Critics, however, tend to be those theorists who are frightened of the possible snags and difficulties that may be involved for them and their practices.

15

Telling the patient the truth, the whole truth and nothing but the truth?

The issues

The following issues are under discussion: How much to tell the patient? What to tell and in what way? What *not* to tell and why? Who to tell – family and who else? When to tell what and how much?

These issues have to be resolved by each physician in his contact with his patients. Each physician must develop his ways of telling the truth as he/she sees it.

The case for telling the patient the truth
Axel Engberg Pallesen

THE TRUTH ABOUT SERIOUS DISEASES

Patients with malignant diseases were previously only told about the true character of the disease in exceptional cases. That was the official policy of doctors and other hospital personnel in our hospitals for many years, a policy which was based on tradition and on the opinion that only very few patients are emotionally strong enough to bear the unembellished truth about their diseases. 'Occasionally healing, often relieving, always comforting' has been the doctor's position since this was formulated by Hippocrates. Since the possibility for cure was rare, and for relief was modest, it was more charitable of the doctor to protect his patient from the brutal and shocking knowledge of the desperate nature of his disease.

271

The medical art became a skill of comforting. Our position in this respect has been a consequence of our meagre capacity, and therefore has been characterized by evasion, false comfort and concealment.

The increasing demand in recent years for a more open availability of information, also in relation to incurable diseases, has brought about a new standpoint in the public, and in doctors and nurses, since a radical breakaway has been made in many areas from concealment, which is now considered unethical and stressful to all parties, not least the ill. This new standpoint should be viewed from the basis that the prognosis for many patients with severe – and previously fatal – diseases has now improved substantially.

The Hippocratic oath and ethical rules adhered to by doctors express the profession's customary recognition of the medical ethical principles and prerequisites of medical practice. Within the ethical rules are en-joined the patient's right to self-determination and the right to be in-formed about his condition, which acknowledges that the patient must have a primary responsibility for his health, and therefore must be included in the treatment of his illness. This is the so-called informed consent, which is recommended by the European Council's Parliamen-tary Assembly in a declaration published in January 1976, and which is endorsed in principle throughout the western world. This obligation to give information can be extremely difficult to observe under certain conditions where the prognosis is unfavourable. Absolute truthfulness must not be the doctor's first duty but should yield to the demand that, first and foremost, he must not harm the patient – *primum nihil nocere* must be the doctor's first commandment. Warmheartedness is more important than a stereotyped requirement always to follow the pledge of truthfulness without regard to the situation.

To deprive a patient of the hope for life is unwarrantable, and to proffer guesses as to how long the patient can live is inadvisable. As long as there is life there is hope, and conversely, as long as there is hope there is life. The will to live is deeply fundamental in human nature.

Most – indeed, maybe all – dying patients sustain a hope which often exceeds all logic, and which is based on man's sense of immortality. This hope extends to the grave, it is said. In any event, the doctor should be cautious about uttering an unequivocal prognosis and should never set a distinct time-limit, which thereby locks out hope for the dying. We must understand clearly that hope is multifaceted, not simply the hope to continue living a long life, but the hope that the disease's symptoms, which at present may be distressing, can be relieved by treatment, the hope that pain can be treated effectively, the hope that all current social problems can be resolved, as well as spiritual and religious hopes. All of these are components of human hope which aid the patient to live as long as he lives. Hope is the best protection against anxiety and fear, and is necessary for the patient to mobilize power to fight the disease. Hope is always present, even when the patient perceives and accepts death as a reality with which he must live.

WHAT DOES THE WORD 'CANCER' MEAN TO A PATIENT?

What is the patient thinking when he asks if he has cancer? What does the word '*cancer*' mean to a medical expert? Malignant disease – cancer – is clothed in many psychological connotations. Cancer is the public's most feared disease, surrounded by mystery, dread and doom. Therefore, a number of special conceptions are associated with cancer, so that one can say that cancer victims and therapists have their own psychology, which is explained by historical and cultural conditions. To this must be added the mystery that surrounds the numerous new forms of treatment, which the public cannot evaluate and which can create an attitude of hopelessness. This is very stressful to all those who work with cancer patients, because it tends to close channels of communication with those patients, so that they become isolated from their surroundings.

The diagnosis of cancer is connected with incurability. It is this disease's sombre outlook that evokes the anxiety associated with cancer. Patients have a rigid, inflexible opinion on the disease's highly variable manifestations, as well as on the technical difficulties connected with diagnosis and prognosis considerations directed toward cancer treatment. Therefore, the individual cancer case is not without further factors which allow a rather certain objective estimation. And 'the truth' about the individual case in the meaning 'it is in agreement with the actual condition' is encumbered with great uncertainty.

'The truth' about a disease is valid only for what the doctor is certain of at the present moment. Therefore, it would appear more expedient for the doctor to share his knowledge of the illness with the patient and to arrange this knowledge and its consequences in the most suitable and humane manner possible.

HOW DO TERMINALLY ILL PATIENTS REACT TO THE KNOWLEDGE THAT THEY SUFFER FROM A FATAL DISEASE?

The process of dying, both for the patient as well as for the relatives, represents an adversity which surpasses the resources of many people and which therefore can be considered as an acute traumatic crisis. This can be examined from our experience of critical situations. To acknowledge the reality of death is a painful and shocking experience which no-one can accomplish without anxiety and without mobilization of a series of defence mechanisms: denial, projection, regression and depression are customarily found. The dying patient is aware much earlier that he suffers from a fatal illness than are those people around him, and the reaction pattern that he develops and performs, the defence that he mobilizes, are on the whole the same whether he has been informed or not. Numerous investigations have confirmed that far fewer dying patients react with fear than those around them had expected, and that the reaction was dependent on the manner in which those around them were prepared to respond to their own fear and anxiety.

WHY DOESN'T THE PATIENT ALWAYS REQUEST A DIAGNOSIS OF HIS DISEASE, AND WHY DOESN'T THE DOCTOR ALWAYS GIVE THIS INFORMATION?

The patient often does not ask for the diagnosis for several reasons. One reason may result from anxiety and fear that his dreaded expectation will be confirmed, or that he still does not possess strength enough to use one of the weapons in his defence mechanism, denial; or he may consider it useless to obtain this information from personnel who perhaps appear harassed.

Equally often the doctor thinks that the patient will break down. Perhaps he does not know what he will say, or he will avoid the conversation that he fears might be a confrontation, which will stimulate anxiety in him and make him powerless. For some doctors it is difficult to have to confess that they are unable to bring about any remedial improvement in the patient's disease. Moreover, many doctors have a pronounced and unresolved fear of death, which means that each confrontation with a dying patient stirs up anxiety within themselves. This type of doctor – or nurse – will always avoid situations which stress them emotionally.

The precondition necessary for obtaining a deeper psychological contact with a dying patient is, naturally, that the patient is motivated and that both parties are capable of establishing an emotional union. Unfortunately, not all dying patients are able to formulate a need to discuss emotional problems.

Some cases from general practice

A 60-year-old man with inoperable cancer of the colon was cared for at home by his wife and two daughters, who had returned home to help their mother. The married couple had always lived a close life, deeply dependent on one another – a symbiotic marriage. The patient was treated by his family, who competed with each other to provide the most care. They all spoke past each other in a completely closed context which isolated the patient, and they established a psychological contact that was dominated by false comfort and suspicion. After her husband's death the wife underwent a prolonged period of deep sorrow.

A man consulted his doctor and asked for his counsel and advice. His wife was in hospital in the last phase of an incurable ovarian cancer, about which she had never been informed. During the course of the illness the couple participated in a dual communication – the husband had been informed by the hospital staff about his wife's serious condition and he was now at a loss as to how he could tell her, as he had never before discussed the future with her.

A 14-year-old girl had her left leg amputated because of bone sarcoma. Twelve years later her doctor voluntarily told her that she had had bone cancer. This information provoked a hysterical outburst in the girl and it required considerable effort to calm her down.

A man was clinically suspected of suffering from liver metastases, and scanning confirmed this opinion. He died later and sections from his liver revealed cirrhosis but no tumour.

A gastroenterostomy was performed on a man because of an inoperable cancer of the stomach. A biopsy verified the diagnosis. The man had no difficulty for 12 years but his condition rapidly deteriorated and he died 13 years postoperatively. At autopsy, cancer of the stomach of the same histological nature detected 13 years previously was found.

A 50-year-old man was found to have malignant lymphogranulomatosis, about which he was informed completely during the treatment period. He took part in instruction on openness in cancer diseases and behaved jovially, always relaxed and unstressed; however, he was taciturn and clearly set himself apart from others. After his death the doctor unexpectedly learned from a conversation with his wife that her husband never at any time discussed his illness with her. He played one role in the hospital and another at home, where his illness was never discussed.

A 79-year-old active and mentally alert woman was hospitalized for acute haematemesis, due to stomach cancer (a 3–4 cm long polypoid broad-based tumour in the large curvature) of the adenocarcinoma type. She was advised against an operation due to her age. After discharge from hospital she said she had been told she had a stomach ulcer which could be cured by medical treatment. After a period at home, where the condition gradually worsened, the patient indicated indirectly several times to her doctor that she wished to discuss with him her illness, which she suspected of being cancer. She became suspicious and aggressive toward the hospital and medical department. She lived with her daughter, who all her life had been terrified of contracting cancer and who consulted the doctor several times to emphasize her opinion that her mother should not be informed. The doctor deduced that the patient had a psychological need to discuss her problems and he told the daughter that he had detected signs in her mother which indicated she wished to talk about her illness. The daughter reacted violently and hysterically, admonishing the hospital for its standpoint and for the information it had given out.

A 23-year-old man had cancer of the testes and died from cancer cachexia. Even at the very beginning of the disease the patient desired absolute openness and information about all phases of the disease and its treatment – this was seen by the patient as his best guard against panic, and allowed him to see beyond the horizon limited by anxiety and to preserve his self-respect. He felt he could improve himself, could chat with his large family, could arrange his thoughts and adjust himself to fear. To him, uncertainty was the greatest hardship. During the entire course of his illness he sustained hope until the very end. He was thankful for all the therapeutic interventions implemented in his behalf, he never felt he had been abandoned, that anything had been left untried. He was able to live productively to the end, to be active and make plans. He was a strongly meditative young man who was capable even in the terminal phase of the disease to mobilize his resources and resolve the problems which awareness of impending death gave rise to. This case is an example of the completely open context between the cancer patient and those in his surroundings, and of the importance of providing honest information as a prerequisite to psychological support to the patient.

These case histories encompass a large number of ethical aspects: have informed consent and the ethical rules concerning investigations and treatment been complied with? Who should decide the question as to who shall/must inform the patient about the diagnosis? How much cooperation should there be between the hospital and the family doctor? What are the difficulties in helping the dying patient who has been maintained in a closed context? How about the immediate family, etc.?

THE LINES AND COURSE OF THE COMMUNICATION PROCESS

The whole question of 'truth disclosure' and the many emotion-laden opinions expressed for and against 'to tell or not to tell the truth' can potentially disrupt the process which takes place between the dying patient and the therapeutic group around the patient. It is obvious that this process – the process of communication – constitutes far more than pronouncing a diagnosis, that it is an active bilateral process which creates comfort and confidence.

There are two phases in this process, one early and one late. In the early phase the dying patient is given a realistic picture of the illness, and in the late phase he is informed that death is imminent.

The communication process with the dying patient can be illustrated as a stage play, with the patient, relatives, doctor and the nurses and hospital personnel as the cast.

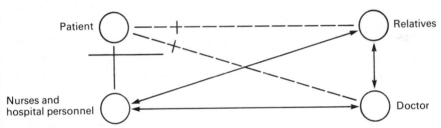

Figure 15.1

If one decides to spare the patient and to carry out honest discussions with the relatives only, a tragicomedy of concealment and evasion is very likely to result that can become a great burden on all parties. It can be seen in Figure 15.1 that exchange of information which excludes the patient, such as from the doctor to the relatives, will have the effect of isolating the patient. On the other hand, if both the patients and relatives are informed at the same time, the sorrow and mutual apprehension will be shared in a valuable united psychological process. Many dying patients are subjected by relatives and the doctor to an atmosphere of false comfort and minimization of the symptoms, talking past one another or playing a game of concealment by avoiding subjects close to the essential problem.

It is important that we all clearly understand that communication takes place on both an intellectual as well as an emotional plane. And it is a fact that verbally conveyed information about the truth rarely occurs under conditions where the psychological contact between patient and doctor is good. The dying patient, either consciously or subconsciously,

always knows he is dying and, consequently, the dialogue between therapist and patient proceeds on all planes, and both comprehend each other.

The right not to be informed

It is a human right that each terminally ill patient be given as much
information about his situation as he himself desires, and which he feels
is necessary at that time for him to evaluate and settle his affairs. This
also implies that each patient has the right *not* to be informed and to deny
the reality of the gravity of his illness, so that he has the opportunity to
resolve problems with which at the moment he is unable to deal. Achieving a balance between these two positions is not always easy.

Many people, not least doctors, have a compulsion to make decisions
for other people. This type of person can easily be inclined to persuade
dying patients to accept his own personal standards and opinions. Therefore, hospital personnel must recognize this side of their personality and
attempt to control their compulsion to dominate. The dying patient must
not be informed – or die – on the basis of conditions of the doctor or other
medical personnel.

Who should take the initiative in the conversation about death?

It ought to be a fundamental rule that the patient should take the
initiative in the discussion about death. Medical personnel must be
attentive to any sign in the patient's behaviour which implies the wish to
discuss his impending death. If in their conduct or behaviour medical
personnel display a reluctance to discuss the patient's psychological
problems, the patient often responds to this by avoiding sensitive subjects.
The patient's wish to be informed must always be the guide as to what
and when information shall be given.

Both Kübler-Ross and the Swedish thanatologist, Loma Feigenberg,
through conversations with dying patients, have confirmed that these
patients wished to manage their dying.

When should the patient be informed?

In most cases this should occur as soon as possible after the diagnosis has
been made. In the early phase the dying patient should be given a
realistic picture of his disease, and in the late phase he should be told that

his death is near. It is quite obvious that it will be difficult to create an openness with respect to the disease if the relationship was begun on the basis of evasion and concealment.

Where should this information be given?

Should it be given in the hospital when the diagnosis is made, in the doctor's office between just the patient and the doctor, or together with the relatives? The answer to this question depends on many circumstances which obviously require time and fulfilment of certain practical conditions.

Who should inform the patient?

It is most often the doctor who is best suited to answer the questions which the patient will ask about the treatment of the disease.

How should the information be given?

We must concede that we arrive at our prognoses from statistics and patient material, but that this particular patient is not a participant in that material. Therefore, we should not become entangled in details and technically complicated explanations which will be interpreted by the patient as beating around the bush.

It is important to allow the patient himself to come forward with his questions and to give him as much information as he can understand and cope with. All information should be given in small portions. Even words and expressions should be adjusted to the patient's situation, to his capacity and experience, to his knowledge and personality structure, and to how far he has advanced in accepting his incurable disease. In practice it is best to inform the patient gently, that is step by step, in order, it is said, 'to help the patient grow accustomed to the truth'. Acceptance of 'the truth' must never be hurried. On the contrary, it is our duty to smooth the way so that the ill patient can intellectually and emotionally arrive at a comprehension of his condition. We must clearly understand that *how* is more important than *what* we communicate.

It is often beneficial for the doctor to ask the patient questions, and in this manner determine what he knows, what he has been able to deduct from the information he has already obtained. Very frequently the patient has a much better understanding of the situation than expected. It is highly preferable to have the patient himself arrive at the conclusion that his disease is desperately grave.

As in all treatment of the critically ill, we must not employ fixed methods or cut-and-dried opinions. The patient should be given an optimistic but not unrealistic version of the truth, and no definite time-limit should be mentioned, if only because it can never be accurately estimated.

THE ENVIRONMENT AROUND THE PATIENT

Different social contexts based on different degrees of open communication are often established around the dying patient. 'Awareness context' has become a concept in communication with dying patients and is defined by Glaser and Strauss (1965) as follows: 'What an interacting person knows of the patient's defined status, along with his recognition of the other's awareness of his own definition – the total picture as a sociologist might construct it – we shall call an awareness context'.

The patient–personnel relationship can be described from the context which characterizes the course of communication in the environment surrounding the dying patient and his relatives. The different types of context rest on a number of different attitudes and preconditions, which we must try to sort out and understand. It is the communication's pattern and human behaviour in the widest meaning. We react incessantly to the interpretation of another person's total communication, both verbal and non-verbal, in an interplay between people on several levels.

Irrespective of the type of context the information process involves the patient, doctor, relatives and personnel in the widest extent. Therefore, it is not simply an interaction between the patient and individuals but includes all the people surrounding him, with a series of consequences from their mutual conduct in relation both to the patient and to each other.

The closed context

The closed context, with respect to the closed environment around the patient, implies that the medical personnel have been told that the patient suffers from a fatal disease and that he has not been informed of his condition. This context depends on a number of preconditions, for example that the patient is falsely informed or the information has been withheld. The family is warned to preserve the secrecy about the nature of the illness, and both medical personnel and family have agreed on what they should say and how the various complaints should be interpreted. The patient is treated with false comfort and his complaints are evaded by various forms of avoidance mechanisms, the explanations being constructed and agreed upon in advance. In practice, it is impossible to circumvent the patient's suspicion. This closed context is marked by instability.

Consequently, the effect of this on the patient means that he withdraws within himself, if he prefers that pattern and if the family and medical personnel can be kept at a distance. Under these conditions the patient does not have the opportunity to arrange his final hours in a reasonable manner and is deprived of the possibility to improve himself at the conclusion of his existence. The family is compelled always to hide and suppress their sorrow toward the patient. A life which perhaps was always characterized by openness and mutual confidence can easily be terminated in an atmosphere of deception and falseness, where everyone is acting a role in a drama. This situation can easily develop into an unworthy, unreal masquerade between a married couple, for example, where their belief in each other will be subjected to great stress.

The doctor and personnel in the closed context usually avoid the dying patient as much as possible by assuming a remote attitude, which at the same time protects them against exposure to a powerful emotional strain, toward which they do not know how they will react.

The atmosphere of suspicion, which is always present in the closed context, will harm nursing personnel particularly, as they are most closely associated with the patient's problems. They feel defensive and exposed to criticism which they cannot answer honestly. A pattern based on fundamental deception gives rise to a ritual drama of mutual shamming around the dying patient, where the relatives and personnel are hindered from working out the psychological problems that invariably occur. That would be against the rules of the game. 'Open suspicion awareness affects continued interaction. The way that staff members handle the patient's suspicions, whether they confirm or deny them, affects whether the patient will choose later to play a mutual pretence game or speak openly of his coming death' (Glaser and Strauss, 1965).

The open context

The open context implies that all parties – the patient, relatives and medical personnel – have been informed about the patient's condition, and this is openly visible in their manner of communication with each other. Communication under these conditions occurs spontaneously and openly, and the personnel are not forced into fixed roles but instead can express themselves honestly and perform their duties in a relaxed manner. The open context allows them the opportunity to support the patient when he is confronted with the knowledge that death is unavoidable, and to create a therapeutic environment around the dying patient which is a precondition to psychological death care:

> A patient who makes it easy for himself also makes his death easier for his family. So far as awareness is accompanied by acceptable dying, it reduces the strain that would otherwise be imposed on kinsmen by closed or suspicion awareness. *If the patient is able to attain a kind of psychological closing of his life before he dies, his kinsmen may be able to share his satisfaction for the remainder of their lives* (Glaser and Strauss, 1965).

The 'open context' is especially preferred by nursing personnel because it allows them to speak openly with the patients, but it demands in return a personal attitude which not all of them have.

DEALING WITH THE TRUTH

In order to penetrate the isolation of anxiety that surrounds the dying patient, we must learn to see truth face to face. And dealing with the truth is more complicated than it is often made out to be.

A few quotations from a discussion between two learned thanatologists can perhaps serve to clarify the dimension of the problem.

> *E:* I don't think it is ethically permissible to attempt to hold a patient in ignorance, regardless of the type of illness. One runs the risk of isolating the patient and making him passive. He is not included in the struggle with the disease. It is doubly unfavourable because the patient usually knows quite well that something is wrong.
>
> *L:* Very often I am asked if I tell the truth, but one must not forget that there isn't anything called truth. My obligation must always be to do what helps, what calms, what best advances the patient's condition today. Tomorrow, it can be something else entirely.
>
> *E:* The much-discussed problem about truth in recent years has created the impression that the essential problem is to speak openly about dying with the seriously ill.
>
> *L:* We doctors usually answer much more than we have been asked. The medical profession commonly uses an enormous power to say more than the patients in reality wish to know.

There is no standard position on the many aspects of truth disclosure. Therefore, one should be cautious about telling the truth as a dogmatic necessity in order for the patient to die a worthy death.

The art of medicine, with respect to this phase of life, is also based on the ability to identify, to listen, to be courteous and to provide human regard. Consequently, the demand for informed consent under all conditions is more complicated than it appears.

Respect for the patient's integrity, creation of confidence and comfort are fundamental properties of true medical art. The obligation to give information to the dying should always rest on the precondition that the patient has available psychological support to resolve all the many problems that the information will evoke. This is most suitably expressed in the old saying: 'Honesty without charity is brutality'.

Disclosure of the truth and psychological support to the dying belong together – they are two sides of the same coin.

Reference

Glaser, B. and Strauss, A. (1965). *Awareness of Dying*. (Chicago: Aldine)

The case against telling the patient the truth
Robin Steel

'What is truth? said jesting Pilate: and would not stay for an answer', wrote Francis Bacon in 1625 in the first of his 60 essays and passed in discussion from 'theological and philosophical truth to the truth of civil business' including as an alternative to truth the 'shadow of a lie' (1902). He compared simple truth to a pearl which is best seen by harsh daylight, but pointed out that the more valuable diamond reveals different aspects in 'varied lights'. Bacon's second and ultimate essays concern Death, 'men fear death as children fear to go in the dark', and although he personally opens by finding it 'the least of all evils' he 'knows many wise men that fear to die' and says 'death arrives gracious only to those that sit in Darkness or grey' or to the 'poor Christian that sits bound in the galleys' but ends he hopes 'I would die together and not my mind often and my body once, not wishing to see the evening of my age a mere return to infancy', but hopes 'briefly death is a friend of ours'.

Death or to die well was important to the ancients, and it has been the stuff of writers, poets and dramatists for centuries. Death was a morbid preoccupation of the Victorians, and suffering an eclipse of interest in two World Wars has emerged from its taboo only recently. *The Hour of Our Death* (Aries, 1981) is a recent book discussing the age of the 'invisible death'. In the cinema, *In for the Treatment* which won the Prix Italia Award of 1979, showed a market gardener aware in hospital that tests reveal bad news by the faces of his visitors; on television Stephen Frears' *Going Gently* contrasted reactions to the realization by patients that their illness is terminal.

The topic of telling the patient 'the truth, the whole truth, and nothing but the truth', is evidently of increasing interest to patients. Physicians, also, possibly accelerated by the recent need to ascertain brain death before transplant donation, or the increasing problems generated by high-technology medicine making once-lethal problems resolvable, but at variable costs. The ability to maintain the length and style of dying, as seen in the death of General Franco were less ideal.

To stimulate continuing debate 'the truth' is being sought as in anglo-saxon Law Courts or at Wimbledon when two tennis protagonists oppose each other before judges. This leads to extreme positions not usually associated with other methods of seeking truth such as the inquisitorial mode of other judiciaries or the scientific mathematical controlled statistical experiments or surveys more familiar to medical scientists.

REASONS FOR NOT TELLING THE WHOLE TRUTH

Reasons why patients should not be told the truth, the whole truth and nothing but the truth may be considered under the following headings:

(1) The doctor is unaware of the truth.
(2) Truth is relative.
(3) The truth may be wrong.
(4) The truth may not be wholly known.
(5) The doctor may have reasons not to tell.
(6) The patient's relatives may forbid the truth to be told wholly.
(7) The patient may not want to know.
(8) Though the patient may have earlier, when well, expressed a wish to know the truth, attitudes alter when ill.
(9) There may be conflict over the ideal way of telling the truth.
(10) The patient may not be capable of being told the truth.
(11) Circumstances may alter and if the whole truth has been told then it can never be untold wholly.

The doctor is unaware of the truth

An academic general practitioner was waiting at an airport to fly back to his home town after a busy committee day in London when a lady he recognized as a former patient approached him. She enquired how he was and then asked if his heart was all right. Having ascertained that they both were well she then recalled how a few years previously, before her husband had moved to London, the general practitioner had performed a life insurance examination telling her husband 'your heart is in excellent condition' adding frivolously 'better than mine'. The lady then revealed that a few months after moving her husband had dropped dead and the post-mortem revealed extensive coronary arteriosclerosis!

Truth is relative

A young soldier wounded after World War II North African tank battles had severe leg wounds. The hard-pressed, overwhelmed, singlehanded medical officer told him 'nothing could be done' and gave him large doses of morphia. He died shortly before the casualty station was captured by the enemy, who set up a small field hospital with facilities that might have been able to save the young soldier's life.

Doctor Lawrence (later a famous diabetologist) as a young doctor in the 1920s developed diabetes and went to the warmth of the Mediterranean for what he had been told was his terminal illness. Whilst there he received a cable informing him of the discovery of insulin and its availability. He survived and went on to lead a full professional life as an authority on diabetes.

A similar success story is told concerning a medical student whose fiancée was dying of myasthenia gravis before he read of a new successful treatment in the medical press.

Who can say what the future holds when treating a patient with multiple sclerosis or motor neurone disease or malignancy? With genetic engineering is alteration of Down's syndrome unthinkable?

The truth may be wrong

A small boy with Down's syndrome also had renal abnormalities susceptible to surgical intervention. At a postgraduate teaching institute a junior surgeon training told the highly intelligent parents that the chromosome result just received had excluded Down's syndrome. There had been a clerical error and a glance at the boy should have alerted the junior doctor to check again on the report's veracity.

The truth may not be wholly known

A successful builder, who had developed from nothing a thriving firm, came to see his general practitioner on a busy Monday and complained that on the previous Saturday after only three games of squash he had become breathless. If the patient had not been so stable, or if the general practitioner had not known him, this could have been dismissed as frivolous. The only physical sign was a small bruise; blood count revealed pancytopaenia, and even after marrow puncture next day this baffled haematologists for several months. A third marrow puncture ultimately revealed features of leukaemia, which eventually became all too obvious. A tendency towards megaloblastosis involved treatment with vitamin B_{12} until the truth was wholly known and the patient informed in appropriate terms.

The doctor may have reasons not to tell

Regrettably some doctors, especially surgeons of the 'old school', can never tell their patients the truth, but talk euphemistically of ulcers, inflammations and removing tissues that could 'turn into cancer'. Possibly it is better to have a technically superb surgeon with poor patient management than a mediocre surgeon with outstanding pastoral skills. A case may possibly be made for maintaining morale in the acute phase, but in many cases the doctor is either old-fashioned, unskilled or even personally disturbed by death. However, in some societies litigation is so prevalent that the doctor who confesses all may find himself (or herself) practising without malpractice insurance cover. Sometimes the 'white lie' is kinder than frank whole truth. A professor of obstetrics saw a student creep late into the back of a tutorial and found he had been taking blood, but without full explanation to the patient. Unfortunately the professor castigated the student before learning that the blood was necessary for a repeat WR test, the routine first one having been lost.

The patient's relatives may forbid the truth to be told wholly

The family physician may find this request one of the most difficult to
handle, and one of the greatest tests of medical skill and experience of the
family. In most circumstances time and the evolution of events allows the
initial panic to evaporate. Sometimes the ban is complete and unalterable
and occasionally, in retrospect, correct. For example shortly after a
couple's golden wedding the wife developed postmenopausal bleeding
due to endometrial carcinoma; the husband was adamant that she was
to be told it was a polypus (because after 50 years he knew her best). A
while later he developed a mole that histologists confirmed as melanoma.
The wife said that the husband was not to be told that the histology was
malignant (as after 50 years she knew him best) unless he developed
secondaries. Both died several years later of other causes, pleased that
each had guarded well their respective spouses and in the opinion of the
family physician most successfully.

The patient may not want to know

Although this can be further rationalization of the doctor's fear of the
task, without doubt some patients cannot be told. It is not usually the
hypochondriac or the neurotic but often the blustery extrovert with a
veneer of being in control. The example of 'Big Daddy' in Tennessee
Williams' *Cat on a Hot Tin Roof* demonstrates the collapse of such a
character. After an involved family argument Big Daddy is told by his
younger son that medical tests have revealed a bad prognosis, not the
all-clear that the doctor in collusion with the family has told Big Daddy.
The experienced family physician, can usually, even with the intention
of never lying to his patients, recall some who will not wish to hear their
personal future discussed. A retired devout administrator, when less than
half his usual weight, pointedly insisted on discussing the colour of next
year's roses and courteously rejected any signals from the doctor that he
was available to talk about the future. Denial is not the worst of ego
defences.

Though the patient may have earlier, when well, expressed a wish to know the truth, attitudes alter when ill

A registered nurse had worked with the family physician before being his
patient. She had remarked socially that if she were ill she would like to

know the truth; following surgery and radiotherapy for breast carcinoma she thanked the doctor for his frankness. However, when she developed liver and bone secondaries she denied the future and was adamant that palliative chemotherapy was going to cure her, though both her friends and her doctor could see her liver swelling.

Similarly, a Worcestershire man who had emigrated to the United States developed disseminated lupus erythematosus with progressive renal involvement so he brought his wife and three sons home to England knowing his prognosis. His opening bargain with his new family doctor was he wished to have monthly blood ureas, and always to be told the results. For a year results were normal and discussed; however, when compensation failed he still came for blood tests but evaded an interest in the results.

It is essential to make sure that the change is not due to depression that is treatable. A family friend, for business reasons, had asked for the prognosis following which he ordered his affairs settled. He developed anorexia and bizarre views on his treatment, but this coincided with early morning wakening, and the excellent response to nocturnal tricyclic antidepressants confirmed that the episode was depressive and highly responsive to treatment. Even dying patients can have other intercurrent illnesses.

There may be conflict over the ideal way of telling the truth

Even if the truth is known the method of telling has to be adjusted to the patient, the family and the regime. It is not a decision to be taken without in-depth thought and knowledge. As an example, a nervous woman had two episodes of what was likely to be multiple sclerosis. Her husband, together with the specialist and family doctor, felt that it was too soon to tell her the symptoms were atypical, and she should only be told if the diagnosis was certain. It was therefore disastrous when the junior doctor, taking the follow-up clinic, asked her how long she had had multiple sclerosis.

There is an old joke about the Wild West Town where the cowboy knocked on the door saying 'does widow Jones live here?' and when he was told it was 'Mrs Jones' replied, 'well, it's widow Jones now ... your old man's been shot'. There is a much to be said for choosing a time to broach the truth, for instance after a convalescent holiday with the family.

The patient may not be capable of being told the truth

Some patients may be unconscious, demented or brain-damaged, others psychotic or mentally retarded. Legally it could be impossible to tell some patients the whole truth and on this the judge would direct the jury to declare this debate for the defence case. William Osler used to teach that a physician should consume his own smoke: in other words, anxiety over the patient's problems should not be transmitted to the patient and his family without thought and appropriate circumstances.

Circumstances may alter and if the whole truth has been told then it can never be untold wholly

The world is full of octogenarians who were given 6 months to live by their medical attendants long since deceased. Some of their statements may have been due to misdiagnosis, some to misunderstanding, and others because in the era before modern therapy giving a poor prognosis protected a doctor's reputation. Nevertheless, well-authenticated spontaneous cures from cancer and other serious illnesses do exist, however uncomfortable this may be to existing medical science. It ill behoves us to have medical delusions of grandeur, and to tell the whole truth without having a loophole or an escape road down which the doctor and the patient may retrack hopefully together if circumstances alter.

A final example may put this in more practical terms. Shortly after the British National Health Service started on the 5 July 1948 a young schoolgirl developed a large swollen liver with a heart murmur and congestive failure. The agreed opinion at the teaching hospital was that she had atypical heart disease with very poor prognosis. When she moved to Worcester her notes routinely followed her (a little-publicized major benefit of the National Health Service). As a late teenager she developed emotional problems and in psychotherapy with her family physician, abreacted that she had overheard from a passing ward round an eminent opinion to the class of clinical medical students she would 'never live to see 20'. In fact, with the passage of time and the evolution of more sophisticated investigations it appeared that she had had a hepatic arteriovenous shunt, which with adolescence spontaneously resolved itself. Her parents, family and friends, and her doctors were well aware the original prognosis was out of date, but locked in this girl's subconscious, like a time-bomb ticking away, was the overheard whole truth substantiated by contemporary NHS hospital letters of the period that she would 'never live to see 20'. This caused extremely disturbing behaviour as 20 approached. It may have been good undergraduate teaching to see things in black and white, but in family practice dark grey is usually better than total blackness.

One of the greatest tests of a family doctor's skill, attitudes, and knowledge, as well as his relationship with the family, is in the handling of terminal illness. Pendulums of medical and public opinion rightly have swung away from blanket 'don't say anything' to the more realistic approach that most patients should be told some of the truth and some patients most of the truth, but the decision to do this is not lightly to be undertaken. It should be done with as much thought as arranging an operation, and needs exploration of the background medically, socially, and psychologically, and when the decision is made, to communicate it to all concerned and adjust its emphasis in the light of events.

Bacon wrote:

> Physicians in the name of Death include all sorrow, anguish, disease, calamity or whatsoever can fall into the life of man: But these things are familiar unto us and we suffer them every hour: Therefore we die daily. ... No man can divine how able he shall be in his sufferings, till the storm come (the perfectest virtue being tried in action). ... Celsus could never have spoken it as a physician, had he not been a wise man withal that a man do vary. ... Physicians are some of them so pleasing and conformable to the humour of the patient, as they press not the true cure of the disease; and some other are so regular in proceeding according to art for the disease, as they respect not sufficiently the condition of the patient. Take a Physician of a middle temper.

These words, spoken 350 years ago, suggest a moderate course and not the extreme. Today's extreme would be rigidly telling the patient the truth, the whole truth and nothing but the truth, which as a practical day-to-day precept is as untenable as the other extreme of telling all patients nothing.

References

Aries, Philippe. (1981). *The Hour of Our Death*, (translated by Helen Weaver). (London: Allen Lane)
Bacon, Francis. (1902). *Essays*. (London: Grant Richards)

Commentary

The two views discussed above are not widely different – they both show the depths and intensities of concern that may be suffered by physicians as well as patients in attempting to decide how best to communicate less than good news. Whatever is told, hope must always remain. Even with the very worst news there has to be hope of relief and comfort if not cure. It is sometimes much worse to tell the 'truth' which may later be disproved because of an error in diagnosis or interpretation.

Observing the physician in the acts of 'telling the truth' provides an excellent demonstration of his/her skills, concern and expertise – it is one of the best measures of his/her professional art.

16 How many patients – more or less?

The issues

Medical practitioners are valuable and expensive public commodities. A medical student who becomes a family practitioner, who prescribes, who cares and who retires will use up over £2 million ($4 million plus) of public money during his/her professional lifetime. It is as important that we do not produce too many doctors as it is important to ensure that we use those that we have to the best advantages.

How many family practitioners do we need per population? Who knows! There are no reliable measures or methods by which community's needs of medical manpower can be estimated – there *is* need for research and trials to estimate how many family practitioners should do how much, bearing in mind that now there is sharing and delegation with other members of the team (see Chapter 13).

Do we need fewer patients per physician, so that he/she can provide more personal care and do more for the patient, such as prevention – but the question has to be asked, *do fewer patients make for better care?* Can we care for more patients per physician, by sharing and delegating work with others – the question that has to be asked is *do more patients make for worse care?*

The case for fewer patients (1)
Stan Schuman

The following are assumptions in the argument (which may or may not be realistic):

(1) The doctor has a choice
(2) The doctor has financial security
(3) Most patients will accept the doctor's style during office visits.

(4) The doctor has the ability to alter his/her style.

(5) A doctor's career encompasses early, mid, and late stages with characteristic styles of practice.

DEFINING THE P:C RATIO

The average consultation (patient–office visit) has been analysed and reanalysed in vivid detail by teachers of family medicine, behaviourists, and time-work experts. From the point of view of this essay, let us consider the axis of time spent for patient *care* versus the time spent for *preventive* services. There is a P:C ratio of time spent per encounter which varies with the condition, age and susceptibility of the patient, and the level of skill and motivation of the physician.

For example, progressive early morning cough with sputum in a young factory worker who is a heavy smoker presents a target for prevention when he comes in for an episode of acute bronchitis. The P:C ratio of this encounter could be 25 per cent prevention (reduced or stop-smoking advice) compared to 75 per cent of the time for diagnosis and anti-biotic treatment (1:3). For an aged patient already a victim of in-operable carcinoma of the lung seen for acute bronchitis, the P:C ratio might be 0:100 per cent since the horse has already bolted from the stable.

For younger patients in particular, the field of accidental injury, poisonings, road accidents, misuse of drugs and sexual experimentation are obvious targets for the doctor who is environmentally aware and prevention-minded. Yet for older patients, a few tips on the lighting of dangerous stairs to prevent unnecessary falls can prevent needless surgery of the hip.

THE 'AGES OF MAN' APPROACH TO A PHYSICIAN'S CAREER

Any physician's career from the end of formal training and residency to the day he retires represents a dynamic process. As in any profession, there is an adaptation of one's skills and offerings to one's community's needs and demands. The physician whose services do not match or grow with the community's needs becomes an antiquated public servant (much like the Dickensian solicitor in his musty office). In the area of traumatic injury alone, skills with horse-and-cart accidents need to be upgraded to cope with high technology burns, chemical injury, and high-speed crashes. Similarly, in the area of multiple choices available for contemporary women, the physician must keep up with the latest information on contraceptive choices and risks.

From my biased viewpoint, it is a sign of growing maturity and wisdom in the physician when he becomes less involved in the immediate gratification of 'hands-on' surgery, emergency orthopaedics, and dramatic relief of cardiorespiratory failure. Such a physician begins to sense the greater challenge of detecting and altering the early course of clinical depression, alcohol abuse, preventable accidental injury in the home and the school playground, and industrial intoxications. Not only has one crossed the threshold into areas of much greater service to the community but often into areas where one lacks special skills. This is a penalty borne by most medical graduates of western schools. 'Let George do it', is the dogma for 'real' doctors involved in the delivery of health services, allowing one to pass the buck to the health department or other agencies. In my experience, the first clue to a previously unrecognized hazard in the workplace, the medicine cabinet, or the hospital is the alert provided by a single medical observer (Francis, 1949; Schuman et al., 1980; Schuman, 1979, 1980, 1982).

This is not to minimize, but rather to reinforce, the power of the 'hands-on' doctor–patient relationship. Somehow, since time immemorial, even the tribal healer has a unique opportunity for prevention at the moment of relieving the pain or anxiety of the immediate condition of the patient: 'next time don't be the first to take on the mastodon's front end during the hunt', or 'next time, check for alligators before trying to fish in the river'. More and more behavioural studies suggest that the efficacy of the physician to curb a patient's smoking is greater than that of concerned relatives including spouses.

POSSIBLE MODELS OF PHYSICIAN BEHAVIOUR IN PRACTICE: THE P:C RATIO

I have come more and more to reflect on each patient/family encounter for episodic care as an exercise in adjusting the P:C ratio of the encounter.

When one starts with a family, such as a newly-wed couple, prevention may seem remote. Nonetheless, the premarital or prenatal visit offers an opportunity for anticipating risk factors (genetic counselling, blood pressure, albuminuria, ABO or Rh incompatibility, or rubella susceptibility). Assuming a tenured relationship with the young parents, a growing bond of trust develops, whereby they are increasingly receptive to a change in the ratio of so-called 'curative' to 'preventive' services. Paediatricians have long endured, and rejoiced in multiple opportunities to allay fears

regarding thumbsucking, nightmares, bedwetting, and short stature –
not a very dramatic or rewarding service for some professionals but
probably highly significant in the daily wear-and-tear of childrearing.

This point was made most effectively by Stevens (1974) in his lecture
to the Royal College. During the course of a single weekend on call, he
saw and treated a variety of conditions by means of home visits. The
details of each household suggest a computer-like diagnostic mind which
is at once sorting out emergency, curative, ameliorative, preventive, and
humanistic considerations. No better example comes to mind than this
narrative of the traditional, yet modern role of one personal physician
making his rounds.

Regarding the P:C ratio as an index of the relative balance between
preventive and curative services during an average physician's career,
straightaway, let us assume that *fewer patients/families under one's direct
responsibility overcomes the primary objection to spending time on preventive services*
including counselling, which may be of unproven, or of unpredictable
efficacy. One may choose to spend the extra time gained from fewer
patients or less sick patients in a variety of pursuits: medical education
(a form of preventive medicine?), medical statesmanship (maintenance
of professional quality), arts and humanities in the community, sports,
recreation, business enterprise and charity.

This argument contends that time is the *excuse* rather than the reason
for omitting or neglecting preventive services. The greatest strain on the
physician is not on his/her time but on one's imagination – a split-second,
really, to ask oneself, how could this be prevented? One may not have
any ready made answer. It may take a visit to the medical library or
several phonecalls with the experts, but once the chain-of-events begins,
the preventive model starts to work. The next very real barrier to repeated efforts at prevention is the frustration of failure, when the advice
goes unheeded. Disappointment and discouragement have an embitter-
ing quality. Should the physician regard a 50 per cent rate of return on
his investment of time for prevention as 50 per cent failure, or 50 per cent
success?

The models presented in Figure 16.1 suggest two possible variations
on the theme of a physician's experience in practice. Physician A leaves
medical training with high hopes for prevention, attacking problems in
the community and in each patient's lifestyle vigorously but with less
than optimal results and satisfaction. Battered and sobered, the physician
gradually reduces his/her efforts from about 50 to 25 per cent at mid-
career. With the serenity of later years, the doctor may return to his/her
first love, prevention, and now more prudently selects targets for change
with renewed efforts (50 per cent).

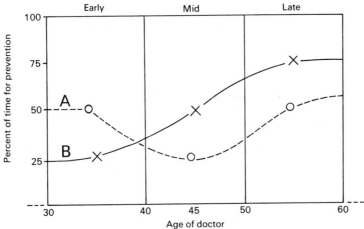

Figure 16.1 Two models (A and B) of changing emphasis in a physician's emphasis in practice. Sequence: for A (○) 50%, 25%, 50%, for B (×) 25%, 50%, 75%

On the other hand, model B tends to fit the ambitious, economically driven US physician in private practice who feels compelled to master his/her skills in therapy and organize an office practice team, in the early years with relatively little time for preventive measures (routine immunizations, cervical (Pap) smears, pre-employment and post-illness physical examinations, etc.) at a level, say of 25 per cent. With time, success, and security, Doctor B begins to find time (about 50–75 per cent?) for implementing preventive measures in the context of office practice.

Perhaps in the later years, fortified with practice-earned insights, one may stretch to do more for one's community and willingly leave the drama of 'hands-on' medicine to younger colleagues. With increased age should come a greater tolerance for half-successes and partial failures. One can accept limits with greater tranquillity without giving up the good fight.

In summary, this is where I stand on the issue of practice size.

(1) More time with fewer patients? Yes!
(2) More time for golf? No! (All right, maybe a little ...)
(3) More time for prevention? Yes! Indeed!

References

Francis, T. Jr. (1949). The family doctor: an epidemiological concept. *J. Am. Med. Assoc.*, **141**, 308

Schuman, S.H., Dobson, R.L., Fingar, J.R. (1980). Dyrene dermatitis. *Lancet*, **2**, 1252

Schuman, S.H. (1982). *Epidemiology for the Clinician.* (Menlo Park: Addison-Wesley Publishers)

Schuman, S.H. (1980). Lessons from the US summer of 1980. *Lancet*, **2,** 529

Schuman, S.H. (1979). Prevention: the vital and unique function of the family physician. *J. Fam. Pract.* **9,** 97

Stevens, J. (1974). Brief encounter. *J. R. Coll. Gen. Practit.*, **24,** 15

The case for fewer patients (2)

Derek A. Coffman

TIME AND POMEGRANATES*

A disciple went to the house of a Sufi physician and asked to become an apprentice in the art of medicine.

'You are impatient,' said the doctor, 'and so you will fail to observe things which you will need to learn.'

But the young man pleaded, and the Sufi agreed to accept him.

After some years the youth felt that he could exercise some of the skills which he had learnt. One day a man was walking towards the house and the doctor – looking at him from a distance – said: 'That man is ill. He needs pomegranates.'

'You have made the diagnosis – let me prescribe for him, and I will have done half the work,' said the student.

'Very well,' said the teacher, 'providing that you remember that action should also be looked at as illustration.'

As soon as the patient arrived at the doorstep, the student brought him in and said: 'You are ill. Take pomegranates.'

'Pomegranates!' shouted the patient, 'Pomegranates to you – nonsense!' And he went away.

The young man asked his master what the meaning of the interchange had been.

'I will illustrate it next time we get a similar case,' said the Sufi.

Shortly afterwards the two were sitting outside the house when the master looked up briefly and saw a man approaching.

'Here is an illustration for you – a man who needs pomegranates,' he said. The patient was brought in, and the doctor said to him:

'You are a difficult and intricate case, I can see that. Let me see ... yes, you need a special diet. This must be composed of something round, with small sacs inside it, naturally occurring. An orange ... that would be of the wrong colour ... lemons are too acid ... I have it: pomegranates!'

The patient went away, delighted and grateful.

'But Master,' said the student, 'why did you not say "pomegranates" straight away?'

'Because,' said the Sufi, 'he needed time as well as pomegranates.'

Shah (1978)

A doctor in any specialty needs to see a certain number of patients in a week in order to gain experience, for so much of our ability is based on personal experiences of dealing directly with patients. This expertise cannot be gained from textbooks but can only be gleaned from direct patient contact. It is my belief that the established family doctor has too many patients and the workload will vary according to a number of factors, many of which he will be unable to influence. He (and I trust my

* Reproduced by permission from Idries Shah's *A Perfumed Scorpion*. pp. 97-98, 1978 (London: Octagon Press).

female colleagues will forgive me for using the male pronoun throughout this text) may practise in an area of high morbidity and there may be a high proportion of elderly patients, many requiring home visits. The urban doctor may be faced with a rapid turnover of patients while the rural doctor may have to travel many miles to visit his patients. Working in a multiethnic area with language problems may also produce further difficulties. Lastly, this workload will depend on the number of patients for whom he cares. Maybe this is the only factor the doctor can influence but even this decision may be affected by governmental as well as other external factors, for the ratio of doctors to patients within a country is related not only to the number of students graduating but to medical immigration and emigration and, of course, to population changes within a country.

The young competent doctor may well be able to cope easily with a large list size. In later years, however, he may feel the need to work at a slower pace, and in the United Kingdom general practitioners practising within the National Health Service are automatically given payment in the form of 'seniority awards' when they have been in practice for a certain number of years. This could be seen as encouraging them to reduce their workload without any financial loss.

HAZARDS AND RISKS OF MEDICAL PRACTICE

Is it not odd, however, that doctors who are so ready to accept responsibility and to shoulder the burdens of others, and indeed advise accordingly, have so many difficulties in managing their own affairs? Capable of making important day-to-day decisions about their patients, many doctors are unable to make similar decisions with regard to themselves and their families. Marital problems leading to divorce, alcoholism, drug abuse, consultations with psychiatrists and suicide rates are all increased within our profession. In England and Wales the death rate from alcoholic cirrhosis is $3\frac{1}{2}$ times that of the general population and admission rates into psychiatric care because of alcoholic dependence in Scotland are 2.7 times higher amongst doctors than individuals in other professional groups (HMSO, 1978; Murray, 1977).

A paper from Massachusetts, United States which, admittedly, may not represent doctors worldwide, is worth relating here (Vaillant *et al.*, 1972). Medical students were followed up with matched non-medical controls for 30 years. At the time that the paper was written the doctors were approaching 50 and were all in good clinical health, but 47 per cent had made poor marriages or had been divorced compared with only 30 per cent of the controls. More than a third of the doctors used night sedation coupled with alcohol, or had taken amphetamines and tranquillisers daily for more than a month compared with only a fifth of the controls, and 34 per cent of doctors had paid ten or more visits to psychiatrists compared with 19 per cent of controls. The authors divided the subjects into two groups according to specialty: firstly, surgeons, administrators and research workers who were considered as 'not having primary responsibility for patient care'. This group had symptom patterns of childhood similar to those of the controls. The second group – the internists, obstetricians, psychiatrists and paediatricians (general practitioners?) – who were considered 'to have direct responsibility for primary medical care', had significantly more emotional difficulties during adulthood and instability during childhood as compared with the other group and the controls. The authors of this paper contend that some doctors may elect to assume direct care of patients to give others the care that they did not receive in their own childhoods. This would stand in contrast to the assumption that clinically involved doctors have more problems because of the physical demands of their work. What may be said, however, is that should doctors have such problems, these can only be exacerbated by excessive workloads. Statistics in the United Kingdom also show unequivocally high rates of suicide in the medical profession compared with other professions. (In the United States, however, this suicide rate is exceeded by dentists and pharmacists. (Rose and Rosow, 1973).

STRESSES OF PRACTICE

It is unlikely that we do actually work harder than many other groups, but there is a constant stress in our daily lives and at times feelings of helplessness, not only because of our inability to relieve suffering but also because of our inability to alter the course of many problems brought to us for solving, thus producing feelings of frustration and inadequacy. Furthermore, patients today are much more questioning about their bodies and their illnesses than previously. This in itself may make a doctor feel threatened for no longer do we have a god-like authoritarian role. The younger doctor, in particular, may constantly feel this threat, and if he is not mature enough to overcome, or grow through these feelings undue stress will result. However, if we acknowledge our own vulnerability to sickness and to life's problems, patients can then begin to relate to us as human beings (as well as doctors); this will enable us to achieve greater understanding and practise more effective medicine. It has been said that a doctor needs to come down from his pedestal of infallibility to reveal that he too is human.

TOO MANY PATIENTS

But how can we lessen this effect of stress? As I have stated at the outset, I contend that, in general, doctors take on too much work and readily care for too many patients. The number of patients for whom one is caring may be felt to be an indication of one's success yet, because doctors tend to be ill-organized, that number of patients can be the very factor to cause stress and distress. However, the doctor caring for a list of 2000 may be considerably more stressed if he is ill-organized, than the well-organized doctor caring for 2500 patients with a practice team which could include receptionists, secretary, district nurse, health visitor, social worker, psychologist, etc. But doctors are not always able to surround themselves with such a team, and so many are unable to delegate the work, be it clinical or non-clinical.

Furthermore, apart from this problem of stress, I believe that not enough doctors make any effort to enjoy their work. In order to practise medicine in a satisfying way certain criteria should be fulfilled. A doctor must be knowledgeable – for this he needs to have time to read journals and to attend refresher courses. He should work from well-equipped, comfortable premises – yet how many doctors have consulting rooms whose comfort level is well below that of their own living room? He should employ ancillary staff, and last but most important, he should have time in order to care. Time to spend with his patients in order that consultations can take place in an unhurried, relaxed and satisfying way. Time for clinical diagnosis; time for psychosocial assessment; time for preventive medicine, and time to educate the patient. Without this time (surely the most difficult of these factors to achieve) he is unable to maximize on the quality that he is able to give to the consultation. We have a specific expertise, but how many of us use it because we are always rushing and leaving no time to implement such expertise?

ENJOYING THE CONSULTATION AND LIFE

For want of a better phrase, we should 'enjoy the consultation' and feel some sense of satisfaction when the consultation is at an end. More importantly, the patient should also feel the consultation has been worth-while.

The end of the working day should leave one with, perhaps, a feeling of fatigue, but nevertheless a sense of fulfilment, and the day following should not be filled with dread, tiredness and, worse still, lack of interest. I believe that as a profession we spend most of our day running when, in fact, we should be walking at a brisk, if not leisurely, pace. Too often we are constantly running, and it is not surprising that not only are we unable to solve any of our patients' problems, but we cannot solve our own. Let us, however, look further. The doctor is not an isolated member of society, but has a part to play within and without the walls and boundaries of medicine. He needs time to be an individual within that society and an individual in his own right, to make a marriage, to bring up a family and have time to relax, for sports and hobbies, and outside interests. Because we frequently run, more and more problems are un-solved, causing increased consultation rates and increased referral rates. The insoluble problems produce even greater frustrations and the busy, tired doctor is much less likely to carry out good consultations than the wide-awake, relaxed, unstressed doctor, and the busy, tired doctor is more likely to be the subject of stress himself.

We should also be asking ourselves why society has put restrictions on the working time of airline pilots and long-distance lorry drivers. Why have trade unions fought for a reduction in the number of hours per week worked by their members, yet no such restrictions are placed upon the doctor? Society rarely questions whether doctors, by overworking, are making hasty and faulty decisions.

I believe that if a doctor has less patients and learns to walk rather than to run, he becomes more contented and less subjected to the many stress diseases of today. More time for his patients will mean more problem-solving. More problem-solving means happier and healthier patients. More time for families means happy families and, what is more important, if the doctor has more time for himself he will be a happier doctor and may even live a little longer.

In summary, therefore, I believe that one of the most important therapeutic tools is time, and because we have too many patients we are normally used to stealing time by working longer and longer throughout the working day, or worse, giving our patients less and less time.

I contend that we should not be stealing time to look after more and more patients, but we should have less patients and thus not overreach ourselves. By having less patients we are able to use our most powerful drug – ourselves. With too many patients there is just not enough of this particular therapy to go around.

References and further reading

Bennett, G. (1979). *Patients and their Doctors*. (London: Baillière Tindall)
Bennett, G. (1982). Sick doctors – ourselves. *Update*, **25,** 9
Murray, R. M. (1977). The alcoholic doctor. *Br. J. Hosp. Med.*, **18,** 144
Rose, K. D. and Rosow, I. (1973). Physicians who kill themselves. *Arch. Gen. Psychiat.*, **29,** 800
The Registrar General's Decennial Supplement England and Wales (1970–72) (1978). *Occupational Mortality*. (London: HMSO)
Vaillant, G. E., Sobowale, N. C. and McArthur, C. (1972). Some psychologic vulnerabilities of physicians. *N. Engl. J. Med.*, **287,** 372

The case for more patients
Eric Gambrill

At times it seems that almost every country in the world feels that more doctors are needed to serve the population. From Soviet Armenia, where one person in every 300 is medically qualified, to some developing countries, where a single doctor may be responsible for up to 100 000 people, the cry is the same. Yet there is very little available evidence on which to base firm proposals for achieving an ideal doctor–patient ratio. What evidence we do have suggests that more doctors will give more care – examine more, prescribe more, operate more, especially in a fee-for-service system – but there is no evidence that all this extra activity leads to better health for the population.

In Central America, Guatemala has more doctors than Jamaica, similar living standards and health problems, but markedly inferior health statistics. Similarly, in Europe, Sweden is relatively underdoctored by the standards of the affluent countries, yet has the lowest perinatal mortality, infant mortality, maternal mortality and the highest longevity figures in the whole world. In contrast, Italy, producing vast numbers of doctors each year from its overcrowded medical schools, is one of the least favoured nations of Europe in respect of its health statistics. It would seem that Ivan Illich may have had a point when he stated that 'doctors may damage your health'.

In view of the fact that doctors are also expensive to educate, train, provide facilities for and pay, it becomes even more important to attempt to match needs and resources in an acceptable manner. For the purpose of this discussion we must avoid the complexities of how many specialists and hospital doctors are required and concentrate on the needs of primary care, family medicine and general practice.

It is my contention that almost all affluent countries already have far more doctors involved in primary care than are required to provide a good service to the population. The reasons for this fall into three categories. Firstly, a large amount of professional time is taken up in managing minor illnesses which could and should be well within the capacity of patients or parents to manage themselves. Secondly, many health problems can be competently dealt with by nurses or other trained health workers, thus freeing the doctor to concentrate on those problems which require his degree of training and skill. Thirdly, many doctors are so poorly organized that they achieve much less in a working day than is within their capacity. Let us now consider these assertions in more detail.

SELF-CARE

Community studies indicate that only a small proportion, ranging from 3–25 per cent, of all symptoms experienced by individuals are presented to a doctor in the United Kingdom. We are beginning to understand a little more why some patients are happy to cope with their own minor health problems whilst others have a much lower threshold for consultation. Basically neurotic personalities measured in a variety of ways are more liable both to experience symptoms of illness and to seek medical care in response to those symptoms. Such patients often have an unrealistic expectation of the doctor's therapeutic powers.

Of course, doctors who respond to self-limiting minor illnesses such as upper respiratory tract infection or diarrhoea and vomiting by prescribing inappropriate antibiotics or ineffective symptomatic remedies are reinforcing the patient's belief that consultation was indeed required. Many valuable opportunities for health-education in the surgery are missed every day. In this instance we are not dismissing the need for consultation where there is a diagnostic problem or the patient has a real fear of the significance of a particular symptom. Nevertheless, a higher level of health education for the general public would help to ensure that they are better able to differentiate between trivial and potentially serious symptoms and also have a better understanding of how their bodies work. More emphasis, too, on prevention, stressing the value of sensible eating, drinking and exercise habits and aiming to eliminate the pernicious habit of smoking would do more to improve the nation's health than any contribution that doctors can make.

Some general practitioners have produced their own handbooks for patients of the practice which explain the personnel involved and the services available and also give guidance on the management of minor illness. It has been shown by Morrell (1982) that a combination of positive efforts towards health education and restriction of prescribing for minor illness is effective in reducing consultation rates for trivial symptoms.

A further source of unnecessary consultations in the British National Health Service is the role of the general practitioner in certification. This irksome chore represents a considerable misuse of medical manpower since certification for short-term illness must, in effect, be self-certification as there are frequently no objective signs of illness. Morrell has shown that frequent short-term absences from work are largely socially determined and not medical in origin, and should be tackled as such by the employers.

ALTERNATIVES TO DOCTORS

One of the factors which make doctors less effective than they might otherwise be in the field of health-education is the social, cultural and professional gap which separates them from many of their patients. Experience in the third world, from China to Tanzania, has shown that the most effective person in this area is the part-time health worker or 'barefoot doctor'. These people are part of the community, they have acceptable other skills which they continue to practise, they may be trained on a part-time basis and they are selected and recompensed directly by the community. Above all, they are seen by the community as one of us – the public, and not as one of them – the professionals. Perhaps we need a few 'barefoot doctors' in our schools, shops, factories and farms. It is already the rule that suitable people are selected for training in first-aid measures and some of them could be encouraged to take on further responsibilities for health education and advice regarding the management of minor illness.

Another group whose contribution to primary care is often unrecognized are the retail pharmacists. They already play a large part in advising the public about the management of symptoms, a role for which they are neither trained nor paid, and providing guidance on self-medication. It is reassuring to see that a recent series of articles in the *Pharmaceutical Journal* has concentrated on these aspects of primary care and it may well be that this area could be expanded with profit to all concerned.

Within the primary health care team, as at present constituted in the United Kingdom, district (home) nurses, health visitors (public health nurses) and midwives already play a large part in prevention and treatment.

Although most of this work is within the mainstream of nursing functions and is not strictly supposed to have a diagnostic component, there is no doubt that every nurse working in primary care is inevitably involved in guiding patients on the management of symptoms and advising them on whether or not it is necessary to see the doctor. If the team concept is working well, then the doctor can often accomplish a great deal through the medium of his nursing colleagues without even seeing the patient. Much of the surveillance function in respect of the very young, the handicapped and the very old can be carried out by the health visitor; much of the routine care of the chronically ill is within the capacity of the district nurse, and most of the care required during pregnancy, labour and the puerperium is well within the capacity of the midwife. The range of responsibilities which a practice nurse, employed directly by the doctor, can undertake provided that she is capable, specially trained in primary care, keeps good records and is legally covered, has been expanding steadily over the last decade. Some of these nurses are involved in family planning, in surveillance clinics for hypertensive and diabetic patients within the practice, in screening patients who arrive without an appointment, in follow-up home visits and even in primary home-visits in suitably selected cases.

In the United States and Canada physician's assistants and nurse-practitioners have been shown to be capable of performing most of the functions of a family physician, albeit at a slower pace, with no evidence of detriment to the quality of care. Indeed, some writers have stressed the advantage of the doctors having to clarify their own thoughts and policies in order to teach their nursing colleagues, and Spitzer et al. (1974) have demonstrated a high degree of patient satisfaction and increased job satisfaction for both nurses and doctors working together in this way.

A relatively new departure in the United Kingdom is the appointment of clinical psychologists and psychiatric nurses (CPN) to posts within the community nursing service. Since there is plenty of evidence of emotional problems and minor psychiatric disorders accounting for perhaps 25–30 per cent of all morbidity in primary care this is a welcome innovation. Although a minority of general practitioners have a special interest in these problems, they are extremely time-consuming and all too often the doctor's response is to prescribe tranquillisers or antidepressants indiscriminately, to refer patients unnecessarily to the specialist psychiatric services and sometimes to admit patients to hospital inappropriately. The CPN in Britain is a registered mental nurse, usually with considerable hospital experience, who has undertaken a further 1-year course on psychiatric nursing in the community. He or she is able to monitor drug prescribing, including administering injections of psychotropic drugs, to intervene psychotherapeutically with individuals, families or groups and to provide a link with the specialist services. Shaw found that the CPN was acceptable in the practice setting and added a great deal to the doctor's knowledge of his patients. In addition, he found a decrease in hospital admissions for mental illness, a decrease in the need for domiciliary visits by a psychiatrist and a dramatic decrease in the prescribing of psychotropic drugs. He considered that the CPN provided time, expertise and economy along with an increase in the quality of care provided and his experience has been borne out by many other general practitioners.

One of the increasing problems for doctors working in primary care is that, because they are generally accessible and well-known to their patients, they are frequently approached for help with problems for which their skill, training and expertise are inappropriate. There is a danger that such problems, be they social, financial or legal in nature may be 'medicalized' and treated inappropriately, dismissed as irrelevant, or tackled ineffectively. For this reason some general practitioners have encouraged lay counsellors, ministers of religion and support groups to operate from their premises and some enterprising social service departments have come to appreciate that attaching one or more social workers to a group practice facilitates referral and enables the social workers to become involved with problems at a much earlier stage than usual, when the chances of successful intervention are maximal.

ORGANIZATION

There have been major advances in the organization of general practice in the United Kingdom over the past 25 years. Almost all doctors now employ receptionists, telephonists and secretaries to perform those essential functions which would otherwise take up a substantial proportion of the doctor's time. Larger practices now usually employ an administrator or practice-manager to perform higher level administrative tasks and supervise the implementation of policies agreed by the partners. Appointment systems allow the doctor to control his workload to some extent and spread the load more sensibly throughout the working week. However, there is still considerable room for improvement in the efficient use of medical time in general practice.

There is a long tradition in British general practice for some doctors to consult at a rate which precludes a proper assessment of all but the most trivial reasons for consultation, and thus the tendency is to bring patients back frequently in order to monitor progress and conduct appropriate examinations or investigations. Apart from inconvenience to the patient this habit tends to increase the total time spent on unravelling a problem.

A considerable amount of follow-up can be delegated to the nurse once the doctor has made an appropriate diagnosis, which is his principal role. At present well over 50 per cent of all consultations in British general practice are initiated by the doctor. Some doctors have introduced new methods of working within the surgery premises which involves the doctor moving between two or three rooms where the patient awaits the doctor, thus reversing the usual arrangement and providing the doctor with physical exercise and a change of scene between patients. For some doctors, at least, this provides a more pleasant and efficient method of working.

Home visiting has traditionally occupied a considerable proportion of the doctor's working time in the United Kingdom. However, in recent years there has been a steady decrease in home-visiting and younger doctors place much less importance on this aspect of their work. Whilst it remains true that the willingness of the general practitioner in Britain to visit patients at home allows some patients to be cared for at home who would otherwise require admission to an institution, it is also a fact that the availability of home-visiting leads to inefficient use of medical time in many cases where the patient could easily be transported to the surgery. Experiments with transport systems organized within the practice have proved rather expensive to finance in a system of medical care where there is no charge to the patient for the convenience of having a doctor visit the home. Although some traditionalists, led by Pereira Gray, have argued persuasively on philosophical, sociological and psychological grounds for the perpetuation of widespread home-visiting their campaign has the flavour of a rearguard action.

The telephone is an instrument which is probably underused in British general practice. In many countries the doctor sets aside a specified period of the day to accept telephone calls or ring patients back. Provided the doctor is aware of the limitations of a telephone consultation he may well save both the patient and himself considerable time and inconvenience without reducing the quality of care. If the doctor makes a point of speaking personally to all patients requesting a home visit he is in a position to advise whether or not a visit is required and, if so, with what degree of urgency.

The organization of out-of-hours cover is another area where unnecessary stress may be reduced by effective rota systems, within or between practices, or by a properly staffed deputizing service. Much out-of-hours care in urban areas could be based on hospital casualty departments or emergency rooms, as is the practice in North America, and there is no reason why the general practitioner on call should not use the department as his base if this seems appropriate for local conditions.

USE OF EXTRA TIME

If it is possible to make extra time available for the general practitioner, how best should this time be used? One suggestion is that much more time and effort should be spent on screening for presymptomatic disease. Before this is accepted we must consider what screening methods have proven value and whether these methods require a doctor to administer them. Space precludes a detailed examination of this topic but there is certainly no good evidence for the value of an annual general medical check-up, even though there is considerable support for this idea among the public, even in the United Kingdom. Screening for phenylketonuria, hypothyroidism, hearing and visual defects in children, the detection of moderate or severe hypertension in adults, and possibly hypothyroidism in the elderly seem to be of value, but it is noteworthy that none of these requires the presence of a doctor to detect them.

More family doctors are becoming involved in teaching and research and, in the process, are becoming aware that their record systems would benefit from a thorough overhaul and reorganization, possibly with the aid of a microcomputer.

In the British context, one possibility would be for general practitioners to become more involved in the care of their patients in hospital. In view of the changes in staffing which will be required in NHS hospitals in order to bring the needs of service to the patients, and training and career prospects for the doctors into more sensible relationship, it could well be that British general practitioners will be increasingly occupied in hospital work in the future.

In practice it seems likely that, as usual, the staffing of both hospitals and community posts will be dictated by the availability of doctors and the need to prevent widespread medical unemployment, rather than by an objective appraisal of the requirements of the nation. Since we in Britain have doubled the number of medical graduates in the last decade, and since traditional emigration escape routes have been blocked by other countries conscious of their impending surplus of doctors, it seems inevitable that list sizes in Britain will fall markedly over the next two decades irrespective of need. This should enable the general practitioner to enjoy a shorter working week and increase his leisure time, in line with economic and sociological predictions of the general pattern of life by the 21st century.

Nevertheless, after a detailed examination of his own practice, with considerable emphasis on patient-satisfaction, Marsh concluded (Marsh and Kaim-Caudle, 1976):

Given a desire to reduce and rationalize workload, given an attitude that patients should monitor their own short-term illnesses, given a delegation-oriented doctor and a team of readily available paramedical workers whose facilities are excellent, given a clinically confident and experienced GP who does not devalue or minimize the training, experience and ability of the members of the team, given a known group of patients and even given an attitude which avoids hospital referral rather than seeks it, it would appear that even in a high morbidity and high mortality area, the workload of a GP can become quite small ...

His sociologist colleague, Kaim-Caudle adds 'yet be compatible with a mere 2 per cent of patients expressing overall dissatisfaction with their primary health care'.

Reference

Marsh, G. and Kaim-Caudle, P. (1976). *Teamwork in General Practice*. (London: Croom Helm)

Morrell, D. (1982). *Management of Minor Illness*. (London: Health Education Council)

Spitzer, W. O., Sackett, D. L., Sibley, J. C., Roberts, R. S., Kergin, D. J., Hackett, B. C. and Olynich, A. (1974). The Burlington randomized trial of a nurse-practitioner. *N. Engl. J. Med.*, **290**, 251

Commentary

Since there are no reliable ways of measuring medical manpower needs there are tremendous ranges of distribution of physicians per population both in different countries and in different areas in the same country. It may be that individual practitioners have differing capabilities of coping and differing enjoyment of high and low workloads. Maximizing work can be achieved through better organization, encouraging more self-care and using alternative resources of primary care services.

It is argued that fewer patients will provide more time for prevention and health promotion as well as better personal care of specific problems. The effects of stress through excessive workloads on individual practitioners have to be recognized. It is suggested that such stresses lead to increased morbidity among medical practitioners, and that fewer patients might make for more enjoyment of work and better health of physicians but this is still hypothetical.

17

Medical check-up – useful or useless?

The issues

The 'medical check-up' is a fine concept. It suggests that regular personal medical contacts and physical examination are sound practice. Certainly medical check-ups are popular with the public and with those practitioners who are well paid for carrying out the procedures.

The issues must be whether, when put to the test of scientific evaluation and trial, the medical check-up is shown to be beneficial in preventing disease, improving health and correcting bad personal health habits.

The case for a medical check-up (1)
E. C. Gawthorn

A century ago no one had heard of antenatal or child care. The work of those fathers of preventive medicine in persuading their colleagues of the value of these measures was long and arduous. Gradually the community came to accept this. Once this was achieved the entrenched doubters in the medical profession came into line. Now we accept routine preventive health programmes for antenatal and child care to the age of 14. This is the age when health care often stops: but surely it is the time when we should actually redouble our efforts to counter the positively unhealthy influences of adolescents and young adults. Sportloving, active children become sportwatching obese adults addicted to alcohol and tobacco while we agonize over the value or otherwise of routine adult health care.

Unfortunately some of the exponents of expensive multiphasic preventive screening have done disservice to those who would advocate a balanced low-cost programme of health promotion and maintenance. The expense has hardened informed opinions, including governments. Medical systems deny the general community the care that it should

311

receive, while the anxious wealthy develop an iatrogenic obsession with their serum cholesterol. On the other hand, despite the proven value of some manoeuvres such as the endocervical smear or continuing preventive immunization against tetanus, how many people in the community fail to have these? Still more hazardous, how many people with diagnosed essential hypertension fail to continue proper preventive maintenance care? In these cases who is to blame: the patient, the doctor, or the attitudes and available health care within the community?

Therefore the *principle* of preventive health screening in adults is not open to question. It is the frequency, the contents, the method, the effectiveness and cost to which we should address our argument. The least expensive, and the best person to undertake the responsibility is the individual's family doctor.

WHY A CHECK-UP?

There are many reasons why people want a check-up:

(1) They just feel that they should have one.
(2) Some constraint is put upon them, for example, an employer, a life assurance company, an organization catering for obese people, a spouse.
(3) They are worried about something. These fall into two categories; either they know what it is and are afraid to tell or they just do not know.
(4) While they are attending the doctor because of some minor problem it seems convenient or conventional at the time.
(5) There are all sorts of other reasons, including those who are converts to programmes of preventive care.

Whatever the reason, having told the doctor of the desire for a check-up, the patient may find himself in several different types of situation. For example:

(1) Because the doctor is educated to treat illness, and because the waiting room is full of such people requiring episodic patient patching, he is too busy to bother. In such a case the poor patient may discover himself ejected from the surgery door like the product of a sausage machine with a perfunctory reading of blood pressure and a not too gentle pat on the back!
(2) There may be a screening routine of varying grades of sophistication.
(3) Or the doctor may actually have time to sit back and listen.

In the latter case the doctor may discover the *real reason* why the patient has attended; but this takes a caring empathetic attitude, it takes skill and it takes *time*. It is only by this pathway that the real usefulness of a medical check-up may be obtained. Now both the patient and the doctor know exactly what goals they hope to achieve in any subsequent routine. And now we are in a position to consider the practical applications of what might follow. No medical check-up should ever proceed without this *initial interview*.

PLANS

As well as specific goals personal to the patient, the following example presents a plan for routine adult care with general goals for differing ages. It is taken from the second Australian edition of a *Manual for General Practice* (1982).

Consultation Plan I

General recommendations

1. Consider the health goals of the age group

2. History: additional to traditional medical data, lifestyle and environmental information is of great importance. Smoking, alcohol, diet – including fast foods and fat intake, physical activity at work and recreation, and personality type, are all important in determining predisposition to disease as well as providing an excellent basis for health promotion.

3. Physical examination including special tests

4. Counselling session
    (a) Explain the information which has been obtained
    (b) Provide health education applicable to age; e.g. self-examination
    (c) Individual counselling and treatment if required

Young adults 18–24 years: Examine once during this time, preferably before employment, university entrance, or marriage*

Health goals
Transition from adolescence to maturity with maximum physical, mental and emotional resources, and full capacity for healthy marriage, parenthood and social relationships

Professional services
1. Full standard examination
2. Height/weight relationship
3. Take blood for VD and cholesterol estimation
4. Advise dental examination
5. Other tests if indicated

Counselling
Diet, exercise, work, sex, smoking, alcohol, drugs, driving, occupational hazards, interpersonal relationships

*Note: Cervical smears and dental checks should be performed every 2 years

Young middle age 25–39 years: Examine every 5 years*

Health goals
Maximization of total potential, prolongation of the period of maximum energy
Prevention of chronic disease by health promotion and early detection and treatment

Counselling
Diet, exercise, smoking, alcohol, emotional aspects of health-related lifestyle
Self-examination: breasts, skin, testes, neck and mouth

Professional services
1. Full standard examination
2. Special tests
   Electrocardiogram
   Take blood (fasting) for cholesterol and triglyceride estimation
3. Advise dental examination
4. Other tests if indicated

Consultation Plan II

Older middle age 40–59 years: Full examination every 5 years with basic screening annually; and that for cervical, breast, and intestinal cancer every 2 years

Health goals
Prolongation of physical capacity and mental and social activity, including adjustment to the menopause
Early detection of any chronic major disease

Counselling
Self-monitoring reinforced by regular annual visits

Professional services
1. Full standard examination
2. Particular attention to cardiovascular disease, notably coronary disease, and its production by diet, inactivity, stress, and smoking
3. Careful screening for neoplastic disease
4. Other tests if indicated

Age 60–70 years: Full examination every 2 years

Health goals
To prolong physical, mental and social activity
To minimize handicapping effect of onset of chronic disease
To prepare for retirement

Counselling
Changing lifestyle, nutrition, absence of family, reduction of income, and decreased physical activity

Professional services
1. Full standard examination
2. As for previous age group, especially to detect early signs of neoplastic or other chronic conditions
3. **Annual** basic screening, influenza immunization, dental and foot care
4. Other tests if indicated

70 years and over: Full examination annually

Health goals
Prolongation of active independent life
To minimize chronic disease

Counselling
Nutrition, activity and living arrangements

Professional services
1. Full standard examination
2. Annual influenza immunization, dental and foot care

Note: All adults should be advised to maintain tetanus immunity

To be useful a check-up must therefore satisfy the following criteria:

(1) It must satisfy the patient's personal needs. Particularly important is the thorough assessment of any problems.
(2) It must be adjusted according to age and sex.
(3) It must not be repetitious. For example, it is useless testing for colour blindness more than once.
(4) It must be convenient to the patient, and possible for the doctor within the parameters of the work routine.
(5) Both patient and doctor must be motivated to the routine.
(6) It must encourage self-help.
(7) Nothing of importance should be omitted.

SUBSEQUENT HISTORY AND PHYSICAL EXAMINATION

Many of the questions which are routinely asked, and some of the things which we do with our patients are steeped in tradition, and require careful evaluation as to effectiveness.

Questionnaires, whether verbal, written or mechanical, must never be allowed to become boring routine, meaning nothing to either patient or doctor. They should be kept simple, must be seen to be understood by the patient, and if necessary explained; meaningful answers should be recorded.

Our recording systems should ensure accuracy of both positive and negative data. It is interesting to check back on a questionnaire, and surprising how often different or more accurate answers emerge from further close questioning.

Patients often have an entirely different set of answers to questions, for example, in a pre-employment medical examination versus application for a pension. Doctors too, appear to be afflicted with duplicity, the best example being different medical evidence for the plaintiff and defendant in legal action.

Written or computer questionnaires should only be used *after* an initial detailed personal history and an explanation to the patient that the routine applies in case something has been omitted or forgotten. Often a printed questionnaire taken home by the patient will prompt their relatives to detail important facts not remembered or known by the patient.

WHAT IS 'FULL STANDARD EXAMINATION'?

The routine is important to consider; what does one do in any particular case? An example is examination of the lungs, where there are some important conditions which cannot be detected except by X-ray or bronchoscopy. There are many examples, however, where physical examinations will reveal important findings in the absence of any history of illness. It is now generally accepted that routine chest X-rays are more dangerous and expensive than is warranted by the number of positive findings that are revealed. But it does not follow that the simple, non-dangerous, inexpensive use of six clinical senses and a stethoscope is rendered illogical and unnecessary. At the very least, if done properly, it draws the patient's attention to the need for preservation and enhancement of pulmonary function; and gives the doctor a solid basis for the later counselling session.

Similar considerations apply to palpation of the abdomen. It is noted in the Canadian Task Force study (1979) that examination of the abdomen and rectal examination have been deleted from recommended procedures. One wonders how many firm livers have been found in patients who confess to alcohol consumption. Certainly there are examples of this finding in people who have denied alcohol intake and later present a more truthful answer. One could argue that the accidental finding of a large secondary hepatic tumour by routine physical examination was too late for curative treatment. But is it? And supposing one does find such a case, is it not timely for the patient to be made aware of the situation? Or would readers want to pursue their own lives in ignorance?

Whatever the studies have shown, and these opinions are open to question, the very 'thoroughness' of a physical examination will in itself promote trust and empathy, and give an opportunity for further discussion.

LABORATORY INVESTIGATIONS

While there has been much argument, very few tests are of proven value in symptom-free people; and informed community opinion has now lessened pressure for multiphasic screening. The only test in adults which was confirmed by the Canadian Task Force (1979) as being of proved value, was mammography in women aged 50–59.

Other tests which are of importance in adults mainly apply to high risk groups. Some examples are:

(1) Haemoglobin estimation (?haemoglobinopathies).
(2) Test for faecal occult blood in persons aged over 45.
(3) Urine cytology.
(4) Tests for sexually transmitted diseases.

Of course it is obvious that testing may be required further to elucidate problems revealed by history and examination.

THE VALUE OF COUNSELLING

We have stated that there may be differing expectations by the patient requesting a check-up, and have stressed the importance of *initial interview*. Of equal importance is the relationship between doctor and patient *after* clinical evaluation and what actually happens at that time. Doctors performing health checks must be trained in counselling skills.

Some important points are:

(1) What are our goals, and have the patient's reasons for requesting a check-up been satisfied?

(2) How are the goals to be achieved? Perhaps the best examples are obesity, smoking, alcohol, or lack of exercise. With these problems how can a climate be created where people will actually lose weight (permanently) or stop smoking? It is the author's experience that we actually need to take *time* at this stage. It is useless spending time and money on identifying a problem, only to send the patient away with something like, 'All the tests are OK; but you had better stop smoking!' as the patient is ushered from sight and the doctor's conscience somehow satisfied.

In cases of obesity are you prepared actually to take *time* to work out the motivations, the eating habits and underlying causes, with your patients? Are you prepared to explain carefully the details of good eating habits, or to refer them to a dietician if you do not have the time? Unless the sort of answers posed by these questions are positive, the whole exercise of a medical check-up is useless. How often do we abrogate our responsibility for patients into the hands of editorial staff of fashionable magazines?

(3) We must recognize that fears may have been created by the mechanisms of questioning and physical testing. These require attention and suitable reassurance. It is important that delays from the time of

initial interview be kept to a minimum, especially if tests are performed. We must guard against the creation of iatrogenic obsession.

(4) The necessity for follow-up of any problems is vital. Patients with problems expect our help and interest. This continuing caring helpful attitude is fundamental.

The logistics of the check-up require study. Assuming 2000 patients on a doctor's list, and an accepted routine of health checks every 5 years, space for 400 annual examinations, or approximately eight per working week would be required. It is important that patterns of practice allow for this, and that the load is spread as evenly as possible. Appointment systems must be designed, and patients educated to make a special booking. The receptionist has a key role to play. Screening should be performed, where possible, when the patient attends, and recording systems should highlight dates of routine tests.

There is no value in perfunctory examinations on demand, when the doctor is too busy attending to illness; but there is value in educating people in the need for preventive medicine, including immunization programmes, and arranging that they can attend when they are motivated and when both the patient and the doctor have time to spend.

The clinic nurse has an important role to play in assisting; but for reasons already stated the patient must have a full opportunity for interview and examination by the doctor.

Leaving aside the individual patient's wants, community resources, customs and expectations require study. It is reasonable to expect changes in community attitudes being influenced by the whole medical profession; but the individual doctor would have little hope. He must therefore take cognizance of the norms of society in the country and district which he serves.

In summary and conclusion, a medical check-up, if properly managed with a strong accent on listening, patient participation, and counselling, especially if coordinated with self-help programmes, is useful.

References and further reading

Allen, D. W. (1979). Preventive care in general practice. *Aust. Fam. Physician*, **8,** 1118–1133

Breslow, L. and Somers, A. S. (1977). The lifetime health monitoring program. *N. Engl. J. Med.*, **296, No. 11,** 601–8

Bruhn, J. G. (1979). The complete health check-up: fad, fiction or fact. *Southern Med. J. (USA)*, **72, No. 7,** 865–8

Canadian Task Force on the Periodic Health Examination (1979). *Can. Med. Assoc. J.*, **121, No. 9,** 1193–1254

Carel, R. S. and Leshem, G. (1980). Evaluation of cost-effectiveness of an automated multiphasic health testing system. *Prev. Med.*, **9**, 689–697

Manual for General Practice. (1982) 2nd Australian edition. Beecham Research Laboratories

The case for screening

Nils Andersen

BASIC ESSENTIALS

In the following pages I use the word 'screening' to mean: to examine a group of the population in order to find precursors to, or manifest disease.

General practice is the natural area in which to screen, probably the only area where it is possible with good reason because it is here that such a varied majority of the population comes in contact with the health system. Also, patients coming to see the doctor are used to being examined. They are therefore more relaxed about the examination-process, for example, checking blood pressures, and the doctor is used to making children feel at ease.

The general practitioner is also in a good position to know the family and local community backgrounds.

Screening is not prophylactic, but when screening-examination is performed the conversation will often touch topics which have a prophylactic aim – 'Isn't my child too fat? Shall I give him/her different food? Is it wise to jog? What shall I eat? Shall I stop smoking?' – the more so as the screening-procedure is usually part of a consultation.

Screening is not a 'medical check-up'. Here a patient asks to have certain examinations done to obtain reassurance and guarantee that he is completely well. That is an absurd situation. Screening, on the other hand, is to detect diseases at early or even preclinical latent stages. Diseases most suitable for screening are those with prodromal features, with clearly defined latent phases, which untreated will lead to manifest disease (Figure 17.1).

In order for screening to be useful abnormal findings must be amenable to positive therapeutic measures, or continuous observation and follow-up. Screening procedures in general practice must be simple using every-day standard equipment, and they must be conducted with minimum trouble or discomfort to the patient. There must be accepted normal values, standardized and inexpensive methods of examinations.

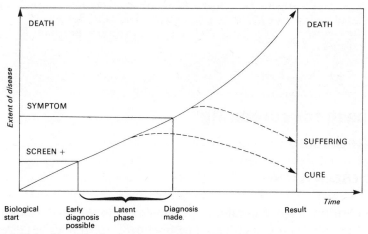

Figure 17.1 Stages in the development of the disease process

EXAMPLES OF SCREENING PROCEDURES

Antenatal care

In Denmark a pregnant woman attends for at least three consultations with her general practitioner. At the first consultation the blood is examined routinely for various factors. The procedures fulfil the criteria for good screening, and their significance is well-known. Later in pregnancy assessment of blood pressure, proteinuria and body weight are equally valuable.

Postnatal examination of children

Shortly after delivery of the baby the following screening is carried out: auscultation of the heart to eliminate congenital heartfailure; examination of the hip-joints to exclude congenital luxation of the hip (a simple procedure, where a positive finding leads to treatment which is almost trouble-free and will effect a complete cure instead of many years with pain and impairment of walking); and the examination of urine for phenylketonuria.

At the age of *5 weeks* most of the consultation will concentrate on checking for CNS defects, excluding them by testing a certain number of reflexes – standard examinations with a common aim. It is important to do these tests at this age because of the importance of early intervention for optimal development of the child. Screening must be directed at a group where positive finding lead to sensible and early treatment.

There is one particular estimation which it is important to carry out at all ages – the measuring of body length and height, which in early childhood is an important indicator of health, and later may also indicate disease. If, for instance, a prepubertal girl does not grow sufficiently, it may be a sign of Turner's syndrome – a rare condition but easy to diagnose, and then initiate vital treatment.

At *2 years old* an evaluation of speech may give a hint of a reduction in hearing, even if hearing tests have been made earlier.

At *3 years old* a vision test should be made. It may be difficult to make the child cooperate at this examination, but there is a good chance as the consultation takes place in familiar surroundings at the general practitioner's. It is important to diagnose visual defects in order to prevent amblyopia.

Preschool examination of children

In Denmark all children are offered regular, free consultations by the district nurse and the doctor at 5 weeks, 5, 10 and 15 months, 2, 3, 4 and 5 years. Even if these consultations are officially called 'prophylactic', they are essentially screening exercises (the doctor is paid fees for these examinations).

Smears – vaginal cytology

This screening procedure is ideal in many ways, but unfortunately there are problems with the implications of the importance of the slight changes in the cells, and the control and treatment that follow the finding of premalignant (suspect) cells in the smear. If, however, malignant cells are discovered, a complete therapeutic cure can be expected.

Blood pressure

Many people have hypertension without knowing it. It is important to check blood pressure in adults at regular intervals, to discover hypertension in its early phase before any complications arise. Early diagnosis leading to early treatment may improve prognosis.

Interpretation of blood pressure values demands personal knowledge of the patient, as many psychosocial conditions play a role. The continuing patient–doctor relationship and knowledge of the family, work situations (unemployment) and local community are important factors.

Breast screening

By teaching the woman to self-examine her breasts and encouraging her to do so every month, any lumps, whether benign or malignant, can be discovered early. This may lead to further examination, and an early diagnosis of operable breast cancer.

The case against a medical check-up
Michael D'Souza

INTRODUCTION

In the United Kingdom anyone wishing to have a full general check-up may have to pay for the service. For a country with a national 'health' service this might seem a somewhat paradoxical situation. Yet I believe that any dispassionate examination of the evidence in favour of such general check-ups would lead one to support a policy decision not to include general health screening as a useful routine procedure within a health service, and in this chapter I hope to be able to explain why.

ORIGINS OF SCREENING

The routine public health use of screening probably first became established in the nineteenth century when, in conjunction with quarantine regulations, it was used to check immigrants, particularly those trying to enter the United States. Its value in controlling epidemics was taken for granted and at no time was its effectiveness seriously questioned, let alone tested.

Also during the late nineteenth century the examination of recruits joining the armed forces was begun. The high levels of ill-health uncovered by this procedure, particularly during the Boer War, had a profound impact on political reformers and led to the screening of schoolchildren being introduced by Act of Parliament in 1907.

Very soon, industry began to use the medical examination both in a pre-employment and follow-up context. In part this may have been a self-defensive use of medicine by employers, the provision of pensions and compensation for war injury and disability having become a feature of life after the Boer War and industrial injury acquiring a similar, potentially costly, status. As a consequence, baseline information on the health of employees assumed new importance. Nevertheless, the most obvious value to industry of pre-employment screening was to select people who were fit for a particular job, while continued screening or health surveillance was seen as being useful in checking that the effects of disease, ageing, or work hazard had not altered this fitness. In many instances, however, such screening examinations came to be seen as a fringe benefit, particularly for the executive classes; screening was being viewed as a valuable service to the employee for ensuring his future health.

At the start of the twentieth century medical examinations began to be used by insurance companies to load the life premiums of poor-risk clients. This practice has grown continuously despite there being no published evidence for the financial value of such screening to the insurance business.

In 1926 a comprehensive experiment in total medical care, the Peckham Pioneer Health Centre, was begun. Essentially this was an experiment to set up a successful medical and social centre in the south of London, which provided not only ordinary general practice medical care and family planning advice, but also a periodic health overhaul for whole families. In addition it promoted 'social health' by establishing sports and gymnastic facilities with recreational and club activities, babysitting, health education, holidays and many other activities. The screening provided by this centre consisted both of formal medical examinations with laboratory tests, and of informal surveillance, particularly of children during their leisure activities. Pearse and Crocker (1943) writing about the Peckham experiment in 1943 after the centre closed during the Second World War, were emphatic that the purpose of their screening was not simply to act as a disease sieve, but rather that this was a natural, though incidental, part of their general aim of promoting health in those attending the health centre. They found that only 10.2 per cent of their urban population were without any abnormality: that 68.5 per cent of those with abnormalities did not know they had anything wrong; and that of the 21.3 per cent who did complain at the time of screening, only half had already taken their complaints to the existing medical services. It is perhaps not surprising that Pearse and Crocker observed then that 'nothing short of periodic health overhaul on a national scale can lead to the rational application of medical science for the elimination of sickness'.

MODERN APPROACHES

In America in 1942, the Kaiser Foundation began a small scale health service plan which later included screening as part of its services (Cutter *et al.*, 1973). Thus, although the earliest experiment in adult health check-ups were undertaken in Britain, it was the United States that pioneered the development of this activity and the bulk of the screening literature has originated from that country. Technical advances such as mass miniature radiography, biochemical autoanalysers and computer data handling have each been exploited by those planning screening programmes and the majority of the reports centred around such technical ways in which screening could be accomplished, rather than any evaluation of their effectiveness in achieving better health – indeed, this is often assumed to be a self-evident outcome of earlier diagnosis. The changing pattern of morbidity in the developed countries, with chronic degenerative diseases replacing the acute infections as the major health problems, encouraged many to believe that screening could produce considerable benefits. It now seems that every developed country is actively spending public funds on providing general health check-ups in some form for its populations.

THE MOTIVES FOR SCREENING

Much discussion as to the motives of screening has appeared in the literature. Sackett (1973) talked of four reasons for screening: (1) to influence the gamble of life insurance; (2) to protect people, other than the patient, as in industrial and public health screening; (3) to obtain clinical baselines; and (4) to do the patient some good – so called prescriptive screening. Clearly, there are other motives for screening such as financial reward, biological research, satisfying public and medical demand and gaining information for administrative purposes. Often an amalgam of these objectives is achieved as a spin-off from the activity rather than as a result of any specific design. Certainly most of the debates on the screening issue have centred around Sackett's last category – namely prescriptive screening. The general aim of prescriptive screening for doing good might encompass several separate medical goals. Most often the notion of secondary prevention is considered in this context of screening, early diagnosis being seen as postponing death or preventing disability.

But in the context of an infectious disease, such as tuberculosis, a public health dimension of 'prevention' is also added, since screening may result in removing the patient from where he would continue to act as a focus of infection in his community. Furthermore, tuberculosis screening also provides the opportunity to cure the patient of the disease, so cure and prevention were clearly definable goals. In more recent times interest has refocused on caring as opposite to curing, particularly on the care of the elderly and disabled. The notion of using screening for identifying people in need of care, or indeed, in itself providing a form of care, is receiving increasing attention. Lowther, Macleod and Williamson (1970) and Anderson (1976) have provided both evidence and opinion in favour of this.

In recent years the phrase 'automated multiphasic health testing' (AMHT) has featured increasingly in the American literature. The basis of this new term is the sophisticated use of the computer as an integral part of the screening operation. Much work has been done on cutting costs and producing quicker results by such devices as the mechanized administration of branching questionnaires by online computers. Improvement of the repeatability and reliability of tests has also been attempted, and the financial and epidemiological implications of a test's sensitivity (ability to identify true positives) and specificity (ability to exclude true negatives) has been extensively discussed and mathematically explored. Ironically, however, despite all this undoubted technical ingenuity, very few American authors have devoted time to evaluating seriously the health benefits of such prescriptive screening to their patients.

THE LITERATURE ON SCREENING

The majority of papers on screening fall into three groups: (1) simple accounts of uncontrolled experiments in screening for different diseases; (2) technological papers devoted to exploring the methodology of screening; (3) philosophical papers discussing the merits and demerits of screening services, tests and ideologies. All three of these groups can be considered as not primarily devoted to the issue of reporting on controlled scientific assessment of the value of screening and, as such, could be termed '*Non-Evaluative*', and will therefore not be as exhaustively reviewed as the much smaller groups of papers in which some form of scientific measurement of the value of screening has been attempted. To date, Australia, Canada, Denmark, England, Holland, Ireland, Israel, Italy, France, West Germany, Japan, New Zealand, Norway, Russia, South Africa, Scotland, Sweden, Thailand, the United States and Yugoslavia have all contributed to the non-evaluative literature on screening. The characteristic of most of these contributions, apart from originating nearly exclusively from wealthy developed countries, is that they share a common view that screening is a self-evident advance in medical philosophy and technology.

SCREENING METHODOLOGY

There is a large number of publications devoted to the evaluation of the tests and other tools used in screening services. For example, Moskowitz *et al.* (1976) present the results of a good study demonstrating the relatively poor efficiency of thermography as a means of screening for carcinoma of the breast. Rautaharju (1977, 1978) discussed the drawbacks of the ECG in the context of screening for coronary disease. Hsieh (1974) however, in reviewing all the screening tests used in a Baltimore Hospital Screening Service, calculated *false-positivity* ratings by comparing initial screening findings with final diagnosis on follow-up. The worst test was tonometry which was 100 per cent false-positive. Others mentioned included vision testing 31.8 per cent false-positive, spirometry 29 per cent, audiometry 23.1 per cent, urinalysis 49.6 per cent, blood pressure 6.2 per cent, X-ray 10.3 per cent, ECG only 0.1 per cent, psychiatric testing 10.2 per cent, visual fields 39.1 per cent, cervical (Pap) smear 42.8 per cent, VDRL 60.0 per cent. *False-negativity* is more rarely examined, though Schor *et al.* (1964) reported that over half the people dying of cancer and heart disease had been passed fit within the last year at their previous annual physical. The view that tonometry is an extremely poor screening test is further supported by other work where the conclusions are that monophasic screening using this test produces a very low yield of pathology, and that the newly discovered glaucomatous patients would have probably presented to the regular services sufficiently early to have made the screening service unnecessary.

For other tests, there is much doubt of their value as screening instruments. Urine testing for instance has been described by Fraser, Smith and Peake (1977) as adding to the cost of a screening service without giving significant benefits.

More interesting has been the work of Bradwell, Carmalt and Whitehead (1974) who showed that 35.5 per cent of 200 patients with abnormal biochemical screening tests were healthy on follow-up 5 years later.

Other tests have been reviewed in great detail, perhaps the most well known being cervical cytology which now has a large bibliography entirely of its own. A recent review of the epidemiological difficulties of assessing the value of this screening procedure in the absence of controlled trials, is given by Gardner and Lyon (1977). They point out that the incidence of carcinoma of the cervix has been steadily decreasing since 1946 irrespective of cervical screening.

THE EVALUATIVE LITERATURE ON SCREENING INSURANCE MEDICALS

Probably the earliest attempt at a measured evaluation of the efficacy of screening was the work of Knight (1921). He reported on follow-up data of 6000 policy-holders of the Metropolitan Life Insurance Company who had been given physical examinations in 1914 and 1915 at the insurance company's expense. After $5\frac{1}{2}$ years 217 had died, whereas, he calculated that 303 deaths would have been expected in 'persons of this class'. He went on to suggest that this 28 per cent reduction in mortality had a monetary value of $126 000 in reduced life insurance claims. Since the examinations had only cost the company $40 000 he expressed the opinion that screening was a cost-beneficial exercise for insurance companies with an over 200 per cent return on capital. This conclusion is highly suspect by today's standards, as it hinges totally on the accuracy of the calculated expected death rate. Recent published data from British insurance sources (*Continuous Mortality Investigation Reports*, 1973) fails to reveal any significant difference between those policy-holders undergoing insurance medicals and those who were issued without screening. Here again, however, there is no way of being certain that one is comparing like with like.

Following up 451 executives who had had periodic health check-ups Thorner and Crumpacker (1961) reported 11 observed deaths over $4\frac{1}{2}$ years compared to 25 expected. But two large Scandinavian studies (Jungblut, Enterline and Danber, 1960; and the Varmland Survey, 1971) concluded that screening had no impact on mortality.

A similar study to that of Knight was reported by Roberts *et al.* (1969) on a population of 20 648 men who were having 'employer-sponsored' periodic health examinations. Again, these authors reported a reduction of the actual to expected deaths, but they were more cautious in their conclusions and recommended that properly controlled prospective studies be undertaken.

MONOPHASIC OR SINGLE DISEASE SCREENING STUDIES

Carefully controlled trials should be able to overcome the shortcomings of the studies mentioned above. Shapiro *et al.* (1973), in a large controlled trial demonstrated that it was possible to delay significantly the mortality from carcinoma of the breast in women aged 50–59 years old by a mass screening programme. However, not only were the capital and manpower required to achieve this success beyond the resources of most countries but there remains controversy over the possible hazards due to the X-rays used in mammography which is probably the best available screening method.

In other studies of single test or single disease screening, results have been less convincing. Brett (1968) evaluated the effects of six monthly chest X-rays on preventing death from bronchial carcinoma and concluded there was no measurable benefit. No adequate controlled studies are available for cervical carcinoma screening, and the only controlled trial on blood pressure screening (D'Souza, Swann and Shannon, 1976) failed to reveal that such screening had any impact on either individual or population blood pressures.

Johnstone and Goldberg (1976) evaluated psychiatric screening in general practice. They administered a general health questionnaire (GHQ) to detect minor psychiatric disorders in 1093 *consulting* general practice patients; 32 per cent were found to have overt psychiatric disorders and a further 11 per cent had latent psychiatric disorders. This latter group with latent disorders was randomly divided into control and study groups. Case detection and treatment were found to be beneficial with a duration of episode of the disorder being much shorter for patients whose disorder was recognized by the general practitioner. For patients with more severe disorders there were significant differences between the two groups 1 year later. The 'detected' group increased their consultation rates for emotional complaints but not their overall consultation rates.

MULTIPHASIC COMMUNITY STUDIES

In the field of multiphasic or general health screening in the community, three major controlled trials have so far been completed, two in the United States (Cutler *et al.*, 1977; and Olsen, Kane and Procter, 1976), and one in Great Britain.

A study has been started in Yugoslavia but has not yet published any results. It will be of great interest as it has been undertaken on a random sample of the town of Titograd where initial results of screening have revealed a relatively high prevalence of tuberculosis (Thorner and Val, 1973). When final results are available they should reveal whether screening is of measurable value in such regions of high tuberculosis prevalence, especially now that the work of Horwitz (1974) has thrown so much doubt on the value of tuberculosis screening in a more developed country such as Denmark.

Kaiser Permanente Study (USA)

As mentioned previously, the screening service undertaken by the Kaiser Permanente Group in California in 1941 was among the earliest to become established. The decision to try to evaluate the medical benefits of this screening was not taken until 1964, over two decades later. By this time, screening had become an accepted part of a commercially successful middle-class medical service (Cutler *et al.*, 1977).

By 1978 reports on comparing screened persons with controls showed no differences in mortality rates and uncertain results for morbidity and cost-effectiveness.

The Salt Lake City Study

Olsen, Kane and Proctor (1976) reported a truly controlled study of the impact of screening healthy subjects, with the evaluation undertaken over a much shorter time period.

Three populations representing three different social and economic groups and systems of health-care were compared. First a random sample of 200 families from a neighbourhood health centre in Salt Lake City was chosen to represent a low-income group enrolled in a prepaid health-care programme. The second group of 200 families was also of low income but was not enrolled in any health-care programme. The third group was a middle-income group of 188 families and were volunteers from employees and families of a local utility company. Within each group, each family member over 18 years of age was initially interviewed for baseline data and then randomly allocated to either experimental or control groups. The experimental subjects were urged by telephone to obtain free multiphasic screening at the health centre.

A year after this screening a second interview was undertaken on both the experimental and control groups. Complete data was obtained in 84 per cent of the original sample. Change in health status between the initial and final interview was assessed using (1) a questionnaire health status index; (2) number of disability days caused by illness; (3) patterns of health care utilization; (4) health knowledge; and (5) a scale of hypochondriasis. In addition, the physicians of the subjects in this study were also interviewed about their knowledge of the abnormalities found at the screening and about what further testing they had ordered. The findings of this study were almost totally negative, with no significant differences between the screening and control populations except that the former actually spent significantly more days in hospital.

THE SOUTH-EAST LONDON SCREENING STUDY

In 1977, the largest truly randomized controlled trial of general health screening was reported (South-East London Screening Study Group, 1977) on the value of introducing prescriptive general health screening for middle-aged men and women. Two group practices in south London took part in the study. Using age–sex registers, all persons aged 40–64 years in 1967 were identified and the families in each general practitioner list were randomly allocated into two equal groups. The screening group, numbering 3297 individuals, was invited to attend a screening clinic which was held in the evenings in a local infant welfare clinic. Table 17.1 shows the screening tests that were performed.

Table 17.1   Content of multiphasic screening

Self-administered symptom questionnaire
Interviewer-administered questions on occupational data
Anthropometry: height, weight, skinfold thickness
Visual testing: near, distant, visual fields
Audiometry
Chest X-ray
Lung function tests
ECG
Blood pressure
Blood tests: haemoglobin, packed cell volume (pcv), blood urea, random blood sugar, protein-
    bound iodine, serum uric acid
Stool for occult blood
Basic clinical examination: skin, mouth, teeth, joints, abdomen for hernias, legs for varicose veins,
    breast and pelvic examination

The initial screening took place in 1967–68, and 2 years later, the screening group was invited to attend a second screening clinic. Together, these two screening sessions constituted the 'treatment' under assessment in the controlled trial. All the information collected at both screening sessions was passed to the general practitioners who decided on the further investigations, diagnoses and treatments that would be appropriate.

From the first day of screening, information was collected at 6 monthly intervals on the following 'outcome measures' of screening: consultations with the general practitioners, hospital admissions, periods of certified absence due to sickness, and deaths. In addition, all individual departures from the study population were carefully recorded.

Because of the relatively high migration rate of the study population from the area (20 per cent over the first 5 years), it was decided to employ an additional assessment of outcome before the residual population became unrepresentative of the original. This took the form of a direct survey of both the screening and control groups 2 years after the second screening.

Results

Response to screening

Of the 3297 individuals invited to the first screening, 2420 (73.4 per cent) attended, while of the 2677 individuals invited to the second screening, 1775 (65.5 per cent) appeared. At the survey (for which especially intensive encouragement was offered), 4026 (82.4 per cent) of the 4887 people invited attended.

Yield and management of disease at screening

At the initial screening an average of 2.3 'diseases' per person was found. Just over half (53 per cent) of this morbidity was previously unknown to the general practitioners. Similar proportions (about 5 per cent) of both the known and unknown abnormalities were considered clinically 'serious'. At the second screening 2 years later, the yield of both total and unknown morbidity was somewhat lower than at the first screening. Minimal new therapeutic action was taken on the basis of the abnormalities revealed with two exceptions: anaemia and high blood pressure. Advice on stopping smoking and weight reduction was given to all for whom it was appropriate.

The controlled trial design of the study permitted comparison of the screening and control groups with respect to the various outcome measures (morbidity findings at the survey, general practice consultation rates, hospital admission rates, sickness absence and mortality rates). The analyses were performed on the data collected over the first 9 years from the start of the study.

Comparisons at survey (1972–73)

The health survey of both screening and control groups revealed no significant differences in either the prevalence of symptoms or disability.

General practice consultation rates

Women consulted their general practitioners more frequently than men, but there were no statistically significant differences in either the overall or disease-specific consultation rates between the screening and control groups.

Hospital admission rates

There were no statistically significant differences between the screening and control groups in either the overall or disease-specific consultation rates between the screening and control groups.

Certified sickness absence rates

There were no statistically significant differences in certified sickness absence rates between the screening and control populations.

Mortality rates

There were no statistically significant differences in the mortality experienced by the screening and control groups. Analysis by cause of death also failed to reveal significant differences. An interesting finding was the consistently higher mortality experienced by those who had refused screening.

The findings of this study confirmed the general pattern of results reported from elsewhere in that the impact of screening a middle-aged population on measurable indices of health is minimal.

SUMMARY OF RESULTS FROM THE LITERATURE

From this review of the literature, while it is important to state that no *final* answer is yet available to the question of whether general health testing in middle age could under ideal circumstances be of value, the consistently negative results found in all the proper controlled studies do suggest that it is most unlikely that any similar service to that employed by them would prove to be of general benefit. Perhaps as a final exercise it might be worth trying to assess the reasons for this and in addition to discuss possible harmful effects that might ensue from the introduction of mass screening.

POSSIBLE REASONS FOR SCREENING BEING INEFFECTIVE

One can speculate about many reasons why screening services can fail to be of demonstrable worth in controlled trials, but there are other issues more profoundly related to the nature of the situation in which screening takes place that may be the real causes for its failure.

The first reason for the likely failure of screening and almost certainly the most important, is related to the effectiveness of modern medicine itself. Serious appraisal of the management of many of the most serious diseases at which screening services are aimed, such as ischaemic heart disease and cancer, would suggest that their treatment generally is in-effective, irrespective of what stage it is commenced, or how thoroughly it is pursued. The high mortality and morbidity rates from these condi-tions are clearly related to our basic ignorance about their aetiologies and pathophysiological mechanisms and require further research.

The second reason for the failure of screening is an equal challenge to research. Although it would appear that where we have epidemiological evidence that certain factors such as smoking and hypertension are involved in the aetiology of important diseases, we are still a long way from developing effective means of modifying patients' behaviour over the long term so that these factors can be consistently reduced.

The final reason relates more specifically to the adequacy of screening itself. There is at present no good evidence to suggest that the methods of screening are as well developed as many people assume. In one study by Schor et al. (1964) in the United States the relative inadequacy of screen-ing at detecting really important diseases was amply illustrated. These workers compared the death certification of people dying 1 year after a periodic health examination with the records made at the time of their screening. Only 58 per cent of those whose death was due to ischaemic heart disease had had this diagnosis made on screening, and only 43 per cent whose death was due to a neoplasm had had this detected at screening. In fact, overall, in only 51 per cent of all the deaths irrespective of cause had the screening service made any relevant ante-mortem diagnosis.

POSSIBLE HARMFUL EFFECTS OF A SCREENING SERVICE

If screening services are at present generally ineffective at improving health, is there any reason to suppose that they might have any harmful effects?

One study by Haynes *et al.* (1978) did provide positive evidence of screening producing a measurable harmful effect. In this study 208 Canadian steelworkers were labelled as hypertensive after screening. Of those, 138 were new cases and 70 had been told previously they were hypertensive. Comparing work records with the year prior to screening, it was found that the newly diagnosed cases showed an 80 per cent increase in days off sick in the year after being labelled hypertensive. This was equivalent to the loss of a whole working week. Apart from this, however, there is little evidence of general health screening having been shown to be harmful. Although there seems little doubt that much anxiety and possibly iatrogenic hazards have been caused by its insensitive application.

CONCLUSIONS

It seems reasonable to conclude that the introduction of a mass health screening service for the middle-aged would be ineffective and unlikely to prove of any general benefit. Although it is possible that some individuals might receive advantages, it seems equally likely that others would be disadvantaged.

The effectiveness of monophasic or single test screening has not yet been adequately studied in routine service in this age-group. However, for breast cancer screening in the over-50s, there has been controlled trial evidence of efficacy, and case-finding for psychiatric disorder may also be of value. Also, hypertension screening (and/or case-finding) seems to be worthy of further study, since there have recently been new developments in therapy and a fresh understanding of the problems of compliance. It is because development of new techniques in both screening and medical therapeutics can be expected, that it is in no way possible to view the current literature as a once-and-for-all condemnation of the worth of screening. Indeed, it is to be hoped that advances will be made which will enable further controlled trials to be conducted which have good prospects of showing measurable benefits in both effectiveness and efficiency from mass screening.

Until such a time I would argue that we should confine our screening to a few well-chosen conditions. Although it has been argued that it does much to allay the anxieties of our patients, as a method of anxiolysis screening is unproven, expensive and potentially meddlesome. It would seem much more sensible to try to prevent anxiety by searching for ways of creating more self-supporting personal communities within our cities, similar to that attempted by the Peckham experiment, and to delay the introduction of general screening until it can be shown to be of use.

References

Anderson, F. (1976). The effect of screening on the quality of life over seventy. *J. R. Coll. Physicians*. **10,** 161–169

Bradwell, A. R., Carmalt, M. H. B. and Whitehead, T. P. (1974). Explaining the unexpected abnormal results of biochemical profile investigations. *Lancet*, **2,** 1071–1074

Brett, G. Z. (1968). The value of lung cancer detection by six monthly chest radiography. *Thorax*, **23,** 414

Continuous Mortality Investigation Reports No 1. (1973). (London and Edinburgh: Institute of Actuaries.)

Cutler, J. L. *et al.* (1973). Multiphasic check-up evaluation study 2: Disability and chronic disease after seven years of multiphasic health check-ups. *Prev. Med.*, **2,** 207–220

D'Souza, M. F., Swan, A. V. and Shannon, D. J. (1976). Screening for hypertension in general practice: The results of a long-term controlled trial. *Lancet*, **1,** 1228–1232

Fraser, C. G., Smith, B. C. and Peake, M. J. (1977). Effectiveness of an outpatient urine screening programme. *Clin. Chem.*, **23, 12,** 2216–2218

Gardner, J. W. and Lyon, J. L. (1977). Efficacy of cervical cytologic screening in the control of cervical cancer. *Prev. Med.*, **6,** 487–499

Haynes, B. R., Sackett, D. L., Wayne Taylor, D., Gibson, E. S. and Johnson, A. L. (1978). Absenteeism from work after the detection and labelling of hypertensives. *N. Engl. J. Med.*, **299,** 14, 741–744

Horwitz, O. (1974). Long-range evaluation of a mass screening program. *Am. J. Epidemiol.*, **100,** 1

Hsieh, R. K. (1974). Multiphasic health testing in a public health service hospital. *Med. Instrument.*, **S,** 5

Johnstone, A. and Goldberg, D. (1976). Psychiatric screening in general practice. *Lancet*, **1,** 605–608

Jungblut, E. J., Enterline, P. E. and Danber, R. T. (1960). Study of the Special Effect of Periodic Physical Examinations on Mortality Rates. Paper presented at the Annual Meeting of the American Public Health Association, November 1

Knight, A. S. (1921). Value of periodic medical examination. *Statist. Bull. Metropolitan Life Insurance Company*, **2,** 1

Lowther, C. P., MacLeod, R. D. M. and Williamson, J. (1970). Evaluation of early diagnostic services for the elderly. *Br. Med. J.*, **3,** 275

Moskowitz, Myron *et al.* (1976). Thermographic diagnosis of breast cancer. *N. Engl. J. Med.*, **295,** 5

Olsen, D. M., Kane, R. L. and Procter, P. H. (1976). A controlled trial of multiphasic screening. *N. Engl. J. Med.*, **294,** 17, 925–930

Pearse, I. and Crocker, L. (1943). *The Peckham Experiment.* (London: George Allen and Unwin)

Rautaharju, P. M. (1977). Value of the electrocardiogram in population studies: can computers help? *Heart Bull.*, **8,** 97–98

Rautaharju, P. M. (1978). Use and abuse of electrocardiographic classification systems in epidemiologic studies. *Eur. J. Cardiol.* **8/2,** 155–171

Roberts, N. J., Ipsen, J., Elsom, K., Clark, T. and Yanagawa, H. (1969). Mortality among males in periodic-health-examination programs. *N. Engl. J. Med.*, **281,** 20

Sackett, D. (1973). Periodic health examinations and multiphasic screening. *Canad. Med. Assoc. J.*, **109,** 1124

Schor, S. S. *et al.* (1964). An evaluation of the periodic health examination. *Ann. Intern. Med.*, **61,** 999–1005

Shapiro, S., Strax, P., Venet, L., and Venet, M. (eds.) (1973). *Proceedings of the Seventh National Cancer Conference.* p. 663. (Philadelphia)

South-East London Screening Study Group (1977). A controlled trial of multiphasic screening in middle age. *Int. J. Epidemiol.*, **6,** 357

Thorner, R. M. and Crumpacker, E. L. (1961). Mortality and periodic examination of executives. *Arch. Environ. Health*, **3,** 523–525

Thorner, R. M., Djordjevic, D., Vuckmanovic, C., Pesic, B., Culafic, B. and Mark, F. (1973). A study to evaluate the effectiveness of multiscreening in Yugoslavia. *Prev. Med.*, **2,** 295–301

Varmland Survey (1971). *Socialstyrelsen Redovisar*, **23,** Stockholm

Commentary

The case *for* the medical check-up is put by two firm enthusiasts who describe how they carry out such exercises in their own practices with satisfaction.

The case *against* the medical check-up is put in a devastatingly argued collection of report upon report that fails to provide any measurable significant benefits.

Regular contacts with our patients are beneficial providing that they have some modest objectives that can be achieved – for example, opportunities for patients to air any personal problems are most useful, as are opportunities to enquire upon and correct bad smoking habits, encourage weight-reduction, if overweight, measure blood pressure (every 5 years or so), carry out cervical smears (every 5 years or so) – but anything else has to be proved that it is cost-effective and therefore viable.

18 Solo practice or group practice?

The issues

The issues here are comparatively clear-cut: solo practice is good for the patient and the physician! Group-practice is even better for physicians and patients!

The case for solo practice
Susi Rottenberg

Single-handed practice has fallen out of favour; it is no longer fashionable. It is disappearing like the corner shop to be replaced by the medical supermarket. The pundits tell us that good medicine can only be practised by groups of doctors working together, preferably in large impersonal health centres. The doctor working alone is derided, scorned and threatened with extinction.

Medicine has changed a great deal over the centuries. Procedures very prevalent at one time have fallen into disrepute. Bloodletting, once a common treatment, is now rarely used. Drugs once universally used have proved to be ineffective, if not actually dangerous to the patient and have been replaced. Medicine is a living, changing science. It is vital to keep an open mind, not to adhere to strong views dogmatically and unflinchingly. At present the pendulum is swinging away from single-handed practice but it may swing back.

I have had experience of working in a group of three doctors, in a partnership with one other doctor and, for the last 13 years, in single-handed practice. Very few doctors working in groups and challenging the right of the single-handed doctor to exist have had such varied personal experience. My information about single-handed practice is all drawn from first-hand experience and is not vague, academic and theoretical.

Doctors are as diverse as their patients. Some doctors prefer working together in groups and would rather retire than work alone, others prefer single-handed practice. An unhappy state of affairs would be produced if a doctor who functions better working alone were forced into group practice. Surely in the wide spectrum of modern primary care there is room for all types of practice and their very variety enriches medicine as a whole. There must be a niche where the single-handed doctor can contribute usefully.

Many patients actually prefer being looked after by one doctor and one doctor alone. Many famous personages in bygone ages have had their own personal physicians and have developed a trusting happy relationship with them. This type of relationship, a mixture of trust, friendship and confidence is not possible if the patient has to be looked after by a whole group of doctors.

The patient is delighted that his own doctor has known him for years, that he knows his past history and that of his family. The patient feels more relaxed and able to confide in his doctor if there is this one-to-one relationship. The views of the patient should be taken into consideration when formulating the structure of general practice. I find the image of the family doctor as opposed to the general practitioner or, worse still, the 'head of the primary care team' very appealing. The doctor who really knows his patient, his family circumstances, his background and environment has a useful peg on which to pin his diagnoses. This knowledge is of inestimable value in assessing a patient's illness, and how the patient and his family will react to it. This knowledge tempers the science of medicine and elevates it into an art. It is one of the real advantages that the general practitioner has over the hospital doctor. I cannot stress too strongly how important it it to have a thorough understanding of the patient as a human being. This familiarity with the patient and his family is vital in deciding how to care for the patient. It is endlessly useful in cases of marital breakdown and in the case of the old and terminally ill.

It is because of his unique position that the solo practitioner has a great advantage in really knowing his patient. The single-handed doctor deals with a small circumscribed group of patients and over many years gets to know them really well. The patient who is looked after by a large group of doctors cannot possibly obtain the same degree of personal care. If four to five doctors work together and look after 12 000–15 000 patients, it is impossible for them to be acquainted to the same degree with such a vast army of patients as is the single-handed doctor looking after 2500–3000 patients alone.

I know most of my patients by name, I know the medical history of most of them, I know their background, their housing conditions, their spouses and their children. I feel a rapport with them that I could not feel working in the impersonal atmosphere of group practice.

About 40 per cent of my consultations deal with emotional, psychiatric or social problems. Many of the problems with which I deal are not really even of a medical nature, and my special knowledge of my patients is very helpful in coping with them.

If one sees the role of the doctor as adviser, teacher, friend as well as physician, these diverse functions are better fulfilled if one has a first-hand knowledge of the patient.

I have questioned many of my patients and they tell me that they enjoy the atmosphere in a surgery where they feel personally known and familiar. They like to be greeted by name, both by doctor and reception-ist. They find this more agreeable than the impersonal atmosphere pre-vailing in large group practice where the patients feel they are a number, a case and not a human being. The main moan of the patients looked after by a large group is the lack of continuity of care, the not knowing which doctor they will see when they come to surgery. This is not a happy state of affairs for the patient.

There are many bonuses for the doctor who elects to work in single-handed practice. He is a complete autocrat. He can decide all practice policy. He can chose all ancillary staff and decide what type of staff would best fit in with his practice. He can chose, refurbish, equip and reorganize the practice premises as and when he wishes without consul-tation with a group of doctors. He can indulge his own special interest in any speciality from gynaecology to dermatology. If he is willing to be available he can do home maternity deliveries. Many groups are reluc-tant to do this. If one works alone one can please oneself. Holiday arrangements are greatly simplified if there are no holiday rotas to be observed. The single-handed doctor decides when and for how long he feels he can go away, and then arranges a locum. There is no haggling with the other partners about who has the Christmas or school holidays. Holiday locums provide no problems if one is well organized. I advertised 8 years ago for a locum and found a doctor working in a large group practice in North England. He was entitled to 6 weeks annual leave but could not afford to be idle for so long; ever since then he has covered 3 weeks' holiday yearly for me. The patients have come to know him and he knows many of them. It works perfectly. In a group a locum is rarely employed. Doctors double up for each other during holiday periods and have to shoulder an increased workload; this is not particularly conducive to good medicine. Similarly, in times of illness I have no alternative but to arrange a locum. In a group practice the illness of one partner is usually covered by the others with, again, an increased workload for the remaining partners.

At a luncheon party recently I was introduced to a well-known medical politician, the senior partner in a group of eight. He told me that single-handed doctors should be abolished. He maintained that single-handed doctors were unable to provide adequate cover for their patients at all times. He looked at me accusingly and demanded who was looking after my practice while I was out enjoying myself. I was able to reply that another doctor who was a member of my rota was doing so. I could have asked who was looking after his patients. Certainly it was a member of his massive rota – one doctor stuck with covering for thousands of patients at weekends. I fail to see why my method of individual general practitioners banding together to form their own rota is in any way different or worse than his. No doctor is capable of working 24 hours a day, 7 days a week. There has to be a rota or a deputy for both the single-handed and the group.

Money is the root of all evil, and is often the cause of disagreements between doctors working together. Financial disputes about how to share out practice and private earnings do not occur if one works alone.

Premises are simpler to obtain and organize for the single-handed. The doctor can either practice from a health centre where all facilities are provided, or he can work from his own premises. It is easier to convert premises if one only has to provide for a single doctor. It is extremely expensive to convert existing buildings for group use. All accommodation must be at ground-floor level, as patients cannot be expected to climb stairs, and lifts are extremely expensive and often impossible to install. Purpose-built premises are ideal but it is a great undertaking to build what amounts to a mini-hospital with staff rooms, dressing rooms, examination rooms, a large waiting area and many consulting rooms. Most existing properties just do not lend themselves to conversion into group practice premises. This is so even more in Central London where I work. Here premises are expensive, land on which to build unobtainable and space very much at a premium.

Every doctor attracts a different type of patient and all practices are subtly different. The doctor working alone can soon establish a practice consisting of patients with whom he has a special rapport; the large group never has this unique ability. Keeping in touch with colleagues and keeping up to date with all recent developments is easily possible for the solo doctor. Although one works alone it is very easy to discuss cases with colleagues in a social setting. There are many medical societies and postgraduate meetings where the doctor can meet colleagues and keep abreast. It is very simple to do a clinical assistantship in the local hospital in the speciality of one's choice and so, although working alone, maintain real contact with new developments. If I have a diagnostic problem with a patient the registrar or consultant at the nearby teaching hospital is only too willing to discuss it and advise me. It is absolute nonsense to say that working alone is synonymous with clinical isolation.

There are many disadvantages to group practice. The main one is the awful problem of fitting in with a large number of other doctors. There must always be a senior partner who organizes the group. This can be a source of friction. The whole organization tends to become a massive un-wieldy arrangement with many doctors and ancillary staff working to-gether in a hospital atmosphere with many unpleasant political rivalries.

At the present time we in Britain are producing 4000 doctors a year. This is a surplus of 1300 to our needs. Already there are 100–500 appli-cants for desirable positions in general practice. With this surplus comes abuse of the newly qualified doctor. This has happened before and may soon become rife again in group practice.

In single-handed practice the doctor cannot abuse or be unfair to himself, but in a group the junior doctor can be very abused, and in a situation of too many doctors chasing too few jobs things will become worse.

When I first entered partnership the agreement I signed was not one of partnership but more one of slavery. My senior partner was allowed 6 weeks annual leave, I was allowed 3 weeks. If he was ill I covered, if I was ill I had to provide and pay for a locum. I did all daytime calls. Parity was to be in 7 years and I received a third share of practice income until that time. Any private practice was shared in the following way, the senior partner kept all the extra money that he earned in private practice, I shared all I earned with him. After a partnership like this, it is no wonder I opted for single-handed practice.

I have a friend who worked hard and devotedly in a group. This consisted of two older doctors and himself. He wanted to reorganize the practice – abolish Sunday morning and Saturday evening surgeries, arrange an appointment system and redecorate the surgery. The older partners disapproved and made life impossible for him, and he eventually left the practice and in early middle-age established himself in a new – single-handed – practice.

Another acquaintance had a large well-organized single-handed prac-tice. She decided it would be pleasant to share the workload which she felt had become too much for her to deal with alone and so took in a lady partner. Disputes soon followed; the partners became jealous of each others, one partner accepted an expensive present from a patient and the other doctor felt this was not a correct thing to do. Soon the receptionists took sides, and the doctors ceased to speak to each other. The atmosphere in the practice became increasingly acrimonious and eventually after months of quarrelling the partners went to arbitration and the partnership was split down the middle. The practice was effectively ruined for both partners.

In another case I know, a group of three doctors is working together. One partner is over 80, not capable of coping with a full workload, the other partner is a woman who has young children and is unwilling to do evening or weekend cover. The whole workload of the group is on the shoulders of the remaining male partner. This group cares for more than 8000 patients; so virtually one man cares for this number and this cannot be deemed to be good medicine.

Groups are often formed so that there is a sleeping partner. A doctor who is a partner in name only, and who spends most of his time in private practice, medical politics or following some other interests. This leaves the remaining members of the group again with an intolerably increased workload.

There are doctors with rather abrasive natures who would never survive life in a group practice. Even the most difficult personality finds it hard to disagree with himself.

I am not condemning group practice. Certainly many groups function well, but there are many that do not, and few outsiders can see beneath the surface and recognize what an iceberg of human misery can exist in some groups.

The single-handed doctor must be self-reliant, confident, and experienced. He must be willing to give a great deal of himself to his work and his patients. It is not a situation that suits every doctor. Life is not black or white, it is mainly grey. There are good groups and bad, but there are also good and bad single-handed doctors. The single-handed doctor has a contribution to make to modern medicine. Most medical politicians work in groups. They would otherwise not have time to sit on committees or indulge in medical politics. They advocate group practice only. The single-handed doctor is too busy doing medicine, looking after his patients, doing surgeries and house calls to have time to spend several afternoons sitting on committees. His voice is not so loud that it can be heard, so his views are not heard to the same extent.

The pressures of solo practice are great but so are the rewards: job satisfaction is enormous, small is beautiful. I prefer to work alone and if I can provide a satisfactory service to my patients and they are happy I feel I should be free to work in a manner that suits me so well and to continue to be a living anachronism.

The case for group practice:
the future practice model in family medicine

Roger A. Rosenblatt

The following exposition is an argument for group practice as the preferential organizational mode for the delivery of medical services by family practitioners. This paper is not, nor is it intended to be, a scholarly analysis of the relevant literature comparing different organizational structures. This piece is opinionated, onesided, and occasionally intemperate. Its goal is to stimulate comment and controversy. I hope the reader enjoys the spirit of the debate and forgives the author any rhetorical excess into which he may tumble while pursuing the argument. In my own defence, I must cite the instructions tendered by this book's distinguished editor: '*No*, it is *not* to be a scholarly piece but more as a tongue-in-cheek exercise ... It should be presented as a debating piece ...'. So, tongue firmly in cheek, I proclaim the undeniable superiority of group practice.

Modern medical care requires that physicians belong to organized group practices. Solo practice is at best a nostalgic adherence to the patterns of a long-dead and unlamented era; at worst, it is a recipe for eccentricity, obsolescence, and incompetence. The rapid flux of medical knowledge, the responsibility for continuing comprehensive patient care, and the uncertainty which permeates medical diagnosis and treatment require that the physician have an ongoing, intimate, and open relationship with his peers. Only by practising in a group setting can these essential components of effective medical practice be assured.

The arguments for group practice rest upon the observation that in medicine the whole is greater than the sum of its parts. In group practice, the individual physician is able simultaneously to meet his responsibilities to his patients and his family, to develop fully his own interests and capabilities, and maintain a healthful and sustaining lifestyle. In the following paragraphs, I briefly explore the different areas in which group practice makes the difference between mediocrity and excellence, stultification and growth.

CONTINUED INTELLECTUAL DEVELOPMENT

Man is a social organism. He flourishes in the companionship of his fellows and languishes in isolation. Social and intellectual interchange is the basis of social stability and progress, and medicine is a prime example of this observation. The art and science of medicine are learned largely in the apprenticeship mode; experienced physicians pass on their wisdom and their skills by teaching at the bedside and in the clinic. Medical expertise is the distillation of shared experiences in the solution of psychological and physiological problems. Continued clinical acuity depends on the ability of the physician to constantly reinforce and refine his knowledge by working closely with his colleagues.

The physician in a group practice has the opportunity and the obligation to subject his clinical acumen to the scrutiny of his partners. Quality assurance in medicine reduces, in essence, to making others privy to the quality, consistency, and practicality of one's clinical decisions. In group practice, each physician must expose his intellectual competence to the review of his colleagues. In the process he is stimulated to maintain and improve his general level of functioning. In solo practice – particularly in settings where the physician rarely works in the hospital – errors of judgement, deterioration of performance, or simple incompetence may proceed undetected. Group practice offers at least a certain minimal assurance of quality of care.

Perhaps more importantly, the physician in a group practice is more likely to grow intellectually. No one person can encompass the breadth of medical practice. Through one's partners, a physician can be exposed to the unusual or perplexing case and can learn the gist of new discoveries or procedures which his partner has stumbled upon. There is a cognitive synergism which occurs in a group setting in which the physicians build upon each others' erudition. The solo practitioner suffers from a type of sensory deprivation and is unable to take advantage of the rich flow of impressions and experiences which occur as part of the metabolism of a group practice.

IMPROVED PATIENT CARE

Patients benefit from group practice. Group practice provides a structure within which patients can reap the advantages of a personal physician without forgoing continuity and comprehensiveness of care. A group practice allows the physician to make himself or his partner available 24 hours a day, without incurring the crushing burden of being unable to sequester free time for himself or his family. By installing shared coverage arrangements, the physician in the group practice ensures that his patient will receive the advantage of being seen by a colleague even when the physician himself is not on call.

Solo practitioners also devise coverage arrangements with colleagues or with on-call services, but the care provided to the patient is almost certainly inferior. In a group practice all physicians sharing on-call responsibility have access to the patients' charts. Moreover, all the physicians are familiar with the approach and philosophy of their colleagues and thus can more closely replicate his desired mode of therapy. The patient has the comfortable experience of being within a familiar framework and in fact may have already become acquainted with the covering physician during a routine visit to the clinic. In group practice the transmission of information is facilitated by the close and frequent physical contact between all the physicians; patients benefit from this interaction.

The patient benefits in a second important way: a group practice can offer a much broader range of service than a solo practitioner. Because a group practice is a collection of physicians with different strengths and interests, the practice as an entity is a reservoir of greater knowledge and experience than can be offered by any single individual. Consultation is readily available in the corridors, and patients are the beneficiaries of the kerbside consultation or the quickly obtained second opinion. One partner may in fact develop a special interest – for example in plastic surgery – which all the patients in the group practice may take advantage of.

Moreover, the group practice can afford to purchase equipment that would be impractical for the solo practitioner. Economies of scale definitely exist in ambulatory medical practice, and a group of physicians can share in the use of an electrocardiograph, or X-ray unit, or certain laboratory and diagnostic equipment that could never be justified in solo practice by the low level of utilization. This of course increases the convenience to the patient by eliminating time-consuming referrals to distant laboratories, thus speeding up the process by which diagnoses are made and treatment initiated.

SUPERIOR PERSONAL LIFE

Medicine is a stressful profession. The physician has taken upon his shoulders the responsibility of acting as healer, priest, and friend to his patients. The weight of this burden has grown in our secular society, which has been weakened by the withering away of the traditional supports of church, family, and neighbourhood. The physician is susceptible to the gradual erosion of his physical and mental reserves if he is unable to protect his own private haven of family and serenity. The impaired physician – alcoholic, suicidal, depressed, or cynical – may be the unfortunate product of a practice style that does not allow room for the personal needs of the physician.

The solo practitioner is at much higher risk for these maladies than his group practice colleague. The solo practitioner is always forced to choose between the needs of his patients and the needs of his own family. Time spent in personal pursuits is time stolen from his patients, and there is no comfortable resting-place where the physician can at the same time discharge his obligations to his practice and respect his obligations to himself. No matter what institutional provision is made for patient care while the solo physician is away, the average solo practitioner walks away from his practice with reluctance and is never sure that in his absence his patients will receive the care which he would wish them to have.

Group practice offers the physician that most precious commodity – an untroubled conscience. The physician is secure in the knowledge that his partner and friend – not some impersonal emergency room or deputizing service – is available to act as his surrogate in the care of the patients they share. Group practices are akin to marriages, and when successful, colleagues in such arrangements mutually adapt themselves to one another's outlook and practice style. Mutual respect emerges from sustained observation and coordination, and the mature group practice has a stability and an identity which is unique to the group itself. Within this framework, the individual physician can confidently plan vacation time, schedule periods for continuing education, and escape from the vicissitudes of patient care with a calm mind.

Group practice conveys an additional advantage with respect to the physician's ability to fully realize his own potential. Group practices lend themselves to division of labour. Even within a general practice, individuals develop special interests and enthusiasms, interests that change with time. In a solo practice setting, one physician must minister to the needs of an entire population; in order to change the focus of his practice, he must exclude certain patients or certain conditions from his purview. This may be difficult or undesirable, unfairly depriving segments of the population from ready access to needed medical services.

In group practice, individual physicians can indulge their enthusiasms by developing medical avocations within the larger vocation of general or family practice. The physician with a bent for gadgetry can learn to operate culposcopes, or operating microscopes, or other of the various illuminated tubes with which we peer into the body's nooks and crevices. A second partner may become skilled in counselling patients with problems involving sexual dysfunction, and become a practice resource for dealing with that particular symptom complex. The dynamic nature of the group practice, and the flexibility it confers, allows this differentiation to occur without threatening the generalist nature of the entire practice.

Moreover, physicians can change these interests over time by negotiating with their partners. They can teach one another these separately acquired skills and hence reduce the need for cumbersome continuing medical education courses. Medical practice is thus subject to periodic revitalization, and physicians can even arrange for mini-sabbaticals or other intensive activities without dismantling the practice or jeopardizing their financial or professional security.

SUMMARY

The physician in modern society is called upon to play many diverse roles. Scientist and healer, confidant and priest, the modern general practitioner must distil and apply the rapidly changing products of the physical and biological sciences without losing his close personal relationship with his patients. The role of the physician has become more complex in a world where rapid change is in itself an aetiological factor in human suffering. Medical practice is in flux.

In order to cope with these stresses, physicians have increasingly chosen to work in group arrangements. By establishing formal co-operative practices, physicians gain flexibility and freedom, improving the quality of their own lives, and at the same time they enhance their effectiveness as physicians. Collective practice arrangements allow physicians to continue to grow intellectually, to maintain their personal equilibrium as individuals and family members, and to offer a broader spectrum of predictable services to their patients. Group practice allows the individual physician to transcend his own limitations and to take advantage of the benefits that accrue to participation in a shared enterprise. Physicians in group practice are able to maintain and augment their technical knowledge without disrupting their practice life, to retain some control over their personal existence without neglecting patients, and to change the content of their medical practice without changing location or speciality.

Commentary

Solo practice was the usual pattern of practice in Britain and North America until 25–30 years ago. Now there has been a rapid move to group practice. However, solo practice is still the customary pattern of work in western Europe, South Africa, Australia and New Zealand. Solo practice is demanding in time and out-of-hours cover, but it does have the advantages of continuity of personal relations with the patient relating to the same physician. It also offers complete autocracy should the physician seek it! It offers the individualist the chance to practise on his/her own without risking problems and differences with partners.

Group-practice, however, provides sharing of time, knowledge, expertise, experience and skills. It offers patients a choice, and it should make for better care through continuing interaction between colleagues.

19 Vocational training for family medicine – useful or useless?

The issues

It has to be accepted that the modern undergraduate medical curriculum does not produce a doctor ready and able at once to undertake independent responsible practice in any field. It does, however, provide a basis on to which further vocational training is essential for family medicine as for any other special field.

Family medicine (general practice) is certainly a special field with its own core of knowledge, its own skills and techniques, its own research and teaching components. Vocational training in family medicine must be related to these special needs involving teaching of the special knowledge, skills and techniques.

The growth of vocational training in family medicine has been dramatic over the past 15 years in many countries. Programmes have tended to include more hospital speciality teaching than family medicine. In Britain vocational training is now mandatory and involves about 5000 trainees and almost 2000 trainers at any one time.

The dilemmas and uncertainties here are concerned with the following questions: What have been the benefits of vocational training for the patient; the physician; the local system of care; and cost-effectiveness? How does vocational training for family medicine relate to the training of other primary care professionals? Finally, if vocational training is essential, can we be satisfied with its present contents and methods – if not, how can it be improved?

The case for vocational training

K. H. M. Young

The resurgence of general practice since the doldrums of the 1950s continues, and matters which were once subjects for mere academic discussion are now much more clearly set out, and in the case of vocational training, now have the, admittedly debatable, support of an Act of Parliament. Prior to February 1981, vocational training for general practice was a purely voluntary matter, both in its duration and content, and a doctor could still freely enter upon a career as a general practitioner without undertaking any special further (and probably costly, in terms of time and income) training for the job. After all, a compulsory year in hospital prior to full registration had been his lot, and he had therefore fulfilled all that was legally required of him.

It was, however, clearly recognized by the members of the newly established Royal College of General Practitioners and other bodies in the United Kingdom that the revival of general practice could only be sustained by nurturing the concept that it existed in its own right, had its own content of skills and knowledge, its own literature and research capability, its own teachers and, not least, its own definable and minimum requirement of training for those aspiring to be good general practitioners. This last was not easy to establish for, quite apart from a majority of established general practitioners who were totally indifferent, there was a goodly number of articulate critics who decried, and indeed continue to decry, the very idea that even the basics of general practice could be taught by any other way than that of the time-honoured path of experience guided by elders and if necessary, strewn with willing, though unsuspecting patients! This last, of course, is an exaggeration, for the young doctor of the past almost wholly hospital trained was not likely to endanger his patient by wrong or excessive treatment. Since he had been trained to base his diagnosis on facts and opinions elicited by a group of experts, a group wherein, unlike the lone general practitioner, he could sink into anonymity if events dictated this course.

To examine the reasons for the almost total dominance of all medical teaching by (hospital) consultants, one must go back to the early eighteenth century when general practitioners were apothecaries or surgeon apothecaries and, like physicians, had full access to the hospitals of the day until they rebelled against the system where patients were going increasingly directly to physicians and surgeons, ultimately winning their claim that all patients should be referred by them. And although this did restore their patients, and income, it meant that they accordingly lost their close association with hospital medicine, thereby abdicating their role in the training of doctors. This fundamental development has, over the years, given rise to a continuing source of contention between general practitioners and hospital specialists, for the hospital is still the keystone of all medical training and patient care, and the repeated efforts of general practitioners to penetrate the ranks of this élite have not met with much success in face of the determined resistance of consultants.

However, even those general practitioners who oppose vocational training as presently constituted have recognized that the proper teaching of general practice is too important, too 'specialized', to be left wholly to consultants, and somehow or other general practitioners must not only take a leading part in the training of embryo general practitioners, but should also play a part in the postgraduate training of specialists. The range of work done by the general practitioner is very wide and continues to grow. It is very cost-effective compared with hospital medicine, and in the hands of the well-trained general practitioner costly investigation and treatment, which in some instances has reached a prohibitive level, would be prudently and carefully used, and that only when clearly needed.

What of the patient, the ultimate beneficiary, the whole and indeed only reason for our being? It is interesting to note how often the needs of the patient are ignored; how they are not allowed to complicate or detract from an interesting discussion about medical training and professional expertise! But a general practitioner must, above all, study and understand both the needs and expectations of his patients, and his own capability of meeting these.

Indeed, when one discusses these matters with both patients and colleagues it clearly emerges, somewhat surprisingly, that the great majority of patients ask for very little. They wish to have easy access to their general practitioner, they expect from him a speedy and positive response for any condition which they, the patients, consider to be urgent. They expect competence, and hope for compassion, but rightly presume as fundamental attributes both courtesy and charity at all times.

How then can these virtues be taught? No doubt the basis is laid in the home and in the school, but even more important, taking the very long view, is motivation and mastery of the fundamentals of the art of primary care.

Sadly enough general practice is still very poorly or sketchily 'taught' to medical students. During the 1950s and 1960s departments of general practice were established in some medical schools, and the hope grew that new medical graduates would begin their preregistration year with a good grounding in general practice, but this trend has not grown as much as was hoped and there are still medical schools where guidance, much less teaching, in general practice is little more than perfunctory, hence the continuing and increasing need to provide such teaching in the early postregistration years, for it is no less important to prepare the general practitioner for his role in life as it is the surgeon or radiologist, for example.

There are those who would urge that the preregistration doctor should only be trained in the general professional sense, and that speciality training should only begin in the postgraduate phase. In the main experience has shown that this is a sound concept if only because general practice means 'one-to-one' relationships with real patients and their families, and this is more easily achieved when the student is actually a doctor, rather than a trainee – a designation, incidentally, which should only ever be used between consenting adult doctors in private!

Most patients hope that their disease will be cured; some, but fortunately very few, demand it; and it is this unremitting pursuit of a 'cure' in all cases which is the hallmark of the inexperienced doctor who is not vocationally trained. The patient also expects the highest possible degree of relief for any pain he is suffering, and something also from his doctor to lift the chill shades of fear; this may only need a few words, or just the presence and behaviour of the doctor, if he possesses the confidence which comes from experience and the mastery of professional technique and (dare we say it) mystique.

All these things the vocationally trained doctor should be able to accomplish more skilfully than his untrained colleague, but it is conceded that the most paramount attribute that the patient requires from his doctor is *caring* in the fullest sense of the word, and this vital ingredient may well be possessed in even greater measure by the untrained, and therefore less confident doctor, than it is by the fully vocationally trained one.

How then is this doctor to be trained? Bearing in mind that the requirement that he be so trained is now backed by the might of British Parliament, it follows that the newly graduated doctor, who aspires to be an NHS general practitioner, cannot opt out. He certainly has a reasonably wide range of options as to content and quality, but none as to duration or the division of the training time between the hospital and the practice; he must spend 24 months in rotating, approved hospital posts, and 12 months in an approved training practice. At first sight the ratio of hospital to practice time may seem to be illogical or even eccentric, especially as the vast majority of general practitioners including those hostile to compulsory vocational training believe that the ratio should be reversed, but may be explained by quoting the old adage that 'he who pays the piper calls the tune'. Less time spent in hospital and correspond-ingly more in practice would increase the cost to a degree unacceptable in the present financial climate because the trainee in the practice setting is supernumerary, and therefore not 'in service', whereas the trainee in hospital is 'in service'.

The suggestion, the merest hint that the trainee in the practice may help out a little from time to time, is usually repudiated with some degree of scorn if not heat! Even the absurdity of the vocational trainee working in the deputizing service is not unknown! But the system appears to be working quite well for it recognizes the trainer as a teacher, and recom-penses him accordingly. It has the advantage too, that it facilitates the continuing education of the trainer, his partners and others in the pri-mary care team involved in the vocational training of the trainee, and this feature may well be the most valuable bonus of all. And further, if the ratio of two hospital jobs to one in the practice were reversed it would become impossible to fill the vacant hospital posts and at the same time find enough trainers and training practices to absorb the extra doctors looking for more time in the practice part of their training.

It should be remembered, however, that many teaching hospitals have taken little interest in the needs of future general practitioners and although we would not go as far as Dr Donald Gould when he said, 'If we want to start educating our future doctors then the sooner we get rid of all our medical schools the better', it is quite clear that we must do all we can to train, support and encourage our *trainers*, so very few of whom have themselves been vocationally trained.

The patient's point of view has been examined in some depth and the mechanics of vocational training have been described, but the question, 'why should the general practitioner be vocationally trained?' has still not been fully answered.

The artist and the craftsman can be taught the fundamentals of his calling. The artist can learn the 'laws' of draughtmanship, perspective and colour, the craftsman the use of his tools and the characteristics of the materials he fashions, but there is no means of knowing if he has learnt anything if he does not try to do what he has been taught by himself; the more he does the more he learns, but only the rare genius will succeed if the groundwork has not been done.

The young doctor entering practice should have acquired sound professional values, he should be accessible and clinically competent, and he should be able to communicate – the depth of his compassion and the sincerity of his courtesy must, of course, be presumed.

The consultation is the nub, the very heart, of his work, and he can only achieve some degree of mastery in its conduct by experience. His material, the patient, will display an impossibly wide range of presentation and behaviour, and he must modify his own behaviour accordingly.

If he possesses the confidence and pleasure in the practice of his art, that only comes from a sound basis of knowledge and training, he will then be able to make the best use of that transaction, the consultation which is the very root of good doctoring.

The art of the consultation cannot be taught, but the process itself can be analysed and understood, and the degree of depth to which this can be taken depends on the sensitivity, motivation, professional knowledge and expertise of the doctor; although these latter two come in the main from general professional training the former can only come from, and be nurtured and developed by, a well-constructed, well-applied system of vocational training for general practice.

The case against vocational training
John Fry

It is comfortable and satisfying to assume that specific teaching and training of young physicians for family medicine is an important, worthwhile, rewarding and beneficial exercise.

So it may be but for whom and on what evidence?

Is it worthwhile, rewarding and beneficial: for patients, to produce better personal care? For health care systems, to produce more effective, efficient and economic care? For young residents/trainees in family medicine, to teach them to become good family physicians? For family medicine teachers and trainers, to provide them with a self-satisfying time-killing occupation that is recognized professionally and rewarded generously with money and self-respect? For family medicine as a speciality with its own core of knowledge, techniques, expertise and research?

The honest answers to these questions have to be full of unproven uncertainties based almost entirely on soft subjective philosophical impressions.

We have no reliable evidence that formal training for family medicine leads to better patient care by those who receive formal training than those who do not.

We have no good information that can show that any supposed improvements can be related to specific items of the specific vocational training programmes – or that such improvements are more likely to occur from better methods of selection of medical students who are more intelligent, better able to learn and apply knowledge and who are more kind, considerate and loving of their fellow men and women.

WHY VOCATIONAL TRAINING FOR FAMILY MEDICINE?

Let us try and examine in more detail what is so special about family medicine, and what it is that we are endeavouring to teach to young future family physicians.

It is significant that over the past 5 years there has been a steady process of a change in nomenclature. 'General practice' and 'family medicine' are being replaced by the new term of 'primary care'. It has been given the accolade of acceptance by the World Health Organization who believes that one of the most significantly important measures for better health for people by the year 2000 will be better primary care.

Primary care is much more earthy and descriptive than general practice or family medicine. Primary care is the first level of health care essential in each and every system. It implies much more than care by vocationally trained family physicians. It includes self-care by individuals and families. It includes care by non-physician primary health workers such as nurses, health-aides, physician-assistants, social workers. It must include public health care to ensure the basic social, sanitation, economic, educational and other supportive elements for good health and disease prevention.

The medical profession's monopolistic tight hold on primary care has ceased. It becomes increasingly difficult to make a strong case for general practice/family medicine as a distinct specialty.

Most medical specialities are narrow 'vertical' specialities with well-demarcated systems or subjects. General practice/family medicine is a broad wide-ranging 'horizontal' speciality that cuts right across all other specialities at the primary care level, but is rarely able to take the more complex and difficult situations upwards in terms of professional experience and expertise.

General practice/family medicine does have its own defined roles and functions, its own clinical content and its own techniques and skills – but what is missing is any large core of scientific knowledge based on reliable research. It is difficult therefore to teach and learn about a speciality without such a scientifically researched core.

Of course it is important that future family physicians should be taught about the consultation process based on good communication and relations between patients and doctors – but then all clinical specialities must be based on the same principles.

Primary care is an essential level of health care. It has to protect the more expensive and intensive level of secondary care from inappropriate cases and to protect patients from inappropriate secondary care.

What is not certain is whether the current forms of vocational training for general practice/family medicine are appropriate and cost-effective.

HOW IS VOCATIONAL TRAINING BEING GIVEN?

Programmes of training have sprouted in Western Europe, the United Kingdom, the United States, Canada, Australia, New Zealand, South Africa and Israel. They all include a time in general practice/family medicine of different lengths and most include some time in special hospital departments.

The methods of teaching vary in detail but tend to be based on one-to-one pupil-teacher relationships plus small group discussions.

The quality of teachers has to be variable. In the United Kingdom more than 1 in 20 of all general practitioners are trainers and 1 in 5 of all general practices are involved as teaching practices. These large numbers cannot all be equally good teachers with equally good teaching facilities.

WHAT BENEFITS?

There is scant objective information on evaluation of the vocational training process. There have been no controlled trials. We are very far from having any direct evidence that the process and products of vocational training for the trainee/residents relate with the behaviour of these same trainees/residents as established practitioners years later.

More search is necessary to determine what factors make the 'good general/family practitioner', and which parts of the vocational training programmes can claim credit.

WHAT EFFECTS?

One effect of the vocational training scheme in the United Kingdom has been that many of the trainees become candidates for the entrance examination for Membership of the Royal College of General Practitioners (MRCGP). Each year some 1000 candidates are examined.

The pass rate for vocationally trained young trainees is about 75–80 per cent, and that for mature experienced practitioners who have not been vocationally trained is about 70–75 per cent – scarcely different.

The vocational training programme in the United Kingdom is big business costing the National Health Service over £10 million annually ($20 million), and providing a sizeable income for the trainers.

CONCLUSIONS

If one tries to stop a rolling bandwagon one is apt to get hurt. The vocational training programme for general practice/family medicine *is* such a bandwagon. It is gathering pace and momentum, but though driven hard it runs on an uncertain road.

The programme is popular and it is assumed to be a 'good thing' but such assumptions have little solid foundations.

Before it is too late to pause and perhaps change direction some pertinent questions have to be posed and answered:

(1) What evidence is there that vocational training has resulted in better patient care and in more satisfied and cost-effective general/family practitioners?

(2) Which parts of the programme are useful and should be retained and which parts are useless and should be scrapped?

(3) Would the same results be achieved through less formally planned programmes self-selected by young physicians interested in a career in primary care?

(4) Are all the efforts and money being spent on vocational training really worthwhile?

Vocational training for family medicine: a critique

W. E. Fabb

Feelings of inferiority are hard to overcome. So is depression and paranoia. If one were to judge from the contributions to the case for and against vocational training for general practice, one could hardly escape the conclusion that general practice still suffers seriously from these conditions, at least in Britain. How else can the introspection and self-flagellation so apparent in these articles be explained?

One wonders how representative are the opinions expressed by the writers. They ask 'Why should the general practitioner be vocationally trained?' (Why train a surgeon?); 'What is good general practice?'

(What is good internal medicine?); 'Is training for general practice appropriate and cost-effective?' (Is training for obstetrics?).

It is healthy to ask such questions; it is unhealthy to ruminate on them with wringing of hands and downcast eyes. But what about the specific issues raised by the writers? They allude to the comparative inappropriateness of hospital training for a career in general practice and point to the need for on the job training in general practice. Would any academic in general practice deny the pre-eminence of training in a general practice setting? Maybe political considerations have foreshortened the period of training in general practice in the United Kingdom and North America. In Australia, the 2 years of hospital training are seen as *complementary* to the 2 years of required training in general practice. In one of the articles it is stated that because general practice is a broad-ranging 'horizontal' speciality, it is rarely 'able to take the more complex and difficult situations upwards in terms of professional experience and expertise'. What is complex – understanding the hydrodynamics of intracardiac blood flow or understanding family dynamics in the presence of chronic childhood illness leading to terminal care, death and bereavement? Is it more difficult to diagnose and manage systemic lupus erythematosus (SLE) than to diagnose the cause of tiredness and manage it in a deprived household beset with malnutrition, unemployment, delinquency and alcoholism?

It is stated that general practice is a discipline without a 'scientifically researched core'. Is it? What about the numerous morbidity surveys carried out all around the world? What about the burgeoning literature on general practice in dozens of journals? General practice seems to have researched what it does and how it does it more than any other discipline in medicine. In the other disciplines, the research is mostly clinical; is this where general practice research is deficient? Is the RCGP study on contraceptives clinical research? What about the studies appearing in almost every issue of general practice journals?

It is easy to ask provocative questions. It is just as easy to suggest in the asking that we do not have the answers. But the answers are there for those who look. They are there in scores of new books on general practice/family medicine, in the hundreds of articles in general practice journals and in the reports of dozens of training programmes in general practice. They are not complete answers, but they are enough to answer many of the questions posed.

There are certainly no answers to be found in contemplative armchairs. But there are plenty to be found in the real world of vocational training, in the literature, and out of the mouths of the young doctors in training and their supervisors and patients.

By all means let us question what we are doing and why we are doing it, but with confidence and the courage of our convictions. All the evidence validates such an approach.

Commentary

The case for specific training for family medicine is that it is a special field of practice with its own special problems and diseases requiring their own special knowledge, skills and techniques that have to be taught and learned. Acceptance of this philosophy has led to widespread introduction of special training programmes for family medicine in North America, Western Europe, South-East Asia, Australia, New Zealand and South Africa.

Training for family medicine has become a large medical educational industry in those countries with colleges, academies and associations supporting and organizing programmes and involved in assessment and examinations. Training for family medicine has been welcomed generally by national governments and steps are being taken for programmes to be internationally recognized and accepted.

Such growth and enthusiasm have to be tempered with some pertinent questions: What evidence is there that the increased training has resulted in better patient-care? Are all the components of the training programmes equally useful? Is there a sufficient core of scientific knowledge of family medicine to merit the teaching being given? Should training for family medicine be mandatory?

20

At least one female family physician in every group practice?

The issues

Social changes have created changing expectations from women and have increased the proportion of female physicians. Many women seek care from female family physicians; women doctors find family medicine a good field in which to combine the responsibilities of a wife and mother with those of part-time family practice.

With such changes and expectations should every practice include at least one female family practitioner?

The case for a female doctor in every group practice (1)

Elan Preston-Whyte

THE BACKGROUND

The Todd Report (1968) 'predicted a grave underproduction of doctors in the future', and successive governments adopting its estimates have therefore expanded the intake of students into medical schools in the United Kingdom. At the same time, the proportion of women entrants has risen and by 1985 is expected to reach 50 per cent (Royal Commission on the National Health Service, 1979) (in Leicester it is already 47 per cent). The figures on the next page illustrate the change that will have occurred over 25 years.

361

	Number of graduates	*Number of women graduates*
1964	1500	375 (25 per cent)
1989	4000 (predicted)	2000 (50 per cent)

A study carried out in the Oxford Region (Swerdlow, McNeilly and Rue, 1980) of the career intentions of 252 women in postregistration posts in 1979 showed that the most popular career choice was general practice (23 per cent) followed by psychiatry and the general medical specialities (both 14 per cent). Parkhouse and Palmer (1979) have confirmed that there is an upward trend nationally in favour of women selecting general practice as a career option.

The implications for vocational training and for general practice manpower planning of these trends is therefore of great importance. In 1975, there were 3258 women doctors at all grades in general practice representing some 14 per cent of all general practitioners; 2754 (84.5 per cent) of these women practised as unrestricted principals, 208 (6.4 per cent) were clinical assistants and 215 (6.6 per cent) were trainees, representing some 30 per cent of all trainees (Department of Health and Social Services, 1975). If we apply the predictions of Todd and Parkhouse to these figures, we may expect to see the number of women doctors in vocational training doubling in 1985. Will there be jobs for them at the end of their training? This question emphasizes the relevance of the present debate on having a women doctor in every group practice.

THE DIFFERENCES BETWEEN MEN AND WOMEN GENERAL PRACTITIONERS

Cartwright and Anderson (1981) looked at differences between men and women general practitioners and found that 'in general, it is the lack of difference which is most notable'. The finding was that they did not differ in their qualifications, the type of practice they worked in or their style of practice. Likewise it was appropriate for people to seek help from their general practitioner with problems in their family lives and they made similar estimates of the proportion of consultations which they regarded as trivial.

The main differences that Cartwright and Anderson found were that women doctors had rather fewer patients; more said they sometimes used a deputizing service and were on call fewer nights on average. Surprisingly, they were less likely than the male doctors to say that they fitted IUCDs when the procedure arose in their practice. These latter findings have not been confirmed by a study (Fraser and Preston-Whyte, 1982) carried out in our practice in which we found that the two female principals saw approximately the same number of patients in each diagnostic group as their four male colleagues, except for genitourinary conditions and prophylactic procedures where they saw almost twice as many patients. When these two groups were looked at in detail, it could be seen that the female principals saw nearly three times as many patients with gynaecological conditions (excluding vaginal discharge) as the male principals, but the largest discrepancy was in the family planning group, where the female principals were consulted thirty times more often for contraceptive advice (other than for the Pill) than their male colleagues.

Cartwright and Anderson found that the proportion of women patients consulting women doctors did not differ significantly from that consulting men doctors. Our study, however, showed that the proportion of females to males consulting the female principals was 74 and 26 per cent compared with that of 57 and 43 per cent for the male principals.

As far as the patients were concerned, Cartwright and Anderson's findings were that there was no difference in their general satisfaction with their care whether their doctor was male or female, but that women who had a female doctor were less likely to say they might consult their doctors about a personal problem that was not a strictly medical one than women who had a male doctor (15 per cent compared with 32 per cent). In our study, however, we were able to show that women do make a positive decision to consult a woman doctor when the problem is a gynaecological one (there was no difference in the consultation pattern for women with vaginal discharge, so that patients were not being negatively influenced in their choice of doctor because they wished to avoid a vaginal examination by a male doctor). This may indicate that women who present with certain gynaecological problems relating to menstruation may expect a woman doctor to understand the way in which these problems affect her marriage or career better than a male doctor. Such patients would not regard their problems as 'purely personal', and this may explain why Cartwright and Anderson, whilst recording that 21 per cent of women would prefer to consult a woman doctor on some occasions, failed to identify the reasons why they might wish to do so, an example of how the answers to questions are of value only if the questions are appropriate.

Inevitably, our study is open to the criticism that this may represent a situation unique to our practice, but, similarly, Cartwright and Anderson's study should be subjected to the same scrutiny. Their sample of 36 women doctors represents only 1 per cent of the total number of women in general practice.

Obviously more research is needed, but there have been other pointers

that this is an area which would be important to explore further. Stub-
bings (1979) identified a need amongst women patients when he wrote
'female trainees in all-male practice often comment on the great amount
of gynaecology they see'. This suggests that when practices consist of
male doctors only, a substantial proportion of their female patients may
decide not to consult their doctor about gynaecological problems because
he is a man.

Further evidence of the patients' gender affecting what the patient
presents and feels in consultations has come from a study of attitudes to
general practice carried out by Sawyer (1979) on a random sample of
1038 patients. This study showed that women patients as a group are
more nervous and are more likely to feel distant from their general
practitioner (whether male or female) than men are; they were more
likely to get the impression that their doctor was not listening or was not
interested in them. Sawyer concluded that 'not only do doctors tend to
hold stereotypical views of their patients but that patients, especially
women, are very much aware of these stereotypes and that this, among
other reasons, accounts for the fact that women appear to be relatively
inhibited in communicating with their doctors'.

An Editorial (1979) in the *Journal of the Royal College of General Practitioners* predicted that 'the general practice of the future will be increasingly concerned with caring rather than curing when the nurturative
image of the female will be more appropriate than the aggressiveness of
the male'. The lesson to be learnt from this and from Sawyer's research
is that women doctors during their undergraduate and postgraduate
training should resist the tendency to conform to a pattern imposed by a
male-dominated profession, and that the lesson for vocational training is
that male trainees should be encouraged to become more like their
women colleagues!

BENEFITS TO THE PATIENT AND THE PRACTICE

In a training practice such as ours, the female partners have a major role
in teaching particularly in those areas, gynaecology, family planning,
cervical cytology, where they have an expertise not shared by the
male partners. The *Report* of the Royal College of General Practitioners
(1981) indicated that trainees should be encouraged to gain gynaecological experience within general practice because of the paucity of
hospital posts and because gynaecological outpatient departments provide little background information and little opportunity for continuity
of care.

Employing a woman doctor can also be financially attractive. Even as a part-time salaried partner with the minimum 20 hours a week commitment she will qualify for the full basic practice allowance, and may enable the partnership to qualify for a group practice allowance. The employment of a woman as an assistant, however, is less profitable as this will attract a much lower Family Practitioner Committee (FPC) contribution towards her salary. The more daring practice may decide to experiment in time-sharing, that is, two women sharing the job and salary of one full-time partner. (The practice will probably reap the benefit as each woman will tend to give more than the half-time equivalent).

I suspect that my adversary in this debate has made much of the fact that women are likely to become pregnant and have interrupted working lives as a result. I do not deny this, for it is the fact that women doctors become mothers which more than any other influences their ability to work. The Oxford study (Swerdlow, McNeilly and Rue, 1980) found that the women doctors with no children, whether they were married or not, had on average worked full-time for virtually all of their careers to date but the great majority of doctors with children had not had uninterrupted full-time careers.

So what are the practicalities for a group practice employing a woman doctor who will be entitled to an unspecified amount of maternity leave. The present regulations entitle a practice to claim reimbursement of locum fees when the remaining partners are left with total lists of 3000 patients or more when a partner takes maternity leave. When some doctors appear to manage list sizes of up to 4000 patients with comparative ease, a list size of less than 3000 should not present extraordinary hardship. However, it would be helpful, perhaps in areas where either because of distances to be travelled or the morbidity of the population, for special dispensation to be granted and reimbursement paid when the list size is less than 3000.

It is crucial, however, in order to prevent misunderstanding and acrimonious dispute, that when a woman doctor enters a partnership, a practice agreement is drawn up which clearly states the criteria for all kinds of leave. Male partners would probably feel less hard done by if they were encouraged to claim the sabbatical leave to which they also are entitled.

In Sweden, a married couple can decide whether it will be the husband or the wife who will take leave after the birth of their baby. It would be interesting to know how many male general practitioners in this country would welcome the opportunity to take over the responsibility of baby and household chores for 2–3 months! If the majority would welcome this

Swerdlow, A. J., McNeilly, R. H. and Rue, E. Rosemary (1980). Women doctors
    in training: problems and progress. *Br. Med. J.*, **281,** 754–758.
Todd Report (Report of Royal Commission on Medical Education) (1968).
    (London: HMSO).

The case for a female doctor in every group practice (2)
George Strube

Modern general practice involves doctors working in a team with other professionals skilled in their own field and each contributing their experience. Doctors trained along traditional lines find this difficult to do and they expect to carry the whole burden of responsibility for the clinical care of patients as well as the organization of the practice. They tend to work alone, keeping anxieties about clinical problems to themselves, and this can build up frustration and emotional exhaustion. A woman doctor is able to work with a team more easily. She is not so concerned with her status and is able to exchange ideas and share problems with others. She is willing to take advice from other members of the team and to learn from them. By keeping a low profile herself, she allows the skills of the other members to flourish. She is sensitive to the stresses and strains within the team and helps it to run smoothly and efficiently. Members of the team are able to share the burdens of difficult problems with each other, and the mutual support decreases the feelings of anxiety and stress which can build up in a worker who struggles on alone.

Communication between members of the team can become a practical problem when everyone is working in different directions. A woman is able to facilitate the informal gossip which is so useful in keeping everyone aware of events. More formal meetings of the team are, of course, necessary if there is to be fruitful exchange of ideas.

Possibly because women are relative newcomers to the medical scene, they are not bound by the traditional methods of working and can often see new ways to solve old problems. Lateral thinking and logic enable them to discard time-honoured but useless procedures and adopt a more fruitful course. This can change the practice policy of management and provide a better service for the patient. This could be regarded as medical audit, but the title is so cast about with doubts, threats and fears, that most general practitioners are reluctant to use this terminology.

General practice is a branch of medicine more concerned with caring for people than treating disease. A woman doctor's natural caring role in a family and the community, affects her style of clinical practice. She is more sensitive to emotional problems which are often concealed by physical symptoms. Patients find her more approachable than a man and are able to confide in her more easily. She is therefore able to help them with emotional symptoms, interpreting them to the patient and together formulating a plan of treatment. The more traditional male doctor is not so sensitive to this delicate process. He tends to ignore a vast emotional area of misery which can cause serious disability and increase susceptibility to physical disease.

Health education is a neglected area of our responsibility. During every consultation the patient is learning from the doctor about managing an episode of illness. If he remembers this the next time he develops similar symptoms, he may be able to cope himself without relying on the doctor. Women doctors are used to teaching their families about health and their style of consultation is largely educational. This is particularly noticeable in the child development clinic when they are run by women doctors. They are able to understand the problems of childrearing and take the opportunity to teach the young mothers general principles and also to discuss their personal difficulties.

Women are the greatest consumers of the medical services, as they live longer than men, have a higher morbidity and are subject to greater emotional stress. They are also in charge of family health and sickness and so seek, receive and interpret health care on behalf of children and the elderly. They feel a mutual understanding or empathy in discussing their health with another woman, so many prefer to consult a woman doctor. Asian women find it difficult if not impossible to consult men due to cultural barriers.

The flexibility of work in general practice makes it easy for a woman to adjust her working hours to the requirements of her family. If she has no children full-time work presents no problem, but if she has young children at home her hours of work in the practice can be reduced without major disruption or financial problems. The system of payment in general practice enables her to draw full salary from the Family Practitioner Committee provided that she receives more than one-third of the senior partner's share and works the basic minimum number of hours a week. Thus the salary she draws from the partnership is very little more than the sum paid into the partnership by the Family Practitioner Committee, so that her cost to the partnership is negligible.

The demand for a woman doctor may remain unrecognized by an all-male partnership, until a woman joins it, possibly as a trainee general practitioner, or perhaps a part-time assistant, or even a full partner. The patients are delighted and her instant popularity may come as something of a surprise. Occasionally the patients will write to the practice to ask for a woman doctor to be appointed. Frequently the demand for a woman doctor exceeds the time that she is able to give, and it may become necessary to engage another woman partner. If patient demand is fully satisfied, possibly the optimum arrangement in a group would be to have equal numbers of men and women partners.

The case against a female doctor in every group practice

Tommy Bouchier Hayes

Women are crabbed as constant companions and have tell-tale faces. They are quarrel-some in company, steadfast in hate and forgetful in love; never to be trusted with a secret, boisterous in their jealousy, sorrowful in an alehouse, tearful or talkative during music, lustful in bed, late in keeping appointments, furious when themselves kept waiting, sulky on a journey; most troublesome bedfellows, craving for delicacies whenever they wake; dumb on useful matters, eloquent on trifles; looking on one another with utter loathing. Happy the man who does not yield to women; they should be dreaded like fire and feared like wild beasts for they are moths for tenacity, serpents for cunning, bad among the good and worse among the bad.

This was how King Cormac of Ireland spoke of women nearly 2000 years ago, and his opinions might be echoed by male chauvinists today. But we more reasonable men, while accepting his views as being at least preju-diced, should guard against the temptation to err in the opposite direction and to overcompensate in the name of equality. Today the law has established that women are equal and must be offered the same oppor-tunities as their male counterparts, and this applies as much in general practice as in any other field of endeavour. However, a general practi-tioner is an independent contractor and it behoves him to choose the most suitable candidate for any job, and not, out of some misguided sense of fairness, to choose a woman who might be unsuitable.

General practice today is a business and the total commitment of all those employed is not only desirable but necessary. Its business is to look after the total wellbeing of the patient, to provide continuity of care and to be available when required. With these factors in mind, the perfect partner has been described (Rouse, 1980) as one who:

> arrives promptly to start his morning surgery despite the fact that he has blackwater fever, despite the fact that his wife eloped just before dawn leaving him to feed and dress five children under the age of four, and despite the fact that he is due at his father's funeral at midday in a town two hundred miles away. In short the Perfect Partner does not allow his personal life to interfere with his duty to his patients or – most important of all – to his partners.

The average female general practitioner, with her position as wife and mother, will inevitably, loud as she may cry out against the notion, find it much more difficult than the average male to achieve this ideal. In the selection between equals for a job in a group practice, the advantages of females remain largely theoretical and women doctors have so far failed to produce hard evidence of their own supposedly special role. Evidence of their disadvantages is more readily apparent, and to find it one does not have to resort to the rather fanciful transports of those such as Dr Lawrence Irwell who wrote in 1896 of the effects of menstruation, 'One shudders to think of the conclusions arrived at by female bacteriologists or histologists at the period when their entire system, both physical and mental, is so to speak "unstrung", to say nothing of the terrible mistakes which a lady surgeon might make under similar conditions.' The arguments against employing women in group practices can be based far more realistically and convincingly on common sense and straightforward observation.

The disadvantages can be divided into four main areas – effects on the woman herself, effects on her family, effects on her patients and effects on her partners. We can look usefully at each of these four major areas in turn.

THE EFFECTS ON THE WOMAN HERSELF

Women doctors have high rates for suicide, alcoholism and drug abuse. It would be unfair to jump to conclusions about cause and effect when in none of these conditions is the aetiology clear-cut, but it cannot be denied that stress is a recognized contributing risk factor in each, and that the stress of effectively holding down two occupations – one in general practice and one in the home – can be considerable. Success in combining the two calls for a high degree of resilience and organization and the woman who is to contribute as a genuinely full partner in a general practice – working the same number of sessions as the other partners, conforming to the practice timetable, participating equally in night and weekend work and being available at short notice in an emergency – must marshal her resources with the degree of precision more commonly encountered in connection with a military operation. Housework, even if it is shared, must either be done before work, during the evenings or at weekends or be delegated to domestic help which not only has to be paid but often fails to come up to expectations. Doing the work oneself effectively disposes of leisure time which could otherwise have proved to be one's salvation, while delegating to others frequently increases rather than decreases tensions and frustrations and makes the financial benefits of working minimal.

Housework at least is inanimate and can be abandoned if necessary, but children cannot. The mother who is a full-time general practitioner must be prepared to sacrifice many of the pleasures of motherhood, missing the opportunity to be a close witness to her children's development and the chance to form close bonds with them and resigning herself to worrying at a distance while others nurse their chickenpox and attend their school plays. Unless domestic help is 100 per cent reliable the working mother will find it difficult to prevent at least some crises interfering with her work, and the constant battle to establish priorities along with the accompanying guilt caused by being forced to abandon one for the other can be both emotionally and even physically draining.

For any general practitioner, male or female, patients can prove to be an enormous drain upon resources, and many are the practices in which the female partner seems to attract more than her fair share of emotionally demanding patients. This gravitation results partly from the widespread misconception, frequently fostered by women doctors themselves, but not objectively proved, that they are somehow inherently more caring and sympathetic. Female patients seek the help of one whom they see as sharing the common experiences of marriage, childbearing and motherhood. The majority of complex and usually insoluble emotional problems are presented to the general practitioner by women, so the woman partner may well find herself the vessel for a great deal of vicarious suffering. For one already stretched by coping with home and working life, the additional stress can be an almost intolerable burden.

Another probably less frequently recognized burden is that of professional insecurity. It is often the pattern for a young female doctor that she completes her compulsory preregistration year then leaves the practice of medicine for a variable length of time to have her family, thereby losing the opportunity to build progressively her diagnostic and practical clinical abilities. When she does return to medicine she may do so in a part-time capacity, or in less demanding posts which will allow her to spend more time with her growing children. This pattern leads in some to a lack of faith in their own clinical abilities which they may overcome, especially now that vocational training is the norm, but which can persist throughout their working lives. This must inevitably lead to a high level of anxiety when they are required to fulfil a commitment to the heavy demands of general practice, and often to an increase in workload because they feel it necessary to review patients more frequently or investigate them more intensively than those who are more sure of their clinical expertise.

THE EFFECTS ON THE WOMAN DOCTOR'S FAMILY

First, let us consider her husband. He will probably belong to social class 1 and will often himself be a doctor or dentist. He may well not yet have reached his final resting place in terms of his career, and major decisions will have to be faced about whether wife should sacrifice her own career to that of her husband or vice versa. It is unlikely that both will find ideal posts in the same geographical area and, even in these liberated days, it will be as hard for a man to pass up the opportunity of a good job in order to avoid uprooting his general practitioner wife from her practice as it is for her to make a similar sacrifice. If some sort of compromise is attempted whereby the family home is situated somewhere between husband's and wife's places of work, an inordinate amount of time may be spent by one or both in travelling, and the female partner may live an unreasonable or even impossible distance from the practice area for the purposes of the on-call duty rota.

In any marriage in which both partners work full-time each has to accept that time spent with the other will probably be more limited than would otherwise be so. In the case of a man married to a full-time general practitioner, however, meetings will at times be reduced to passing on the stairs when surgeries start early in the morning or extend into the evening, and night and weekend duties interrupt the family timetable. Sleep will be disturbed, social activities will be severely curtailed and organizing a weekend away or a family holiday can prove a major hurdle when the requirements of the practice and its other members have constantly to be taken into consideration. All the hazards are of course doubled when the husband is himself a full-time general practitioner.

While even the most pampered male will eventually accommodate himself to the idea that having a working wife requires more effort and tolerance on his part if the partnership is to work, children find it more difficult to understand why mummy is rarely around when they leave for school or arrive home, can never attend school activities or stay at home when they are unwell, and often disappears at unlikely times during nights and weekends. The quote from a female general practitioner's 6-year-old daughter who wailed 'I wish you were just a lady like other mothers' is most telling. Some children will discover to their cost that they know the au pair or childminder better than they know their mother, and the kudos to be gained from having a parent who is a doctor will hardly make up for their loss. Mother's lack of opportunity to exert ordinary discipline may result in compensation either in the form of overindulgence or as unnecessarily harsh disciplinary measures. Neither is to be recommended to the already harrassed mother hoping to produce a happy well-adjusted child. I am quite prepared to believe those general practitioner mothers who leap forward to tell me of their confident self-reliant paragons of virtue, but those who have to lay claim to spoiled brats or rebellious youths will be less likely to offer their views.

THE EFFECT ON PATIENTS

As I have already mentioned, a certain number of female patients, particularly those with emotional or psychosexual problems, will seek out a female doctor in the expectation of finding one who will deal particularly sympathetically with their plight. There is in fact no proof that women doctors are any more understanding or adept in these situations than are their male colleagues and some patients must go away disappointed. In general, studies have shown that the majority of patients see a doctor as a doctor and not as a 'male doctor' or a 'female doctor'. Very few women now, except for cultural or religious reasons insist upon seeing only a woman doctor, while there remains a small core of men who refuse to see them if at all possible. The full-time general practitioner should have little problem in providing an adequate service to the patients she does see, though the tendency of a few to investigate intensively and review frequently has already been noted. For the part-timer, however, the situation is different. If, for example, she sees a patient and wishes to review him in a certain number of days, the review may well coincide with a day when she is absent from the practice. This will result in the patient either being reviewed by another doctor, and therefore suffering from a loss of continuity of care, or in his being reviewed at a time which is not optimal from the point of view of ideal management. Similarly, patients have a tendency to become attached to a particular doctor and if 'their' doctor is part-time they are likely to be frustrated or distressed if they find that their care is in fact often shared or if the doctor is not available on days or at times when they wish to make appointments.

THE EFFECT ON THE PARTNERS IN THE PRACTICE

If the female in the practice works full-time, contributes equally and expects no privileges there is no reason why they should find her any more difficult to work with than a male partner. Emotional arguments about premenstrual tension and fragile tempers hold little water. Arguments about lack of complete participation, however, do. Any partner who is less than a full contributor throws an extra burden in terms of time and effort on the other partners. If her contract stipulates part-time employment, other members of the practice at least understand and accept the arrangement from the beginning and are presumably willing to accept an extra share of the responsibilities, as well as the fact that in financial terms she is likely to gain more from the practice than she earns for it. But if privileges outside the bounds of the contract are expected – if she is unable or unwilling to do night or weekend duties, if she takes time off for her children's illnesses or must take her leave during school holidays – the other partners are entitled to be upset. I am not suggesting that a female doctor deliberately seeks to take her partners for a ride but rather that a woman with a home to run and a family to bring up is bound to find it difficult at times to avoid conflict between her domestic and professional responsibilities. When balance cannot be achieved, everyone – the woman herself, her family, her patients and her partners – suffers. Not all women of course will bring these problems with them, but how are we to distinguish who will before we employ them?

At the beginning of this chapter I quoted King Cormac only to disclaim his views as somewhat extreme. I must, however, in considering the choice of partner for a group practice, admit some sympathy for Professor Henry Higgins who asked

> Why can't a woman be more like a man?
> Men are such decent, reasonable chaps.

References

Rouse, Robert (1980). *World Med.*, June 28, 47

Commentary

It is likely that in the future most practices will include at least one female partner because of the logistics of more and more women doctors seeking jobs. Considering unemotionally there should be no real differences between male and female family practitioners, but in practice there are. Attitudes, interests, feelings and concerns differ as do physical potentials and work inputs. With such likely differences it will be necessary for each practice to achieve sufficient flexibility and understanding to offer female family practitioners opportunities to play their parts in this branch of the medical profession.

21 Prevention – realistic or not?

The issues

Prevention ideally *is* better than cure – but it is necessary to consider what is preventable and who should be receiving it. Any major improvements in health in the future are likely to be achieved through prevention rather than through more and better modern medical miracles.

Prevention of our major chronic disease problems – coronary artery disease, strokes, cancer and accidents – lies more in the hands of the public and in the social policies of governments than within the responsibilities of the medical profession. The issues must now be to meet the challenges of the social changes required to alter habits and improve living standards and conditions in order to prevent diseases.

The case for realistic prevention
John Fry

'Prevention is better than cure' is a well-worn cliché that has become a comfortable platitude. Everyone accepts it as a desirable objective but few have taken steps to question its validity, applications and real potentials in practice.

To add another well-worn cliché to the debate – 'to cure sometimes, to relieve often, to comfort always – and to prevent hopefully' – is more realistic because it exposes our limitations both for curing and preventing.

Of course prevention *is* better than cure if it is possible. My case will demonstrate that while there are many enthusiastic hopefuls the real challenges for prevention of disease in the future are those for society as a whole, rather than for the medical profession alone.

377

WHAT IS HEALTH?

Health has been defined by the World Health Organization as: 'a state of complete physical, mental and social wellbeing and not merely an absence of disease'. Such a utopian state must be the experience of few normal persons during fleeting moments in their lifetime.

However, the definition does stress that a healthy state involves much more than prevention of physical ill-health – the usual understanding of a disease. Social and mental factors are strong influences underlying non-health.

WHAT IS NON-HEALTH?

Taking a world view it is startling to discover that one half of all deaths affect infants and toddlers in developing countries and are related to poverty, malnutrition, unsafe water and ignorance. The killing diseases of developed countries, heart diseases, strokes and cancers, account for less than 20 per cent of all current deaths in the world.

Health problems in developed societies in order of frequency are:

(1) Mortality
   (a) heart diseases, especially myocardial ischaemia
   (b) strokes
   (c) cancer
   (d) accidents
(2) Morbidity
   (a) respiratory infections
   (b) psychosocial disorders
   (c) gastrointestinal diseases
   (d) skin conditions
   (e) rheumatism

Arguably, it is questionable how many of the above are readily preventable.

Social factors of non-health

A global historical analysis of control of disease reveals that the two factors that have reduced mortality and improved health have been reduction in deaths from infections and reduction in birth rates.

Lest we assume that such events have resulted from medical advances it must be pointed out that the reductions in deaths from infections antedated the introduction of immunization and antibiotics by at least 50 years, and decline in birth rates in developed societies began long before modern effective contraceptives.

Good health demands an adequate range of food, plentiful safe water, and warmth and shelter. Lack of these basic human necessities is intimately related to poverty. Poverty, whether it occurs in developing or developed countries, carries higher local rates of death and disease. The worst health indices in Britain, the United States, the USSR and western Europe are in those areas where there is evidence of relative poverty.

Control of infections occurred and is occurring chiefly because social conditions improved and these led to adequate food, safe water and better housing. Malnutrition lowers immunological competence. But better nutrition, better hygiene, and lower birth rates are the most urgent factors to improve health in developing countries today. Immunization, drugs, modern medical technology and personal medical care are of less importance in improving health of most of mankind even in the 1980s.

Personal factors in non-health

The aetiologies of the problem diseases of developed countries are multifactorial and unclear.

The causation of ischaemic heart disease, for instance, is somehow related to ageing and living – the condition is probably already pathologically there in childhood and early teens but its clinical manifestations do not appear until middle age onwards. Amongst the suggested causes are cigarette smoking, faulty diets and foods, lack of exercise, stresses and genetic predispositions.

The causation of most types of hypertension is unclear, but raised blood pressure in the young and middle-aged does predispose to strokes; relationships in the elderly are unproven. Cancer of the lung is associated with long-term smoking, but there are no clear definable causes of other cancers. In theory all accidents are preventable, but how many really are?

Thus, personal habits and misdeeds are probably major factors in the causation of diseases in developed countries, but how many are amenable to change?

WHAT IS CURABLE?

Are most diseases non-curable? Strictly speaking, many infections and some surgical procedures are curable. Most common diseases are amenable to control, balance, relief and comfort – for example migraine, rheumatism, diabetes, epilepsy, dyspepsia, depression, and so on.

Nevertheless, therapeutic actions with drugs and other intervention procedures do offer something that a beleaguered medical profession faced with public demands to 'for god's sake do something!' can do and be seen to be doing. It is very fortunate that many human diseases, dysfunctions and disorders have such great tendencies to natural improvement and resolution, for which doctors often receive the credit.

WHAT IS PREVENTABLE?

Now we come to the crux of the issue. What is preventable? Or, more commonsensically, what is amenable to prevention in family practice conducted in the usual manner?

First, there are the *primary preventable* procedures to prevent infections through well-planned and well-executed programmes of immunization of all children and at-risk adults. The family doctor has the tasks of organizing such programmes. *Secondary prevention* is aimed at effective therapy to control established diseases such as diabetes, high blood pressure, cancers and others and to prevent complications – this is part of standard modern medicine. *Tertiary prevention* aims to alter and improve on personal habits and social community deficiencies in order to create better conditions for health for individuals and the mass public.

It is this tertiary prevention which has so many opportunities for improving future health of the people, but which also is so difficult to achieve. It is also the field on which rest most doubts and uncertainties about its feasibility.

WHOSE RESPONSIBILITIES?

With a public that is better educated and informed than ever before; with politicians and public administrators better advised professionally than ever before; and with more medical, public health and social workers than ever before – where and with whom do responsibilities for disease prevention and health promotion lie?

The public

The public is well aware of the basic rules of health maintenance and disease prevention:

(1) no smoking
(2) no excessive eating
(3) no excessive drinking of alcohol
(4) weight control
(5) regular physical exercise
(6) care on the roads and in the home
(7) sensible use of available medical facilities and services
(8) adequate sleep, avoidance of stresses, worries, etc.

Politicians and administrators

The politicians and administrators are well aware of the needs for adequate health resources and services, for good safe roads, for safe water, adequate food supplies at reasonable costs and distribution, for adequate housing, and for full employment, income and social security.

The politicians also know the risks and hazards of smoking and drinking – are they prepared to restrict their consumption for the sake of better public health by punitive taxation or even prohibition?

The medical profession

The medical profession knows that faulty personal habits are at the roots of many modern diseases – is it prepared to take on greater responsibilities and ensure that a sizable part of each consultation should include prevention?

WHAT IS POSSIBLE AND USEFUL?

Assuming that most family doctors are human, with all the human frailties and emotions, it is not surprising that they should go for the soft option of attempting to cure, relieve and comfort their patients in their times of need. Prevention has not been a major part of the medical curriculum. Medical school clinicians are more and more technologically orientated to correcting the products of disease processes. Few have time or inclination to introduce prevention into their specialities. Medical students receive almost all their clinical teaching from medical school technologists.

How much prevention, then, is possible and useful in family practice? In theory much is possible, but in practice little seems to be useful – apart from traditional primary immunization procedures. Unless and until much more reliable and practical evidence is produced that prevention through hopeful education of the patient produces results, most family doctors will not take it too seriously. For them to take a more positive involvement in prevention they will also expect more evidence of interest, concern and participation by the public itself, and by politicians, health planners and administrators.

The case for more prevention
Rae West

In a recent public talk in Auckland, Dr Ma Haide, the American-born medical advisor to the (mainland) Chinese government, related how decisions were made about priorities in health care after the revolution. It was obvious that, because of a lack of finance, a choice had to be made between preventive and curative care. The decision was made for the former and time has proved, to Dr Ma's satisfaction, that it paid off. Because of the technology explosion in medicine, most western countries have now reached the same dilemma and I suggest that the same decision must be made.

Preventive care, except in very highly educated circles, is a public rather than a private responsibility. Where finance ministers have fixed a total sum for the health vote they must decide in which direction the emphasis must go. The political lifetime of a government is unfortunately too brief for many to choose a path with long-term rather than short-term goals.

I hope to demonstrate that, in the range of general practice activities, much preventive care may be added to, rather than substituted for, curative care. I hope we feel that we *must* do it and that it is practicable to do so.

Preventive measures in family practice may be divided into four separate areas:

(1) Preventive procedures for specific disorders.
(2) Detection and care of the early stages of organic diseases for which there are effective and practical interventions available.

(3) Demonstration of health risks known to lead to specific diseases.
(4) Detection of and education about the predisposing causes of diseases which arise from the living activities and environments of people.

PREVENTIVE PROCEDURES FOR SPECIFIC DISORDERS

Specific immunization procedures are well established for diphtheria, pertussis, tetanus, poliomyelitis, and morbilli. The procedures are accepted by both public and profession. However, we have a clear responsibility to improve our coverage and follow-up. The mechanisms are available and we have no excuse for not achieving 100 per cent coverage of those willing to benefit.

The position with rubella immunization will remain obscure until we know the duration of protection conferred. Meantime effort *must* be made to protect all susceptible women and girls, with a flexible and realistic approach to the immunization state of young children who may transmit the disorder to susceptible mothers. Unless we are to resign our responsibilities, family doctors must accept the challenge to make all pregnant women safe. Prevention of the severe handicaps of congenital rubella is within our grasp when we observe the success story of smallpox eradication.

The prevention of skin infections secondary to itching disorders and direct contact are amenable to direct patient education. As the public contacts occur in the very sites where children and parents meet, this aggregation provides easily accessible sites for education and intervention. May I suggest that the combination of public education and implementation by general practitioners be supplemented by the follow-up facilities of government health agencies.

EARLY STAGES OF ORGANIC DISEASES

The practicalities of detection of early stages of organic diseases such as cancers, hypertension and diabetes have been designated as worthy of screening programmes by the World Health Organization (1968). The most helpful recent advance was fully reported by Spitzer *et al.* (1979) in a Canadian study of periodic health evaluation. Readers are referred to the original papers or the summary table in the appendix of this paper concerning those disorders found under various ages to be practical to detect and susceptible to effective intervention. We may not agree entirely with the priorities given in this study. I suggest that our local studies should include a look at regional causes of death, hospital admissions and consultations with doctors to give a lead to conditions which may not have had the same importance in Canada. Otitis media with effusion is a condition not accorded high priority in Canada but must be a subject of importance in Auckland if severe social disability is to be avoided.

It is now an academic argument whether to apply the recommended procedures of detection and care – we have an obligation to do so.

The case for case-finding in general practice against community screening surveys in producing better compliance with therapy has been well proven (Rakel, 1977).

HEALTH RISKS LEADING TO SPECIFIC DISEASES

It is well known that certain specific health risks are causes of diseases, for example, cigarette-smoking leading to cancer of the lung and chronic obstructive respiratory disease. If we look at the latent period of development of such chronic diseases we can observe, in 20 or 30 years, a stage of health risk, a stage of presymptomatic disease, and then a stage of irreversible organic disease. Many causal relationships are now proven between exposure to risks and development of disease. Some recent studies, by linking life expectancies to certain occupations have suggested causes which remain to be proven (Office of Population Censuses and Surveys, 1970–72). It is our responsibility to be aware of these relationships and to relate them to the specific occupations of our patients. It is unlikely that public or governmental action will, for instance, protect children from the risks of lead poisoning in the vicinity of old painted houses undergoing renovation, or unrestrained car travel. The provision and reinforcement of information given by respected family physicians makes a direct contribution to saving life and reducing disabilities – but only if we are alert to the risks our patients run and are very assertive in giving advice. The decline in home visiting by family doctors has reduced our capacity to develop such awareness.

HEALTH RISKS IN DAILY LIVING ACTIVITIES

Everyday living activities are of the greatest importance to future health. For many years the principles of prospective medicine as expounded by Robbins and Hall (1970) have been conceded by most doctors. The method of intervention suggested by the authors, by changing specific living activities, is claimed to change life expectancy with mathematical certainty. To prove this exactitude may be difficult, and to accept such a change in living activities may be almost impossible to a person locked in rigid social habits. It is possible that relationships between the usually recognized health attitudes and practices on the one hand, and disability and survival on the other, may be a reflection on generally healthy behaviour rather than indulgence in activities having specific causal influences. The evidence for a 'package' cause of better survival is becoming stronger. The combination of health attitudes and practices related to alcohol, tobacco, eating, sleeping, exercise and weight control has been shown to be more strongly related to survival in the following decade than is the disease history (Belloc, 1973; Belloc and Breslow, 1972; Belloc and Enstrom, 1980; Belloc, Breslow and Hochstim, 1970). It is surprising that insurance companies have not implemented this lesson (perhaps to our financial disadvantage!). Belloc, Breslow *et al.* have given a strong lead, and the work of my own research group in New Zealand has indicated that having healthy attitudes to all six life activities puts a mother into the socioeconomic/demographic group with a very low disability level. Other characteristics which are clearly related to low disability rates, at least in populations of European extraction, are general education and income levels. (More work has yet to be done to elicit clear interpretations of relationships in other ethnic groups.)

DISCUSSION

The information we already have is sufficient to change the health status of our population substantially. We have been tied to an absolute priority for curative medicine too long. Both our ethical system and the provision of government subsidies for patient consultation have encouraged overwhelming emphasis on curative care over preventive medical functions. In a fee-for-service system of primary care, patients are unwilling, unless well-educated and well-informed concerning health and the use of health services, to pay for preventive care. It is the responsibility of governments to see that it is paid for. I believe the established, consumer-recognized, neighbourhood system of health care is the proper channel for implementation and that the family doctor is central to this system. We can, however, only effect the change if we have the ability to measure results in a practical way and conduct our campaigns, be they for immunization or education about daily living activities, with the facilities necessary to make sure of reaching *all* the people concerned in the programme.

Is it practicable for busy general practitioners to introduce comprehensive case-finding and full preventive cover?

The evidence from the sparse surveys of populations (rather than patients presenting to doctors) suggests that doctors use the 'presenters' as their denominators in assessing completeness of preventive health cover. They ignore the problems and lack of cover of the non-presenting population. Those of us who work in a fee-for-service system without obligatory registration of patients find it difficult to define who our patients are, and are chary of intruding on the free choice of doctor we often champion.

It is essential to have an age–sex register to begin the process. When it has been operating for some years it will provide a list of patients of over 80 per cent accuracy. Patients can be asked about the allegiances of other members of their families to improve it further. A supplementary recording of family socioeconomic characteristics supplies certain indicators of health behaviour, while enquiry into the health attitudes and practices of mothers gives a reasonably accurate guide to health awareness and practice.

The time we need to take to make us aware of health risks and living conditions and activities is time that we take from more financially rewarding tasks. It is probably not good economy to employ doctors, the products of expensive education and supportive services, to elicit histories with a low yield of productive information. We can however motivate our patients to use their own time and to submit to the enquiries of health workers of less costly employment. It is possible to formulate concise questionnaires directed to obtain indicators of specific health risks and the details of living activities. Such questionnaires do not give us diagnoses, they provide us with the means of directing more sensitive, facilitating discussion towards the areas of life which can profit by our education and advice. If we have the means of looking objectively at the health needs of our people, and the means by which our people promote fulfilling activities, our own motivation to do this will be greatly enhanced.

How do we educate the people whom we look after? Much has been done in educational circles to define the specific effects of mass education. It would seem, from observed responses to media information about smoking and obesity that the gap between understanding health influences and acting on them by changing lifestyles is too difficult for many people to cross. Only by family and peer pressures can the desired result be achieved – unless a severely disrupting life event makes the change inevitable. We see this process happen after myocardial infarction and sometimes after childbirth. We cannot initiate such life events but we can use them when they present and profit by the opportunities to see the family together, united by a common goal or threat. Changes seen as a result of applying health interventions often take a generation to become apparent. The marked drop in smoking by doctors has resulted from initial understanding of the message reinforced and acted upon in small steps over many years. We can rely on this process only if we have a convincing argument, a subject of logical frame of mind, and an environment which provides consistent reinforcement.

I believe we must be responsible for most of these changes, by example, by our status in the community, and by our skill in defining needs, in facilitating logical discussion and in giving both patients, families and the public the advice they have the right to expect.

APPENDIX

Useful procedures in periodic health evaluation

The procedures specified refer to: A = evidence compelling that screening is effective: B = evidence fair; and C = evidence poor but recommended for other reasons.

During the antenatal period

A: rubella, gonorrhoea, syphilis, hypertension, blood group incompatibility
B: asphyxia, neural tube defect, Down's syndrome, alcoholism, diabetes, bacteriuria
C: Parenting problems, recurrent spontaneous abortion, breastfeeding, postpartum depression

At birth and during the first week of life

A: Congenital syphilis, ophthalmia neonatorum, neonatal hypothyroidism, phenylketonuria (PKU), blood group incompatibility
B: Postnatal asphyxia, haemorrhagic disease, congenital dislocation of the hip (CDH), Ventricular septal defect (VSD), problems of growth and development, strabismus, hearing defects, cystic fibrosis
C: Accidents, iron-deficiency anaemia, parenting problems

2–4 weeks

A: Congenital syphilis
B: Congenital dislocation of the hip (CDH), problems of growth and nutrition
C: Lower urinary tract anomalies, parenting problems, accidents

3 months

A: Diphtheria/pertussis/tetanus and polio (immunization)
B: Problems of growth and nutrition, strabismus, VSD
C: Developmental delay, parenting problems

5 months

A: Diphtheria/pertussis/tetanus and polio (immunization)
B: Physical growth problems, hearing impairment
C: Developmental delay, parenting problems, accidents

9 months

A: Diphtheria/pertussis/tetanus and polio (immunization)
B: Physical growth problems
C: Developmental delay, parenting problems, accidents, iron-deficiency
     anaemia

12–15 months

A: Measles (immunization), mumps (?immunization)
B: Physical growth problems
C: Parenting problems

18 months

A: Diphtheria/tetanus and polio (immunization)
B: Problems of physical growth
C: Behavioural and developmental problems

2–3 years

A: Dental caries
B: Physical growth problems, strabismus, hearing impairment
C: Refractive errors

4 years

A: Dental caries
B: Physical growth problems
C: Behavioural problems

5–6 years

A: Diphtheria/tetanus (immunization if not complete), polio, dental caries,
     tuberculosis (at-risk patients)

B: Physical growth problems, strabismus, refractive errors, hearing impairment, orthodontic conditions
C: Behavioural and developmental problems, accidents

10–11 years

A: Rubella (immunization of girls), dental caries
B: Physical growth problems, hearing impairment, orthodontic conditions
C: Behavioural problems, refractive defects, accidents, use of alcohol, smoking, sexual development problems

12–15 years

A: Dental caries
B: Physical growth problems, orthodontic conditions, cancer of cervix (when sexually active), muscular dystrophy (at risk)
C: Accidents, use of alcohol and tobacco, sexual development, malnutrition (at risk)

16–44 years

A: Tetanus (immunization), hypertension, dental disease, rubella (at risk) tuberculosis (at risk), sexually transmitted diseases (STD)
B: Hearing impairment, cancer of cervix, muscular dystrophy (at risk), thalassaemia (at risk), malnutrition (at risk), cancer of skin (at risk), cancer of bladder (at risk)
C: Alcoholism, smoking, motor vehicle accidents, family dysfunction, iron-deficiency anaemia

46–64 years

A: Cancer of breast, tetanus, hypertension, dental disease, tuberculosis (at risk), sexually transmitted diseases (at risk)
B: Cancer of colon and rectum, cancer of cervix, muscular dystrophy (at risk) malnutrition (at risk), cancer of skin (at risk), cancer of bladder (at risk)
C: Retirement problems, hypothyroidism, alcoholism, smoking, motor vehicle accidents, family dysfunction, iron-deficiency anaemia

65–74 years

A: Tetanus, ? influenza, hypertension, dental disease, tuberculosis (at risk)
B: Hearing problems, cancer of colon and rectum, cancer of skin (at risk), cancer of bladder (at risk), cancer of cervix (at risk)
C: Malnutrition, hypothyroidism

75+ years

A: Tetanus, ? influenza, hypertension, tuberculosis (at risk)

B: Hearing, cancer of colon and rectum, progressive incapacity of ageing, cancer of skin (at risk), cancer of bladder (at risk), cancer of cervix (at risk)
C: Oral cancer, hypothyroidism

References

Belloc, N. B., (1973). Relationship of health practices and mortality. *Prev. Med.* **9,** 469

Belloc, N. B. and Breslow, L. (1972). Relationship of physical health status and health practices. *Prev. Med.* **1,** 409

Belloc, N. B., Breslow, L. and Hochstim, J. R. (1970). Measurement of physical health in a general population survey. *Am. J. Epidemiol.*, **93, 5,** 328

Breslow, L. and Enstrom, J. E. (1980). Persistence of health habits and their relationship to mortality. *Prev. Med.*, **9,** 469

Spitzer, *et al.*, (1979). Canadian task force on the periodic health evaluation. *Can. Med. J.*, **121,** 1193–1254

Office of Population Censuses and Surveys (1970–72). *Occupational Mortality.* England and Wales decennial suppl. Series DS No. 1. (London: Office of Population Censuses and Surveys)

Rakel, R. E. (1977). *Principles of Family Medicine.* (London: W. B. Saunders)

Robbins, L. C. and Hall, J. H. (1970). *How to Practice Prospective Medicine.* (Indianapolis: Methodist Hospital)

World Health Organization (1968). *WHO Public Health Paper 34*

Preventive care in family practice: a critique

John P. Geyman

The preceding two papers illustrate well the extent and nature of the debate, especially in primary care circles, surrounding the role and effectiveness of preventive care in everyday medical practice. This has been a confused area which traditionally has been poorly taught and comparatively neglected in medical education. Physicians have been conditioned in most developed countries to value more highly the curative aspects of medicine, and prevention has been relegated by many to a low priority area within the personal health care system, some even preferring that other agencies take the major role for prevention (for example, health departments in the public health sector).

The problems of integrating preventive health care into primary care are considerable and varied. The public is often disinterested in prevention, resistant to needed changes to decrease risks of disease, and unwilling to pay for preventive care. In most countries there are financial disincentives to providers for preventive care, with many important activities (such as counselling and health maintenance procedures) not covered by reimbursement systems. Many practices are poorly organized to provide preventive care, so that this kind of activity is often perceived by physicians as wasteful of time and resources.

There has been only limited study of the cost–benefit of many preventive procedures, and research in this area has usually received relatively low priority.

Despite these problems, however, there is reason for optimism that a useful role for preventive care can be defined as an effective part of the family physician's practice. The state of the art in prevention has increased greatly in the last 10 years concerning available knowledge of the cost–benefit of many preventive procedures. The report of the Canadian Task Force on the Periodic Health Examination (1979) provides the most comprehensive literature review and assessment of cost–benefit of specific preventive procedures yet available, and should be part of every family physician's personal library. The recently published book, *The Practice of Preventive Health Care* (Schneiderman 1981) provides an excellent and practical guide to preventive procedures of documented value, and also is a 'must' for a practice library. A special issue of the *Journal of Family Practice* (Eggertson, Schneeweiss and Bergman, 1980) is another useful reference in this area, including descriptions and evaluations of preventive programs in various family practice settings and descriptions of practical medical record systems to facilitate this care.[4] In the area of pediatric health screening, a useful office protocol has recently been described based upon an exhaustive literature review with recommendations for specific procedures of demonstrated value (Eggertson, Schneeweiss and Bergman, 1980).

Preventive procedures need to be critically assessed before they are incorporated into everyday family practice. The following criteria, derived partly from those adopted by the National Conference on Preventive Medicine, Task Force (1976) and partly from the work of Frame and Carlson (1975) in rural family practice, are helpful in this selection (Breslow and Somers, 1977):

(1) The procedure is appropriate to health goals of the relevant age group (or groups) and is acceptable to the relevant population.

(2) The procedure is directed to primary or secondary prevention of a clearly identified disease or condition that has a definite effect on the length or quality of life.

(3) The natural history of the disease (or diseases) associated with the condition is understood sufficiently to justify the procedure as outweighing any adverse effects of intervention.

(4) For purposes of screening, the disease or condition has an asymptomatic period during which detection and treatment can substantially reduce morbidity or mortality or both.

(5) Acceptable methods of effective treatment are available for conditions discovered.

(6) The prevalence and seriousness of the disease or condition justify the cost of intervention.

(7) The procedure is relatively easy to administer, preferably by paramedical personnel with guidance and interpretation by physicians, and generally available at reasonable cost.

(8) Resources are generally available for follow-up diagnostic or therapeutic intervention if required.

Preventive care and health maintenance represent essential elements of family practice as a specialty. What is included in everyday practice must justify the expenditure of time and resources in terms of cost–benefit and positive health outcomes. More research is needed in this area, and family physicians need to review critically this research and adopt practical approaches in the same way that they select among diagnostic and therapeutic alternatives. In addition, they need to organize their practices so that preventive procedures which are considered useful can be readily provided within the constraints of a busy practice. As a minimum, this will most likely include the use of a prevention-oriented medical record, age–sex and high-risk disease registers, delegation of selected tasks to office assistants, risk assessment procedures, mechanisms for patient recall, and protocols for management of high-risk groups.

References

Breslow, L., and Somers, A. R. (1977). The lifetime health-monitoring program: a practical approach to preventive medicine. *N. Engl. J. Med.*, **296,** 601

Canadian Task Force on the Periodic Health Examination (1979). The Periodic Health Examination. *Can. Med. Assoc. J.*, **121,** 1193

Eggertson, S. C., Schneeweiss, R. and Bergman, J. J. (1980). An updated protocol for pediatric health screening. *J. Fam. Pract.*, **10 (1),** 25

Frame, P. S. and Carlson, S. J. (1975). A critical review of periodic health screening using specific screening criteria. *J. Fam. Pract.*, **2,** 29, 123, 189 and 283

Geyman, J. P. (ed.) (1979). *Preventive Care in Family Practice.* (New York: Appleton-Century-Crofts)

National Conference on Preventive Medicine, Task Force (1976). Theory, practice and application of prevention in personal health services; and, Quality control and evaluation of preventive health services. In *Preventive Medicine USA. Task Force Reports for the National Conference on Preventive Medicine, Bethesda, Maryland, 1975.* (New York: Prodist)

Schneiderman L. J. (ed.) (1981). *The Practice of Preventive Health Care.* (Menlo Park: Addison-Wesley Publishing Company)

Commentary

Prevention certainly is better than suffering a disease and attempting to cure it, but it is uncertain how many diseases really are preventable.

It is becoming evident that with control of many of the 'older' infective diseases the scope for improving health and increasing longevity in the future must be in changing potentially bad personal habits that may lead to disease. Changing lifestyles and habits such as smoking, alcohol, diet, overweight, indolence and lack of exercise, and general stresses and strains is not easy. It involves individual actions and responsibilities.

The family practitioner's role here must be to increase his or her scope of care. Good care must involve attention to individual lifestyle habits that may be potentially dangerous to health. It must also include definition and surveillance of special at-risk groups of patients who need regular support and supervision such as diabetics, hypertensives, depressives, those with thyroid disorders and postgastrectomies, and social vulnerables such as elderly isolates and those recently bereaved. Good care must also include population care as well as individual care. There has to be close local collaboration with schools, with industries, with sports activities and other groups.

Prevention presents primary care of the future with many challenges and opportunities, which must be accepted by family practitioners with sensitivity and sensibility. Excessive enthusiasm may be as damaging as inaction.

Index